CELL CYCLE INHIBITORS IN CANCER THERAPY

CANCER DRUG DISCOVERY
AND DEVELOPMENT

BEVERLY A. TEICHER, SERIES EDITOR

CELL CYCLE INHIBITORS IN CANCER THERAPY

CURRENT STRATEGIES

Edited by

ANTONIO GIORDANO, MD, PhD

Sbarro Institute for Cancer Research and Molecular Medicine,
College of Science and Technology,
Temple University, Philadelphia, PA

and

KENNETH J. SOPRANO, PhD

Department of Microbiology and Immunology,
Temple University School of Medicine, Philadelphia, PA

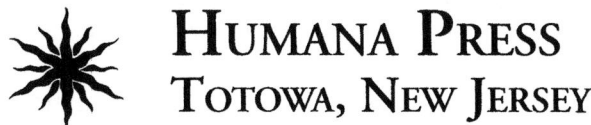

HUMANA PRESS
TOTOWA, NEW JERSEY

© 2003 Humana Press Inc.
999 Riverview Drive, Suite 208
Totowa, New Jersey 07512
www.humanapress.com

Due diligence has been taken by the publishers, editors, and authors of this book to assure the accuracy of the information published and to describe generally accepted practices. The contributors herein have carefully checked to ensure that the drug selections and dosages set forth in this text are accurate and in accord with the standards accepted at the time of publication. Notwithstanding, as new research, changes in government regulations, and knowledge from clinical experience relating to drug therapy and drug reactions constantly occurs, the reader is advised to check the product information provided by the manufacturer of each drug for any change in dosages or for additional warnings and contraindications. This is of utmost importance when the recommended drug herein is a new or infrequently used drug. It is the responsibility of the treating physician to determine dosages and treatment strategies for individual patients. Further it is the responsibility of the health care provider to ascertain the Food and Drug Administration status of each drug or device used in their clinical practice. The publisher, editors, and authors are not responsible for errors or omissions or for any consequences from the application of the information presented in this book and make no warranty, express or implied, with respect to the contents in this publication.

This publication is printed on acid-free paper.⊚
ANSI Z39.48-1984 (American National Standards Institute) Permanence of Paper for Printed Library Materials.

Production Editor: Kim Hoather-Potter.

Cover design by Patricia F. Cleary.

Cover Illustration:Immunohistochemical analysis of retinoblastoma-related protein pRb2/p130 expression in Burkitt lymphoma. Photo supplied by Dr. Antonio Giordano, Dr. Lorenzo Leoncini, and Dr. Caterina Cinti.

For additional copies, pricing for bulk purchases, and/or information about other Humana titles, contact Humana at the above address or at any of the following numbers: Tel.: 973-256-1699; Fax: 973-256-8341; E-mail: humana@humanapr.com or visit our Website at www.humanapress.com

Printed in the United States of America. 10 9 8 7 6 5 4 3 2 1

Library of Congress Cataloging-in-Publication Data
Cell cycle inhibitors in cancer therapy: current strategies / edited by Antonio Giordano and Kenneth J. Soprano.
      p. cm. -- (Cancer drug discovery and development)
  Includes bibliographical references and index.
  ISBN 0-89603-930-7 (alk. paper)
    1. Cancer -- Chemotherapy. 2. Cell cycle -- Effect of drugs on. 3. Cancer
  cells -- Growth -- Regulation. I. Giordano, Antonio, MD. II. Soprano, Kenneth J. III.
  Series.
  RC271.C5 C367 2003
  616.99'4061--dc21

                                                 2002027315

Preface

A precise tuning of cell replication is mandatory for organismic and cellular homeostasis. Indeed, numerous aspects of human pathology can be thought of as malfunctions of the cell cycle. Cancer is unquestionably among these.

In the past, an accelerated mitotic rate traditionally has been considered to be a major characteristic of either benign or malignant neoplastic diseases. For this reason, cancer growth historically has been considered the epitome of a disease caused by loss of control of the strategies that regulate the cell cycle. Although the complex and intricate mechanisms that drive malignant transformation are now better understood, nonprogrammed cellular replication still plays a key role in the theoretical schemes we use to understand, prevent, diagnose, and cure cancer.

Modern medicine now moves swiftly toward novel, and previously unsuspected, fields. The molecular approach to disease is ultimately providing a tremendous amount of knowledge that continuously produces revolutionary changes in our abilities to diagnose and cure most diseases. In this exciting scenario, where health care professionals, as well as graduate and medical students, are continuously asked to deal with radically innovative approaches, the role of the scientific literature is to provide constantly up-to-date information on the many recent advances in molecular medicine. In addition, this information should be communicated in a way that is user friendly and comprehensible.

Cell Cycle Inhibitors in Cancer Therapy: Current Strategies has been conceived as a scholarly book with the aim to provide state-of-the-art information about the molecules involved in cell cycle control. Such a book will deliver, in a clear language, fundamental information derived from the basic sciences to the medical community, where it can have a direct impact on diagnostics, prognostics, and therapeutics.

We feel there is a tremendous need for such a book as this, which is designed to educate physicians in cell cycle and cell growth control. In effect, *Cell Cycle Inhibitors in Cancer Therapy: Current Strategies* will bring current findings from the research laboratory directly into clinical practice. Finally, we also aim to provide an opportunity for feedback in which high-level clinical practice can stimulate basic science investigators to develop new insight into the many diseases that still constitute difficult medical problems.

Each thematic issue in *Cell Cycle Inhibitors in Cancer Therapy* is therefore designed to provide the latest research information and demonstrate its clinical relevance to our understanding of many of the most prevalent diseases afflicting our society today.

Antonio Giordano, MD, PhD
Kenneth J. Soprano, PhD

CONTENTS

CONTRIBUTORS

CRISTIANA BELLAN, MD, PhD • *Institute of Pathologic Anatomy and Histology, University of Siena, Siena, Italy*

MIKHAIL V. BLAGOSKLONNY, MD, PhD • *Medicine Branch, National Cancer Institute, NIH, Bethesda, MD*

CATERINA CINTI, PhD • *Institute of Normal and Pathological Cytomorphology, Consiglio Nazionale delle Ricerche (CNR), Bologna, Italy*

GIULIA DE FALCO, PhD • *Sbarro Institute for Cancer Research and Molecular Medicine, College of Science and Technology, Temple University, Philadelphia, PA*

WAFIK S. EL-DEIRY, MD, PhD • *Howard Hughes Medical Institute, University of Pennsylvania School of Medicine, Philadelphia, PA*

ARMANDO FELSANI, PhD • *CNR, Istituto di Neurobiologia e Medicina Molecolare, Rome, Italy*

ANTONIO GIORDANO, MD, PhD • *Sbarro Institute for Cancer Research and Molecular Medicine, College of Science and Technology, Temple University, Philadelphia, PA*

WILLIAM F. HOLMES, MS • Departments of Microbiology, Immunology, and Biochemistry, Fels Institute for Cancer Research and Molecular Biology, Temple University School of Medicine, Philadelphia, PA

ANDREW KOFF, PhD • *Program in Molecular Biology, Memorial Sloan-Kettering Cancer Center, New York, NY*

LORENZO LEONCINI, MD, PhD • *Institute of Pathologic Anatomy and Histology, University of Siena, Siena, Italy*

JANE B. LIAN, PhD • *Department of Cell Biology, University of Massachusetts Medical Center, Worchester, MA*

VALERIA MASCIULLO, MD, PhD • *Department of Pathology, Anatomy, and Cell Biology, Jefferson Medical College, Philadelphia, PA*

ROB J. A. M. MICHALIDES, PhD • *Division of Tumor Biology, The Netherlands Cancer Institute, Amsterdam, The Netherlands*

LUCIO MIELE, MD, PhD • *Department of Biopharmaceutical Sciences and Cancer Center, University of Illinois at Chicago, Chicago, IL*

MARCO G. PAGGI, MD, PhD • *Department for the Development of Therapeutic Programs, Center for Experimental Research, Regina Elena Cancer Institute, Rome, Italy*

JOANNA K. SAX, BS • *Laboratory of Molecular Oncology and Cell Cycle Regulation, Departments of Medicine, Genetics, and Pharmacology, and the Cancer Center, Howard Hughes Medical Institute, University of Pennsylvania School of Medicine, Philadelphia, PA*

ADRIAN M. SENDEROWICZ, MD • *Molecular Therapeutics Unit, Oral and Pharyngeal Cancer Branch, National Institute of Dental and Craniofacial Research, National Institutes of Health, Bethesda, MD*

ANNA SEVERINO, PhD • *Department for the Development of Therapeutic Programs, Center for Experimental Research, Regina Elena Cancer Institute, Rome, Italy*

CATHERINE SOPRANO • *Sbarro Institute for Cancer Research and Molecular Medicine, College of Science and Technology, Temple University, Philadelphia, PA*

DIANNE R. SOPRANO, PhD • *Departments of Microbiology, Immunology, and Biochemistry, Fels Institute for Cancer Research and Molecular Biology, Temple University School of Medicine, Philadelphia, PA*

KENNETH J. SOPRANO, PhD • *Departments of Microbiology, Immunology, and Biochemistry, Fels Institute for Cancer Research and Molecular Biology, Temple University School of Medicine, Philadelphia, PA*

GARY S. STEIN, PhD • *Department of Cell Biology, University of Massachusetts Medical Center, Worchester, MA*

JANET L. STEIN, PhD • *Department of Cell Biology, University of Massachusetts Medical Center, Worchester, MA*

PAUL J. VAN DIEST, MD, PhD • *Department of Pathology, Vrije Universiteit Medical Cener, Amsterdam, The Netherlands*

ANDRÉ J. VAN WIJNEN, PhD • *Department of Cell Biology, University of Massachusetts Medical Center, Worchester, MA*

DONGMEI ZHANG, PhD • *Departments of Microbiology, Immunology, and Biochemistry, Fels Institute for Cancer Research and Molecular Biology, Temple University School of Medicine, Philadelphia, PA*

SIJIE ZHANG, MD, PhD • *Departments of Microbiology, Immunology, and Biochemistry, Fels Institute for Cancer Research and Molecular Biology, Temple University School of Medicine, Philadelphia, PA*

1

Cdk Inhibitors
Background and Introduction

Giulia De Falco, PhD, Catherine Soprano, and Antonio Giordano, MD, PhD

Contents

1. CELL CYCLE AND CYCLIN-DEPENDENT KINASES

The cell cycle is the series of events which regulate the life of the cell. Two main events characterize the cell cycle: S phase, in which the cell duplicates its genome, and M phase, in which the cell splits into two daughter cells. It is necessary that these two crucial events are regulated and coordinated to occur in an ordered fashion at precisely the right time (for a review *see* refs. *1,2*). This regulation and coordination results from a combination of several signals from different regulatory pathways that are activated in response to the presence of specific stimuli (for a review *see* ref. *1*).

The cell cycle has a central role in controlling cell growth and proliferation: it frequently becomes the target of genetic alteration, the accumulation of which may lead to the deregulation of these ordered events and may be related to the onset of cancer (for a review *see* ref. *3*).

From: *Cancer Drug Discovery and Development:*
Cell Cycle Inhibitors in Cancer Therapy: Current Strategies
Edited by: A. Giordano and K. J. Soprano © Humana Press Inc., Totowa, NJ

Progression through the cell cycle is ensured by particular protein complexes, the cyclin/Cdks. The Cdks are a family of highly conserved serine/threonine kinases, which share a high homology in a particular region, called PSTAIRE. Cdks may control the cell cycle by phosphorylating different targets, which may in turn be activated or inactivated (for a review *see* ref. *4*). Monomeric Cdks have a very low kinase activity and they require the binding of regulatory subunits, referred to as cyclins, as an initial step in their activation process *(5)*. Cyclins are so called because they are cyclically synthesized and destroyed during cell cycle. Thus they are present only when their function is required. Cyclin protein levels are strictly controlled; they are subject to proteolytic destruction by the ubiquitin-dependent pathway (for a review *see* refs. *6,7*). They are less conserved than Cdks, and they share homology only in an internal sequence, called the "cyclin box" *(8,9)*.

2. CDK REGULATION

There are several mechanisms that ensure cell cycle control. Passage from one stage to another is regulated tightly by transcription, degradation of cyclins and modification of the kinase subunits by phosphorylation. When first synthesized, the Cdk has no detectable activity. Its activation occurs in a two-step process, the binding to its cyclin partner and the phosphorylation by a multimeric enzyme complex, CAK (Cdk-Activating Kinase), which in animal cells is composed of Cdk7 and cyclin H *(10,11)* and by another more recently identified component, MAT1 *(12–14)*.

Another regulatory mechanism involves phosphorylation of Cdks on specific Ser/Thr residues, which may lead either to their activation or inactivation *(15,16)*. Changes in structure or cellular localization may occur in response to a change in phosphorylation state *(17)*. Moreover, the subcellular localization of Cdks and their regulatory proteins may represent an additional phase of regulation. By changes in localization, cyclins are able to modify the substrate specificity of their Cdk partners or allow access to different subsets of substrates (for a review *see* ref. *18*).

3. THE CDK INHIBITORS

Regulation of Cdk/cyclin activity may also occur through other regulatory proteins, referred to as Cdk Inhibitors (CKIs) (for a review *see* refs. *16,19–22*). The expression of these inhibitors may be induced by stimuli such as senescence *(23)*, contact inhibition *(24)*, extracellular anti-mitogenic factors like transforming growth factor (TGF) *(25)* and cell cycle checkpoints like the p53 DNA damage checkpoints *(26)*. Their role in controlling cell cycle is crucial. In several forms of cancer, CKIs such as p16 *(27–29)* and p27 are mutated. Also, they have been found to be degraded in several types of cancer; low levels of p27 levels are

Table 1
Targets of CKIs

CKIs	Cycline/CDK complexes
p15	Cyclin D1/Cdk4,6; Cyclin D2, D3/Cdk2,4,6
p16	Cyclin D1/Cdk4,6; Cyclin D2, D3/Cdk2,4,6
p18	Cyclin D1/Cdk4,6; Cyclin D2, D3/Cdk2,4,6
p19	Cyclin D1/Cdk4,6; Cyclin D2, D3/Cdk2,4,6
p21	Cyclin E/Cdk2; Cyclin A/Cdk2; Cyclin A/Cdk1; Cyclin B1, B2/Cdk1
p27	Cyclin D1/Cdk4,6; Cyclin D2, D3/Cdk2,4,6; Cyclin E/Cdk2
p57	Cyclin D1/Cdk4,6; Cyclin D2, D3/Cdk2,4,6

correlated with poor clinical prognosis *(30)*. These inhibitors can be upregulated when required, thus blocking the activation of the Cdk by a cyclin. This arrests the cell in a particular part of the cell cycle until conditions are such that it can continue towards proliferation or, if necessary, be steered towards cell death.

The CKIs are able to associate in vivo with the Cdk subunit, the cyclin or the cyclin/Cdk complex, thus inhibiting their activity. This inhibition may occur in different ways: inhibition of the Cdk kinase activity, interference with CAK-mediated Cdk activation or competition with cyclins in binding to the catalytic subunit (for a review *see* ref. *31*). The inhibitory process can be carried out by one or a combination of these mechanisms. Table 1 summarizes CKIs target molecules.

There are two families of CKIs. The first family includes the INK4 proteins (inhibitors of Cdk4), so named for their ability to specifically inhibit the catalytic subunits of Cdk4 and Cdk6. This family includes four proteins, p16[INK4a] *(27)*, p15[INK4b] *(32)*, p18[INK4c] *(33,34)*, and p19[INK4d] *(34,35)*. These proteins are composed of multiple ankirin repeats and bind only to Cdk4 and Cdk6. The latter family is composed of the members of the Cip/Kip family, and includes p21[Cip1] *(26,36–40)*, p27[Kip1] *(24,41,42)* and p57[Kip2] *(9,43)*, all of which contain characteristic motifs within their amino-terminal moieties that enable them to bind to both cyclin and Cdk subunits *(44–48)*.

Members of the Cip family bind to and inhibit the active cyclin/Cdk complex (for a review *see* ref. *21*). On the other hand, members of the INK4 use an indirect strategy. They bind to the isolated Cdk and prevent its association with the cyclin and thus its activation. However, they can also bind to and inhibit the preformed cyclin/Cdk complex without dissociating the cyclin, suggesting that they may have multiple mechanisms of action (for a review *see* ref. *49*). The INK4 inhibitors are specific for G1 phase Cdks, whereas the Cip inhibitors have a broader Cdk preference.

4. THE INK4 FAMILY

p16 was identified in a two-hybrid screening using Cdk4 as a bait *(27)*. p16 can block Cdk4 and Cdk6 function by sequestering the catalytic subunit, or by blocking the kinase activity of preassembled complexes *(27)*. p16 overexpression induces G1 arrest in diverse cell lines, but has no effect in pRb negative cell lines *(22,50)*. p16 maps to the 9p21 chromosomal region, a locus frequently associated with human tumors because of mutations in the coding sequence or transcriptional repression by methylation *(51,52)*. Due to the fact that several human cancers are associated with loss of p16 function, this gene was proposed as a tumor suppressor in vivo.

p15 is induced by TGF treatment and is expressed ubiquitously *(32)*. This gene maps in the vicinity of p16. Both these genes are frequently deleted in human cancers. This may suggest that the loss of both genes may be significant in the development of certain types of tumors. Both p18 and p19 are widely distributed in different cell types and tissues *(33,34)*. In some cell types, p19 levels oscillate during the cell cycle, undergoing induction when cells enter S phase *(34)*. p19 may function by regulating the activity of cyclin D-dependent kinases as cells exit G_1 phase. All four inhibitors share similar properties and may respond differently to anti-proliferative signals. Members of the INK4 family appear not to be redundant, since they have distinct biologic functions. The consequences of their functional inactivation might be quite different, with the loss of only certain ones being critical in carcinogenesis.

5. THE CIP/KIP FAMILY

p21, p27, and p57 belong to the Cip/Kip family. p21 was cloned by different approaches: in a two-hybrid screening, using Cdk2 as a bait *(37)*, a component of the cyclin/Cdk complex *(36,53)*, as a protein induced in senescent cells *(40)*, and also as a target of transcriptional activation by the p53 tumor suppressor gene *(26)*. p21 can act as a potent and universal inhibitor of Cdk activity; it inhibits Cdk2, Cdk4, and Cdk6 kinases and is capable of inducing cell cycle arrest in G_1 when overexpressed *(26,36,37,40)*. In normally cycling cells p21 is in complex with cyclin/Cdk. p21/cyclin/Cdk complexes retain the kinase activity that is extinguished by the addition of more p21 *(37,54)*. Conversion from active complexes to inactive ones is achieved by changing the ratio of p21 complexed with cyclin/Cdk, so that active complexes contain a single p21 molecule, whereas inactive ones include multiple p21 subunits. In normal fibroblasts, it appears associated in a quaternary complex which contains cyclin/Cdk/p21 and the proliferative nuclear antigen (PCNA), a subunit of DNA polymerase that functions in both DNA replication and DNA repair *(55)*. p21 has two characteristic regions: the N-terminal half of the protein is responsible for the Cdk inhibitory activity, whereas the C-terminal domain binds to the PCNA *(44–46,56,57)*.

p27 was identified in a series of studies on growth inhibitory activity induced by TGF *(41)* and in another study was isolated by a two-hybrid screening, using Cdk4 as a bait *(42)*. p27 is structurally related to p21 and inhibits Cdk2, Cdk3, Cdk4, and Cdk6 complexes in vitro *(56)*. Its greatest homology to p21 resides in the amino-terminus, which contains the cdk inhibitory domain *(41)*. In some cases, p27 binds with a higher affinity to the cyclin/cdk complex than to Cdk alone *(41)*. p27 mRNA levels remain constant throughout the cell cycle, while protein levels change, probably due to translational and post-translational regulation *(58)*.

p57 has been isolated on the basis of its homology with p21 and p27 *(9,43)*. p57 binds to and inhibits several cyclin/Cdk complexes and its expression seems to be tissue-restricted *(9,43)*. p57, like p27, appears not to require p53 and pRb for its function. p57 maps to the 11p15 chromosomal locus, which undergoes frequent deletions or rearrangements in many forms of human cancer *(43)*.

6. A MODEL FOR STRUCTURAL BINDING BETWEEN CKIS AND CDKS

All these processes regulate Cdks at the molecular level and they occur through conformational changes. These recurring structural changes indicate that Cdks possess an intrinsic structural flexibility *(59)*. It may be hypothesized that the monomeric Cdk has not yet completed its folding. When the cyclin binds, it rebuilds this flexible structure. However, the assembly of the active Cdk structure is not complete until after phosphorylation. Even when it is completely assembled and active, the Cdk can still undergo further structural changes, as the Cdk inhibitors can bind to it and refold it into a different structure. The intrinsic structural flexibility of the Cdk plays a central role in allowing the Cdk to be regulated in many different ways (for a review *see* ref. *60*).

7. A ROLE FOR CKIS IN CANCER

Several types of cancer are associated with a deregulation of these CKI proteins. For example, low expression of p27 occurs frequently in many types of human tumors. This reduction correlates strongly with tumor aggression and denotes a poor prognosis (for a review *see* ref. *61*), first demonstrated for breast and colon carcinoma and, more recently, for other tumor types *(30,62,63)*. Low levels of p27 are likely to be causally related to tumorigenesis, as evidenced by studies performed in transgenic mice *(64)*.

Cyclin D1 overexpression and p16 loss have been related to the onset of cancer *(52)*, due to a deregulation of the cell cycle. Tables 2 and 3 summarizes the main tumor types which involve CKI deregulation.

Table 2
The CIP/Kip Family and Cancer

CKI	Tumor type	Alteration
p21	Hepatocellular carcinoma	Upregulation
	Colorectal carcinoma	Downregulation
	Cervical carcinoma	Altered expression
	Leiomyosarcoma	Upregulation
	Pancreatic Intraepithelial neoplasia	Upregulation
	Gastric carcinomas	Altered expression
	Breast cancer	Altered expression
p27	Breast cancer	Downregulation
	Colorectal carcinoma	Downregulation
	Prostate carcinoma	Downregulation
	Bladder carcinoma	Upregulation
	Head and neck carcinoma	Upregulation
	Diffuse Large B Cell Lymphomas (DLBCL)	Downregulation
	Non Hodgkin's Lymphoma (NHL)	Downregulation
	Large B Cell Lymphoma (LBCL)	Altered expression
	Squamous Cell Carcinoma (SCC)	Upregulation
	Leiomyosarcoma	Upregulation
	Digestive endocrine tumors	Upregulation
	Ovarian Cancer	Altered expression
	Mucoepidermoid carcinoma	Downregulation
	Cervical carcinoma	Altered expression
	Oral Squamous Cell Carcinoma (OSCC)	Downregulation
	Non-Small Cell Lung Cancer (NSCLC)	Downregulation
	Lung adenocarcinoma	Upregulation
	Clear cell renal cell carcinoma	Upregulation
	Hepatocellular carcinoma	Upregulation
p57	Leiomyosarcoma	Upregulation
	Pancreatic adenocarcinoma	Upregulation
	Bladder carcinoma	Downregulation
	Gastric cancer	Downregulation

8. CHEMICAL INHIBITORS OF CDKS

In addition to CKI proteins, chemical Cdk inhibitors have been characterized. There are six families of chemical inhibitors, each of which is either a natural product or a derivative of one with a distinct chemical structure. All occupy the ATP-binding pocket of the enzyme and are competitive with ATP (for a review *see* ref. *65*). These chemical inhibitors are under investigation as potential weapons in cancer treatment. To date, only the chemical inhibitor, flavopiridol, has reached clinical trials and it has yet to be proven whether its effects are caused

Table 3
The INK4 Family and Cancer

CKI	Tumor type	Alteration
p15	Acute Lymphoblastic Leukemia (ALL)	Genetic loss
	Acute Myeloid Leukemia (AML)	Genetic loss
	Non Hodgkin's Lymphoma (NHL)	Genetic loss
	Myeloma	Genetic loss
	Hepatocellular carcinoma	Genetic alteration
p16	Lung cancer	Genetic loss
	Mantle Cell Lymphoma (MCL)	Inactivation
	Melanoma	Inactivation
	Acute Lymphoblastic Leukemia (ALL)	Genetic loss
	Acute Myeloid Leukemia (AML)	Genetic loss
	Non Hodgkin's Lymphoma (NHL)	Genetic loss
	Chronic Myelocytic Leukemia (CML)	Genetic loss
	Ovarian cancer	Genetic loss
	Diffuse Large B Cell Lymphoma (DLBCL)	Altered expression
	Bladder carcinoma	Inactivation
	Nasopharyngeal Carcinoma (NPC)	Inactivation
	Hepatocellular carcinoma	Genetic alteration
	Extrahepatic biliary tract carcinoma	Downregulation
	Thyroid cancer	Genetic alteration
	Non-Small Cell Lung Cancer (NSCLC)	Genetic loss
p18	Oligodendroglioma	Upregulation
	Meningioma	Genetic alteration
	Acute Myeloid Leukemia (AML)	Upregulation
p19	Acute Myeloid Leukemia (AML)	Upregulation

by Cdk inhibition. Cdks represent a key part of cell cycle, their deregulation may be involved in tumorigenesis. This suggests that modulators of Cdk activity are good potential targets for intervention. Specificity of these compounds is crucial for their function, so further studies will be necessary in order to generate new and more specific molecules.

9. CONCLUSIONS

Cdks, cyclins, and their positive and negative regulators appear to be the main components of the cell cycle. Although much is known about the cell cycle and its components, several questions remain to be answered. Further studies on their cellular localization, and on the stimuli to which they respond will help to better elucidate the cell cycle regulatory machinery. In addition, the deregulation of these proteins appear to be associated with the onset of cancer. Gaining a better understanding of how these factors work in the cell represents an exciting future challenge.

REFERENCES

1. Sherr CJ. G1 phase progression: cycling on cue. *Cell* 1994;79:551–555.
2. Nurse P. Ordering S phase and M phase in the cell cycle. *Cell* 1994;79:547–550.
3. Sherr CJ. Cancer cell cycles. *Science* 1996;274:1672–1677 (1996).
4. Morgan DO. Cyclin-dependent kinases: engines, clocks, and microprocessors. *Annu Rev Cell Dev Biol* 1997;13:261–291.
5. Connel-Crowley L, Solomon MJ, Wei N, Harper JW. Phosphorylation independent activation of human cyclin-dependent kinase 2 by cyclin A in vitro. *Mol Cell Biol Cell* 1993;4:79–92.
6. Deshaies RJ. The self-destructive personality of a cell cycle in transition. *Curr Opin Cell Biol* 1995;7:781–789.
7. Hochstrasser M. Ubiquitin, proteasomes, and the regulation of intracellular protein degradation. *Curr Opin Cell Biol* 1995;7:215–223.
8. Kobajashi H, Stewart E, Poon R, et al. Identification of the domains in cyclin A required for binding to, and inactivation of p34cdc2, and p32cdk2 protein kinase subunits. *Mol Biol Cell* 1992;3:1279–1294.
9. Lee MH, Reynisdottir I, Massaguè J. Cloning of p57KIP2, a cyclin-dependent kinase inhibitor with unique domain structure and tissue distribution. *Genes Dev* 1995;9:639–649.
10. Fesquet D, Labbè JC, Derancourt J, Capony JP, Galas S, Girard F, et al. The MO15 gene encodes the catalytic subunit of a protein kinase that activates cdc2 and other cyclin-dependent kinases (CDKs) through phosphorylation ogf Thr 161 and its homologues. *EMBO J* 1993;12:3111–3121.
11. Solomon MJ. Activation of the various cyclin/cdc2 protein kinases. *Curr Opin Cell Biol* 1993;5:180–186.
12. Fisher RP, Jin P, Chamberlin HM, Morgan DO. Alternative mechanisms of CAK assembly require an assembly factor or an activating kinase. *Cell* 1995;83:47–57.
13. Devault A, Martinez AM, Fesquet D., Labbè JC, Morin N, Tassan JP, et al. MAT1 ("menage à trois"), a new RING-finger protein stabilizing cyclin H-CDK7 complexes in starfish and Xenopus oocytes. *EMBO J* 1995;14:5027–5036.
14. Yee A, Nichols MA, Wu L, Hall FL, Kobajashi R, Xiong Y. Molecular cloning of CDK7-associated human MAT1, a cyclin-dependent kinase-activating kinase (CAK) assembly factor. *Cancer Res* 1995;55:6058–6062.
15. Nurse P. Universal control mechanism regulating onset of M-phase. *Nature* 1990;344:503–508.
16. Nigg E. Cyclin-dependent protein kinases: key regulators of the eukaryotic cell cycle. *Bioessays* 1995;17:471–480.
17. Dunphy WG. The decision to enter mitosis. *Trends Cell Biol* 1994;4:433–442.
18. Pines J. Cyclin from sea urchins to Helas: making the human cell cycle. Colworth Medal Lecture. *Biochem Soc Trans* 1996;24;15–33.
19. Peter M., Herskowitz I. Joining the complex: cyclin-dependent kinase inhibitory proteins and the cell cycle. *Cell* 1994;79:181–184.
20a. Lees E. Cyclin dependent kinase regulation. *Curr Opin Cell Biol* 1995a;7:773–780.
20b. Lees EM, Harlow E. Sequences within the conserved cyclin box of human cyclin A are sufficient for binding to and inactivation of Cdc2 kinase. *Cell* 1995b;81:149–152.
21. Sherr CJ, Roberts JM. Inhibitors of mammalian G1 cyclin-dependent kinases. *Genes Dev* 1995;9:1149–1163.
22. Elledge SJ, Winston J, Harper JW. A question of balance: the role of cyclin-kinase inhibitors in development and tumorigenesis. *Trends Cell Biol* 1996;6:388–392.

23. Alcorta DA, Xiong Y, Phelps D, Hannon G, Beach D, Barret JC. Involvement of the cyclin-dependent kinase inhibitor p16 (INK4a) in replicative senescence of normal human fibroblasts. *Proc Natl Acad Sci USA* 1996;93:13743–13747.

24. Polyak K, Kato J, Solomon MJ, Sherr CJ, Massaguè J, Roberts JM, Koff A. p27kip1, a cyclin-cdk inhibitor, links transforming growth factor-β and contact inhibition to cell cycle arrest. *Genes Dev* 1994a;8:9–22.

25. Reynisdottir I, Polyak K, Iavarone A, Massaguè J. Kip/Cip and Ink4 inhibitors cooperate to induce cell cycle arrest in response to TGF-beta. *Genes Dev* 1995;9:1831–1845.

26. el-Deiry WS, Tokino T, Velulsescu VE, Levy DB, Parson R, Trent JM, et al. WAF1, a potential mediator of p53 tumor suppression. *Cell* 1993;75:817–825.

27. Serrano M, Hannon GJ, Beach D. A new regulatory motif in cell cycle control causing specific inhibition of cyclin D/CDK4. *Nature* 1993;366:704–707.

28. Kamb A, Gruis NA, Weaver-Feldhaus J, Liu Q, Harshman K, Tatvigian SV, et al. A cell cycle regulator potentially involved in genesis of many tumor-types. *Science* 1994;264:436–440.

29. Nobori T, Miura K, Wu DJ, Lois A, Takabajashi K, Carson DA. Deletions of the cyclin-dependent kinase 4 inhibitor gene in multiple human cancers. *Nature* 1994;368:753–756.

30. Porter PL, Malone KE, Heagerty PJ, Alexander GM, Gatti LA, Firpo EJ, et al. Expression of cell-cycle regulators p27 Kip1 and cyclin E, alone and in combination, correlate with survival in young breast cancer patients. *Nature Med* 1997;3:222–225.

31. Arellano M, Moreno S. Regulation of CDK/cyclin complexes during the cell cycle. *Int J Biochem Cell Biol* 1997;4:559–573.

32. Hannon GJ, Beach D. p15 INK4b is a potential effector of cell cycle arrest mediated by TGF-β. *Nature* 1994;371:257–261.

33. Guan K, Jenkins CW, Li Y, Nichols MA, Wu X, O'Keeffe CL, et al. Growth suppression by p18, a p16 INK4aMTS2-related CDK6 inhibitor, correlates with wild-type RB function. *Genes Dev* 1994;8:2939–2952.

34. Hirai H, Roussel MF, Kato J, Ashmun RA, Sherr CJ. Novel INK4 proteins, p19 and p18, are specific inhibitors of cyclin D-dependent kinases CDK4 and CDK6. *Mol Cell Biol* 1995;15:2672–2681.

35. Chan FKM, Zhan J, Chen L, Shapiro DN, Winoto A. Identification of human/mouse p19, a novel cdk4/cdk6 inhibitor with homology to p16 INK4. *Mol Cell Biol* 1995;15:2682–2688.

36. Gu Y, Turek CW, Morgan DO. Inhibition of CDK2 activity in vivo by an associated 20K regulatory subunit. *Nature* 1993;366:707–710.

37. Harper JW, Adami GR, Wei N, Keyomarse K, Elledge SJ. The p21 Cdk-interacting protein Cip1 is a potent inhibitor of G1 cyclin-dependent kinases. *Cell* 1993;75:805–816.

38. Xiong Y, Hannon GJ, Zhang H, Casso D, Kobajashi R, Beach D. p21 is a universal inhibitor of cyclin-dependent kinases. *Nature* 1993a;366:701–704.

39. Dulic V, Kauffmann WK, Wilson SJ, Tlsty TD, Lees E, Harper JW, et al. p53-dependent inhibition of cyclin-dependent kinase activities in human fibroblast during radiation-induced G1 arrest. *Cell* 1994;76:1013–1023.

40. Noda A, Ning Y, Venable SF, Pereira-Smith OM, Smith JR. Cloning of senescent cell-derived inhibitors of DNA synthesis using an expression screen. *Expl Cell Res* 1994;211:90–98.

41. Polyak K, Lee MH, Erdjument-Bromage H, Koff A, Roberts JM, Tempst P, Massaguè J. Cloning of p27Kip1, a cyclin-dependent kinase inhibitor and a potential mediator of extracellular antimitogenic signals. *Cell* 1994b;78:59–66.

42. Toyoshima H., Hunter T. p27, a novel inhibitor of G1 cyclin/cdk protein kinase activity, is related to p21. *Cell* 1994;78:67–74.

43. Matsuoka D, Edwards MC, Bai C, Parker S, Zhang P, Baldini A, et al. p57kip2, a structurally distinct member of the p21CIP1 Cdk inhibitor family, is a candidate tumor suppressor gene. *Genes Dev* 1995;9:650–662.

44. Chen J, Jackson PK, Kirschner MW, Dutta A. Separate domains of p21 involved in the inhibition of cdk kinase and PCNA. *Nature* 1995;374:386–388.

45. Nakanish M, Robertorge RS, Adam GR, et al. Identification of the active region of the DNA synthesis inhibitory gene p215di1CIP1WAF1. *Embo J* 1995;14:555–563.
46. Warbrick E, Lane DP, Glover DM, Cox LS. A small peptide inhibitor of DNA replication defines the site of interaction between the cyclin-dependent kinase inhibitor p21WAF1 and proliferating cell nuclear antigen. *Curr Biol* 1995;5:275–282.
47. Lin JC, Reichner C, Wu X, Levine AJ. Analysis of wild-type and mutant p21WAF-1 gene activities. *Mol Biol Cell* 1996;16:1786–1793.
48. Russo AA, Jeffrey PD, Patten AK, Massaguè J, Pavletich NP. Crystal structure of the p27kip1 cyclin-dependent kinase inhibitor bound to the cyclin A-cdk2 complex. *Nature* 1996;366: 704–707.
49. Serrano M. The tumor suppressor protein p16INK4a. *Exp Cell Res* 1997;237:7–13.
50. Otterson GA, Kratze RA, Coxon A, Kim YW, Kaye FJ. Absence of p16INK4 protein is restricted to the subset of lung cancer lines that retains wild-type RB. *Oncogene* 1994;9: 3375–3378.
51. Sheaff RJ, Roberts JM. Lessons in p16 from phylum Falconium *Curr Biol* 1995;5:28-30.
52. Serrano M, Lee HW, Chin L, Cordon-Cardo C, Beach D, Depinto RA. Role of the INK4a locus in tumor suppression and cell mortality. *Cell* 1996;85:27–37.
53. Xiong Y, Zhang H, Beach D. Subunits rearrangements of the cyclin-dependent kinases is associated with cellular transformation. *Genes Dev* 1993b;7:1572–1583.
54. Zhang H, Hannon GJ, Beach D. p21-containing cyclin kinases exist in both active and inactive states. *Genes Dev* 1994;8:1750–1758.
55. Xiong Y, Zhang H, Beach D. D-type cyclins associate with multiple protein kinases and the DNA replication and repair factor PCNA. *Cell* 1992;71:505–514.
56. Harper JW, Elledge SJ, Keyomarse K, Dynlacht B, Tsai L-H, Zhang P, et al. Inhibition of cyclin-dependent kinases by p21. *Mol Cell Biol* 1995;6:387–400.
57. Luo Y, Hurwitz J, Massaguè J. Cell cycle inhibition mediated by functionally independent CDK and PCNA inhibitory domains in p21CIP1. *Nature* 1995;375:159–161.
58. Hengst L, Reed SI. Translational control of p27Kip1 accumulation during the cell cycle. *Science* 1996;271:1861–1864.
59. Russo AA, Tong L, Lee JO, Jeffrey PD, Pavletich NP. Structural basis for inhibition of the cyclin-dependent kinase Cdk6 by the tumor suppressor p16INK4a. *Nature* 1998;395: 237–243.
60. Pavletich NP. Mechanisms of cyclin-dependent kinase regulation: structures of Cdks, their cyclin activators, and Cip and INK4 inhibitors. *J Mol Biol* 1999;287:821–828.
61. Tsihlias J, Kapusta L, Slingerland J. The prognostic significance of altered cyclin-dependent kinase inhibitors in human cancer. *Annu Rev Med* 1999;50:401–423.
62. Catzavelos C, Bhattacharya N, Ung YC, Wilson JA, Roncari L, Sandhu C, et al. Decreased levels of the cell-cycle inhibitor p27kip1 protein: prognostic implication in primary breast cancer. *Nature Med* 1997;3:227–230.
63. Loda M, Cukor B, Tam SW, Lavin P, Fiorentino M, Draetta GF, et al. Increases proteasome-dependent degradation of the cyclin-dependent kinase inhibitor p27 in aggressive colorectal carcinomas. *Nat Med* 1997;3:231–234.
64. Fero ML, Randel E, Gurley KE, Roberts JM, Kemp CJ. The murine gene p27kip1 is haplo-insufficient for tumour suppression. *Nature* 1998;396:177–180.
65. Garrett MD, Fattaey A. CDK inhibition and cancer therapy. *Curr Opin Gen Dev* 1999;9:104–111.

2

p27, A Prognostic Indicator Reflecting ...?

Andrew Koff, PHD

CONTENTS

1. SUMMARY

Over the last five years, the expression of p27kip1, a cyclin-dependent kinase inhibitor, has proved to be a strong prognostic indicator for long-term survival of patients with tumors of the colon, breast, prostate, lung, pituitary, and many other tissues. Tumors arising in these organs that were not expressing p27 protein tended to be more aggressive and patients had a poorer clinical outcome. However, it is not clear why p27 was such a strong prognostic indicator in multiple tissues. Furthermore, before p27 is brought into widespread clinical use, prospective studies will be required to validate, in advance, a clinical course or response to therapy. Without the essential knowledge of what low p27 prognosticates, vis a vis the evolution of the tumor, validation will be difficult. Because there is no possibility of determining directly how low p27 expression facilitates tumor development in humans, we have turned to developing mouse models.

From: *Cancer Drug Discovery and Development:*
Cell Cycle Inhibitors in Cancer Therapy: Current Strategies
Edited by: A. Giordano and K. J. Soprano © Humana Press Inc., Totowa, NJ

However, we had to first ask the following questions: Does p27 deficiency contribute to tumor development in the mouse? If p27 deficiency contributed to tumor development, does it mimic the human condition, i.e., were tumors more aggressive? Then, if they were more aggressive, what was the mechanism underlying this? Before we begin to discuss these issues, I apologize to the many investigators whose work will be either uncited or cited only by review.

2. CHANGES IN p27 ACTIVITY/ABUNDANCE ARE PROGNOSTIC IN MANY TUMORS

The diagnosis of tumor stage and grade is quite subjective and largely depends on the experience of the pathologist with that specific lesion. Even among experienced pathologists, there are disagreements about clincial stage and grade. The intermediate tumors, those that are clearly more advanced than just hyperplasia but not yet obviously aggressive, present a substantial problem. Because treatment is based on the severity of the disease and the likelihood of its progression to a more severe disease, it is important to remove the ambiguity surrounding diagnosis and prognosis. Well-developed and well-understood molecular markers of disease stage and prognosis will succeed in this endeavor.

Over the last five years the expression of p27kip1, as determined by immunohistochemistry, proved to be a strong prognostic indicator of patient survival of tumors of the colon, breast, prostate, lung, pituitary, bladder, and glioma (reviewed by *1–4*). Generally, tumors where low p27 expression was prognostic for severity were of intermediate grade. However, there were exceptions. For example, in Burkitt's lymphoma, increased p27 was associated with increased aggressiveness *(5,6)*. Furthermore, cytosolic localization was observed in ovarian cancers of low malignant potential *(7)* and Barrett's associated adenocarcinoma *(8)*. While these differences are organ/tumor type specific, they probably underlie the complexity of the regulation of p27 abundance (Fig. 1).

Stabilization of p27 in Burkitt's lymphoma was associated with an increase in cyclin D3 *(5,6)*, which is consistent with the inactivation of p27 by sequestration as originally proposed *(9,10)* and the observation that myc induced accumulation of D-type cyclins leads to p27 sequestration *(11)*. However, the mechanism by which cyclin D3-cdk association stabilizes p27 remains to be determined—does it block the phosphorylation of p27 on T187 preventing ubiquitin-dependent protein degradation, or does it block the interaction of p27 with the skp2-containing E3?

Cytosolic localization of p27 was observed in BAA *(8)* and ovarian tumors of low malignant potential (LMP) *(7)*, as well as in a diverse number of sarcomas (P. Capodieci, C. Cordon-Cardo, AK, unpublished data), and even in a 3T3 cell line *(12)*. However, the molecular mechanism remains a mystery. Candidate proteins that might affect p27 localization and that could be mutated in human tumors abound. These include jab1 *(13)*, Nup50 *(14)*, and TSC2 *(15)*.

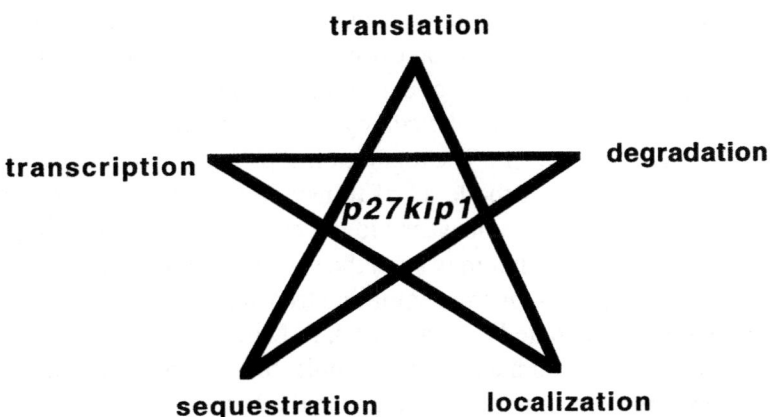

Fig. 1. Processes that regulate the activity and/or abundance of p27kip1. Current investigations are focused on the elucidation of the molecules involved in each of the processes, and the biologic significance of any one of them has not been determined.

The mechanisms leading to the lack of p27 staining are unclear. The absence of p27 protein has rarely, if ever, been attributed to loss of the chromosomal location of the gene (12p13; *16–18*), nor has the absence of protein been well-correlated with loss of mRNA *(1–4)*. However, recent evidence from studies on carcinogen-induced tumor development in p27+/– mice *(19,20)*, and in tumor progression in p27+/– mice intercrossed with Rb+/– mice *(21)* indicated that gene dosage was an important factor. Thus, unlike many genes that require LOH to be implicated as encoding tumor suppressors, p27 is haploinsufficient, and the conclusion that mRNA does not change may need to be re-evaluated keeping in mind that a 50% reduction may not have been readily determined by the most widely used techniques.

On the other hand, it is generally accepted that the inability to detect p27 is due to post-transcriptional changes in protein abundance, and in some cases, it has been suggested to be due to increased ubiquitin-dependent proteolysis *(22–25)*. The strength of this conviction is apparent in the sense that reviews often offer no other alternative *(1–4)*. However, the data supporting this conclusion was derived from experiments generating protein extracts from tumor samples and measuring p27 ubiquitination *(23,24)* or the loss of protein *(25,26)*. This only allows a comparison of proteolytic activity in tumors to that seen in normal tissues. Because p27 degradation is associated with commitment to the cell cycle and entry into S-phase, wouldn't tumor extracts have an increased amount of activity? To overcome this concern, there are a number of studies showing that p27 expression in a tumor was not correlated with proliferation as measured by either Ki67 or MIB reactivity (for example *see* refs. *27–29*) and that these markers together may be more informative than either alone. This reduced the possibility that the prognostic significance of p27 would be associated solely with proliferation, but it does not indicate that proteolysis is the reason for low p27 expression.

Tumors arise as a consequence of cells inappropriately executing the decision to proliferate or withdraw from the cell cycle, they are not simply a decision to continue through the cell cycle. The regulation of p27 abundance between cycling and noncycling states is at the level of translation (30,31). As most cells in a tumor are not proliferating, at least as judged by Ki67 or MIB staining, they are not in the cell cycle, but rather may be in the transition of G_0-to-G_1. A molecular understanding of the mechanisms regulating translational control of p27 mRNA is only now being elucidated (32; A. Vidal, S. Millard, AK, unpublished data).

Perhaps when our understanding of the molecular mechanisms regulating p27 abundance is complete, or better defined than the current synthesis, degradation, and location, we would understand what the loss of p27 represents. Nevertheless, even if we do not know the mechanism that accounts for the loss of p27, a reduction in the amount of functional nuclear p27 protein is prognostic.

3. TUMORS ARE THE SUM OF PROLIFERATION AND OTHER CHANGES IN THE CELL

Recently, reviews on the changes that occur during progression from normal cell to tumor mass were scribed by Hanahan and Weinberg (33). There is very little to add to this, however, it is important for this discussion to review some of the landmarks of tumor development. First, cells must be proliferating. Second, the proliferating cell must not be undergoing apoptosis. Third, the proliferating and living cell must suspend or bypass mortality controls. Of course, even given all these changes, a tumor does not develop in a homogenous environment like a tissue-culture dish, rather it develops in an organism and is affected by its interactions with other cells and on environmental factors. Thus, tumors must induce angiogenesis, and tumor cells often alter their interaction with neighboring cells, alleviating the ability of normal cells to maintain the tissue in a clear, but as of yet molecularly undefined, homeostatic state. Finally, tumor cells that have migrated to distant site must also evolve mechanisms of coping in these strange and often hostile environments.

Not all tumors have the need for angiogenesis or develop metastatic potential; however, all undergo changes in proliferation, apoptosis, and senescence. As we are focusing on p27 and the role that it might play in tumor development, it is helpful to consider how cells move from quiescence into the cycle, and back again.

The effect of mitogenic and anti-mitogenic signals on progression through G_1 phase, and the choice between either commitment to the cell cycle and eventual DNA replication or withdrawal from the cell cycle and perhaps acquisition of a differentiated phenotype, is made by controlling the activation status of the cyclin-dependent kinases. Entry into S-phase requires the activation of two cyclin-dependent kinases, cdk4 and cdk2, which participate together in the inactivation of Rb and the induction of E2F-dependent transcription (34). Although the activation of these kinases is necessary for S-phase entry, it is important to note that there is no evidence in primary cultures of mammalian cells to suggest that this is sufficient to account for all the functions of mitogens required for S-phase entry. Some targets of the cyclin-cdk complexes include pocket-proteins, such as Rb; the cdk inhibitors, such as p27 (35–40); and molecularly defined targets within the centrosome (41). The consequence of target phosphorylation is quite varied. Rb phosphorylation alters gene transcription through changes in HDAC-association and E2F1 association (42). p27 phosphorylation alters its stability. The role of phosphorylation in the centrosome is unclear.

Mitogenic signals, often through the RTKs, induce the synthesis of cyclin D1, inhibit the degradation of cyclin D1, and foster the assembly of cyclin D1 with cdk4 (43–45). Additionally, mitogens can suppress the translation of p27 (30). With an increase in steady-state accumulation of cyclin D-cdk4, the availability of p27 to bind to cyclin E-cdk2 is limited, and thus cyclin E-cdk2 activity could begin to accumulate (10). Once cyclin E-cdk2 accumulates it phosphorylates p27 and initiates ubiquitin-dependent degradation of the protein (35–38,40). This appears to be sufficient to allow for an irreversible commitment to cdk activation in the presence of mitogen.

Anti-mitogenic signals can impact the decision to proliferate by directly increasing the amount of Ink4-type inhibitors. For example, transforming growth factor-β (TGF-β) can induce p15 accumulation, p15 complexes with cdk4 preventing the formation of cyclin D-cdk4 complexes. This prevents sequestration of p27 and the amount of p27 will be sufficient to inhibit cyclin E-cdk2 (46). Likewise, antimitogenic signals can directly induce p27 translation by interfering with the rho-dependent mitogenic signal-transduction pathways that suppress it (A. Vidal, S. Millard, AK, unpublished data). In both examples, the anti-mitogenic signal would antagonize the mitogenic signal; however, the final decision would depend on the equilibrium established between cyclin D-cdk4/ p27 and cyclin E-cdk2.

There are a number of cdk inhibitors akin to p15 and p27, the Ink4 class (p15, p16, p18, p19) and the Kip class (p21, p27, p57), respectively. These proteins are expressed in a cell-type specific manner, and it is generally assumed that they carry out similar roles in mediating growth arrest. However, if that was true, then one would expect that the individual cki-deficient mice would have quite similar phenotypes, i.e., problems in the differentiation of cells that express that particular cki, but this does not appear to be the case (47). The reasons for this are not clear; however, there is cell-type and signal specificity to their accumulation and function in promoting growth arrest. There may be additional functions in differentiated cells, or as regulators of growth arrest in response to DNA damage or nucleotide pool perturbation, or in the assembly of cyclin D-cdk complexes *(48,49)*.

4. HOW CHANGES IN CELL CYCLE REGULATORS MIGHT IMPACT TUMOR GROWTH

For a number of years we have known that the length of time that a cell spends between mitosis and DNA replication can affect its response to the signals that ultimately control its proliferative fate. This was first shown in the response of the simple yeast, *Sacchromyces cerevisiae*, to mating pheromones and was instrumental in uncovering cln3 *(50,51)*. Cancer is a disease where the cell has reduced its dependency on mitogenic signals and no longer responds correctly to anti-mitogenic signals. A few examples from an extensive literature of many mammalian cell types serve to illustrate the fact that G_1 duration affects response: the overexpression of specific D-type cyclins can prevent granulocytic *(52)* or muscle *(53)* differentiation. Cyclin overexpression in fibroblasts will accelerate S-phase entry, but will not prevent growth arrest in response to contact inhibition or complete abolish the need for mitogen. Enforced expression of cdk inhibitors, such as p21 can induce muscle *(54)* or myeloid *(55)* differentiation. In some cases there is no differentiative effect, only a proliferative one. For example, expression of p27 in primary rat oligodendrocyte precursor cells leads to growth arrest but not differentiation *(56)*. Thus we can conclude that mutations that affect G_1-duration have a phenotype similar to one that would affect a growth inhibitory signaling pathway. However, these were all in single cell organisms, explanted cells, or cells grown in culture. Is the same true in a multi-cellular organism?

Mouse genetics has made it possible to examine what overexpression of a cyclin, mutation of a cdk, the absence of a cdk inhibitor, or the mutation of proteins that regulate cdk activity (i.e., cyclin D_1, cyclin E, cdc25, or cdc37), do with regard to tumor development, both spontaneous and carcinogen-induced. There are a large number of these reports on a wide variety of tissues *(57–75)*. The phenotypes of the different cdk inhibitors are discussed individually and have been reviewed *(47,76)*. The phenotypes of the cdk4R24C mutation and the cdk4 knock-out are described in the appropriate references *(77,78)*. Overall, however, individual changes in cdk activity had a relatively modest effect. That might be due to the necessity of activating two cdks, cdk4/6 and cdk2, to drive cells into S-phase *(79,80)*, but even that is not entirely clear, as the activation of cyclin E-cdk2 should bypass the need for cdk4/6 expression by the current model (Fig. 2) and the observations made when cyclin E was knocked-in to the cyclin D_1 locus *(81)*.

Another interpretation is that mutation of the cell cycle, specifically with respects to the proliferation of tumor cells, is kept innocuous by the homeostasis provided by an animal. Proliferating, oncogenically activated cells may be

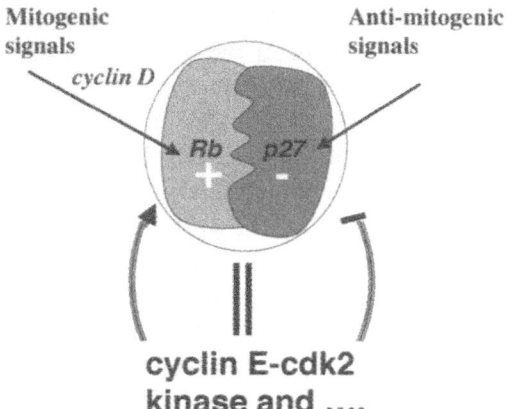

Fig. 2. Cyclin D-cdk complexes and p27 conspire to regulate cyclin E-cdk2. The decision to commit to S-phase correlates well with the activation of cyclin E-cdk2 kinase. Once activated, cyclin E-cdk2 kinase, insures that a strong positive feedback loop is initiated that leads to the increase of cyclin E mRNA, through further inactivation of the Rb-E2F complex, and the elimination of p27kip1, through ubiquitin-dependent proteolysis. Cyclin D-cdk complexes mediate the passage of mitogenic signals to cyclin E-cdk2 through their effects on Rb-E2F complex, and anti-mitogenic signals through their effects on p27.

undergoing apoptosis or senescence continually in the animal. In contrast to the cell cycle changes, when mice were engineered to overexpress or to express mutated forms of many molecules upstream of the cell cycle, i.e., ras, myc, or the her2 receptor, they were obviously tumor prone. Each of these molecules has effects on cell cycle regulators, but also affect proteins that participate in apoptosis and senescence. For example, growth factor cytokines, such as IL-2 *(82)* or c-kit *(83)*, acting through their receptors, often tyrosine kinases, have roles regulating cell proliferation and cell survival, often mediated by interactions through the ras- and PI3-kinase signaling pathways, respectively *(84,85a)*. However, activated ras will induce senescence, presumably through Arf and p21 *(86–88)*. Ras will also intersect the cell cycle: through raf controlling the abundance of the cyclin D-cdk4 complex *(43)*, and through rho controlling the abundance of p27 (A. Vidal, S. Millard, AK, unpublished data). PI3 kinase suppresses apoptosis by activating Akt *(84)*. PI3 kinase activity also can regulate p27 abundance *(85b)*. Additionally, the proliferating cell normally induces a p53 response, which is implicated in apoptosis and/or cell cycle arrest *(86–89)*. The dual nature of p53 rests, at least in part, on its ability to induce p21 *(88,90)* and bax *(91)*, a suppressor of proliferation and an inducer of apoptosis, respectively. Of course, apoptosis and growth arrest can also be p53-independent *(92–95)*.

One way of interpreting this cornucopia of data is that changes in the cell cycle are associated with abnormal proliferation, but are not sufficient to cause abnormal proliferation. Nevertheless, changes in these regulators specifically impact on the ability of the cell to respond to anti-mitogenic signals. Consistent with this possibility, the tumor phenotypes occurring in these mice expressing myc can be enhanced by overexpression of cyclin D_1 *(63,96)*. Those expressing ras can cooperate with cyclin E *(61)*. Keratinocytes lacking p21 and expressing oncogenic ras form aggressive tumors in nude mice, more so than if they lacked p27 or were wild-type *(97)*. Furthermore, mutation of cdk4 makes cells refractory to the actions of Ink-class inhibitors and the overexpression of cyclins would titrate Kip-class inhibitors. This would also seem to be consistent with the finding that only a few mutants in the cell cycle regulators gave rise to "cancer-like" phenotypes. Specifically those in p27-deficient mice, p18-deficient mice, Ink4a-deficient mice, and E2F1-deficient mice were informative, displaying tumor growth properties. Both E2F1 and p27 (see below) are implicated in regulating the transition between cycling and noncycling cells.

However, a word about the Ink4a locus, as this may be due to a non-cell cycle effect. The Ink4a locus is incredibly complex, It encodes both the cdk4 binding protein, p16, and an alternative reading frame, p19Arf1, which share a second exon and have alternative first exons *(98)*. Deletions often, but not always, remove both reading frames *(99)*. Arf1 interacts with and negatively regulates the p53-mdm2 pathway and myc participates in this process, albeit there is still some disagreement over the exact nature of these interactions *(88,100–104)*. Thus mutation in a single locus would affect both the Rb and p53 pathways and has brought into question what the role of p16 deletion in human tumors really is. At this time, this question is unanswered. There are mutations in the p16 ORF identified in tumors that do not affect the p19 ORF, at least by sequence analysis, suggesting that p16 may be a tumor suppressor. However, in mice, the p19Arf1 deletion fully recapitulates the growth and transformation properties of cells and the tumor development property of mice observed with the p16-/-p19-/- mouse (the original Ink4a deletion) *(105–107)*. The rest of this review will studiously ignore the Arf complexity as this has been described recently *(108,109)*.

Consequently, I would raise the proposal that many of the mutations in cell cycle regulators do not drive cell proliferation, but rather make proliferating cells refractory to the consequence of the signals telling them to stop. The goal then became a direct test of the hypothesis, specifically in relationship to p27, rather than culling the data for the consistent observations.

5. p27 AS A PROGNOSTIC INDICATOR: A CELL REMOVED FROM THE CONSEQUENCE OF ANTI-MITOGENIC SIGNALING

The phenotype of p27 deficient mice was quite striking *(110)*. Our mice expressed an amino truncated protein (Δ51, deleted amino acids 1-51) that failed to bind and inactivate cdks, and two other groups created nullizygous mice *(111,112)*. These lines displayed identical phenotypes. Although p18 deficiency can recapitulate some of the phenotypes below, it appears to be more dependent on strain background *(79,113)*. The mice were larger than their wild-type littermates, had no measurable increase in the serum level of growth hormone (GH), insulin-like growth hormone (IGF-1), or IGF-2, and there was an increase in the S-phase fraction of cells in organs in which proliferation was occurring, such as thymus. However, there were very few discernable developmental defects associated with increased proliferation in p27–/– mice except for deafness *(114,115)* and female infertility *(116)*. These data suggested that p27 was involved in the regulation of cell proliferation in many tissues, but did not directly address how.

Evidence from a number of laboratories suggested that p27 was an input for anti-mitogenic differentiation inducing signals, transducing these to the core cell cycle component, cdk2. This was most clearly demonstrated in our studies of the growth and differentiation properties of oligodendrocyte precursor cells isolated from the brain cortex of neonatal mice *(117–119)*, and the granulosa-to-luteal cell transition following hormone induced ovulation *(116)*. Similar results have been shown in the Organ of Corti and in osteoblasts *(114,115,120)*. In each case, a cell-autonomous increase of p27 protein was correlated with differentiation. Thus in cells where it is expressed, p27 clearly has a role in cell cycle withdrawal induced by differentiation signals. The defects we and others reported in the withdrawal program of p27-deficient cells may have been due to a direct response altering their ability to interpret the anti-mitogenic signals, or an indirect response, i.e., these p27–/– cells may have a shorter G_1 period. On this note, although p27 deficiency does not alter G_1 duration in mouse embryo fibroblasts, it has not been examined in any of the cell types above.

As might be expected from the model that cell cycle mutation alleviates cellular response to anti-mitogenic signals, but does not promote proliferation, p27 deficient mice also developed a number of spontaneous abnormal growths—very low grade tumors. These mice spontaneously develop benign prostatic hyperplasia *(121)*, low-grade C-cell carcinoma of the thyroid *(21)*, and a pituitary intermediate lobe hyperplasia or adenoma *(21,110–112)*. Additionally, carcinogens were able to induce tumor development more efficiently in knock-out and heterozygous mice than in wild-type counterparts *(19,20)*. However, it should be noted that heterozygous mice did not spontaneously develop tumors suggesting that haploinsufficiency at this locus is enough to exacerbate a tumorigenic event, but by itself is not tumorigenic.

Now, in order to test the hypothesis that cell cycle regulators, and p27 specifically, might act to prevent anti-mitogenic response of developing tumor cells, we set out to create a mouse model. Our choice to couple the Rb+/– mouse to a p27–/– background seemed reasonable as much was understood about tumor development in the Rb+/– mouse and the tissues affected were similar to that of the p27–/– mouse. Furthermore, if one had to speculate how an oncogenic event would affect cell proliferation, one needs only examine the linkage between ras and Rb. Thus, we speculated that loss of heterozygosity at the Rb locus would provide the oncogenic event and allow us to determine if p27-deficiency would increase the aggressiveness of the resulting tumors.

Rb–/– mice die between embryonic d 14 and 15, depending on the specific disrupted allele and background of the animals (122–124). Death is associated with apoptosis in neural tissues and a lack of fetal hematopoiesis. Rb+/– mice are viable and lead unremarkable lives early in the postnatal period. However, as the animal ages, there is a remarkable incidence of pituitary adenocarcinoma involving the melanotrophs, and C-cell carcinoma of the thyroid (125,126). Remarkably, this is the same tumor spectrum observed in p27–/– mice. Not surprisingly, both p27 and Rb protein accumulate in the mouse melanotroph (21,125). The highly aggressive pituitary adenocarcinoma is thought to be responsible for death of these animals at approx 10–14 mo of age, depending again on genetic background and the specific mutant allele of Rb.

The natural history of the pituitary adenocarcinoma arising in the Rb+/– animal is quite interesting. All the tumors underwent LOH of the Rb locus. This occurred very early in postnatal development with 94% of the animals having undergone an LOH event by day 90 (125). These Rb–/– cells then re-entered the cell cycle, however those cells innervated by the dopaminergic neuron underwent apoptosis. Dopamine is a potent negative growth regulatory signal for the melanotrophs. At some point during the transition from the early proliferates to tumor, the cells acquire a mutation(s) that allows them to develop into an adenocarcinoma. Because these Rb–/– melanotrophs retained the dopamine receptor, it suggested that the other mutations either prevented innervation or the death due to the "oncogenic activation" of Rb LOH coupled with innervation. These mutations might alter the dopaminergic neuron interaction or the ability of the dopaminergic neuron to signal effectively. Whatever the cause, these tumors acquired resistance to innervation and proliferated uncontrollably, or perhaps even proliferated in a manner that now prevented their innervation.

The aforementioned possibilities suggested that signals that disrupt proliferation-induced apoptosis might alter the latency period of this tumor. As indicated this could occur either by disruption of the negative regulatory signals controlling proliferation, or an inability to activate the apoptosis inducing machinery (Fig. 3). Three crosses of Rb+/– mice to other genotypes led to an exaggeration

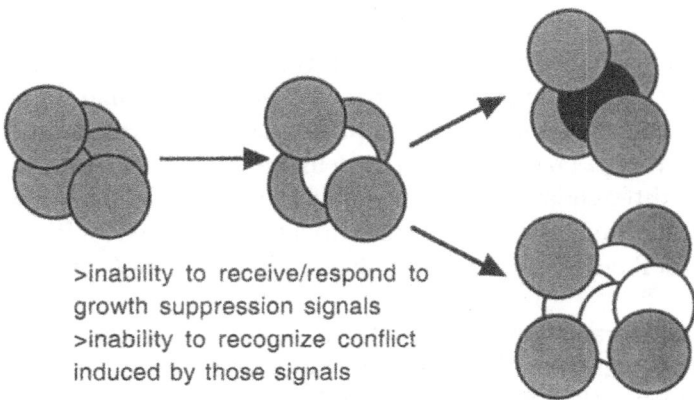

Fig. 3. Possible ways to overcome oncogene induced apoptosis. Following an oncogenic event and the induction of cell proliferation, the cell will either die or senesce before causing any significant tumor to form (top). However, if the cell mutates such that it cannot recognize negative growth regulatory signals from surrounding cells, or cannot initiate an apoptotic pathway perhaps initiated by these conflicting signals, it will continue to proliferate and eventually form a tumor mass.

of tumor phenotype as measured by the classical criteria of a shorter latency period. These included the crossing onto a p53-deficient background *(127)*, a p21-deficient background *(128)*, or a p27-deficient background *(21)*. Although p53 mutation was observed in the original Rb+/– model, the data is consistent with a model wherein the dopaminergic neuron induced death is occurring because of oncogene induced apoptosis, where loss of Rb is the oncogenic event. Likewise, the ability of p21 deficiency to accelerate the tumor may be similar. But what of p27 deficiency?

One possibility is that the loss of p27 prevents the dopaminergic neuron signal from being strong enough to induce p53-dependent apoptosis. In this model, one would have to assume that the cell simply does not recognize the conflict that leads to oncogene-induced apoptosis. However, there is another alternative. The loss of p27 may allow the rate of cell proliferation in the tumor to exceed the rate of apoptosis induced by the dopaminergic neuron. In this scenario, the cells would more rapidly escape the apoptosis-inducing effects of proximity to the neuron. Only now that this model exists can we examine these mechanisms for the aggressiveness associated with low-p27. However, other models are on the horizon. These involve p27 intercrosses to other tumor suppressors such as Pten and inhibin. The findings of these models, with the findings in the Rb model, may shed light on why p27 is a prognostic indicator. Isn't that what it is all about?

CONCLUSION

The aforementioned arguments are built on many assumptions, many of which run contrary to the general belief. However, what is unarguable is: 1) that p27 is a strong prognostic indicator, 2) that p27 status is not correlated with proliferation, and 3) that p27 participates in the withdrawal of cells from the cell cycle in response to differentiation-inducing signals. Furthermore, mice now exist where the prognostic indication of p27 is recapitulated in cancers: for Rb+/– mice in the pituitary, for Pten+/– mice in the prostate, and for inhibin–/– mice in the gonadal tissues.

What is important now, is to decide why low-p27 is prognostic: does it reflect enhanced mitogenic signals, the escape from anti-mitogenic signals, or an escape from senescence *(85)*. When we answer this question, low-p27 expression could join in the pantheon of useful markers. At this time, the three events all coordinate or impact on many levels, not the least of which is the sacrosanct gate-keeper of cell cycle, pRb. However, extrapolation of the ras-mediated changes espoused by Hanahan and Weinberg *(33)*, would be consistent with the notion that ras = mitogen, low-p27 = anti-mitogen, and p53-mdm2-arf-cyclin D-Rb may be related to apoptosis and senesence and the integration of the three events.

ACKNOWLEDGMENTS

I wish to thank David Shaffer, Diana Gitig, Anxo Vidal, Michele Park, and Carlos Cordon-Cordo for comments regarding this review. I also thank the members of the Breast Cancer SPORE of Memorial Sloan-Kettering Cancer Center for opinions on the role that loss of p27 might play in human cancers, and the funding for the creation of the Rb-p27 model. Work in the laboratory is supported by grants from the NIH, Pew Foundation, and Irma T. Hirschl Trust.

REFERENCES

1. Tsihlias J, Kapusta L, Slingerland J. The prognostic significance of altered cyclin-dependent kinase inhibitors in human cancer. *Annu Rev Med* 1999;50:401–423.
2. Lloyd RV, Erickson LA, Jin L, Kulig E, Qian X, Cheville JC, Scheithauer BW. p27kip1: a multifunctional cyclin-dependent kinase inhibitor with prognostic significance in human cancers. *Am J Pathol* 1999;154:313–323.
3. Sgambato A, Cittadini A, Faraglia B, Weinstein IB. Multiple functions of p27(Kip1) and its alterations in tumor cells: a review. *J Cell Physiol* 2000;183:18–27.
4. Slingerland J, Pagano M. Regulation of the cdk inhibitor p27 and its deregulation in cancer. *J Cell Physiol* 2000;183:10–17.
5. Barnouin K, Fredersdorf S, Eddaoudi A, Mittnacht S, Pan LX, Du MQ, Lu X. Antiproliferative function of p27kip1 is frequently inhibited in highly malignant Burkitt's lymphoma cells. *Oncogene* 1999;18:6388–6397.
6. Sanchez-Beato M, Camacho FI, Martinez-Montero JC, Saez AI, Villuendas R, Sanchez-Verde, L, et al. Anomalous high p27/KIP1 expression in a subset of aggressive B-cell lymphomas is associated with cyclin D3 overexpression. p27/KIP1-cyclin D3 colocalization in tumor cells. *Blood* 1999;94:765–772.

7. Masciullo V, Sgambato A, Pacilio C, Pucci B, Ferrandina G, Palazzo J, et al. Frequent loss of expression of the cyclin-dependent kinase inhibitor p27 in epithelial ovarian cancer. *Cancer Res* 1999;59:3790–3794.

8. Singh SP, Lipman J, Goldman H, Ellis FH Jr, Aizenman L, Cangi MG, et al. Loss or altered subcellular localization of p27 in Barrett's associated adenocarcinoma. *Cancer Res* 1998;58:1730–1735.

9. Polyak K, Kato JY, Solomon MJ, Sherr CJ, Massague J, Roberts JM, Koff A. p27Kip1, a cyclin-Cdk inhibitor, links transforming growth factor-beta and contact inhibition to cell cycle arrest. *Genes Dev* 1994;8:9–22.

10. Soos T J, Kiyokawa H, Yan JS, Rubin MS, Giordano A, DeBlasio A, et al. Formation of p27-CDK complexes during the human mitotic cell cycle. *Cell Growth Differ* 1996;7:135–146.

11. Bouchard C, Thieke K, Maier A, Saffrich R, Hanley-Hyde J, Ansorge W, et al. Direct induction of cyclin D2 by Myc contributes to cell cycle progression and sequestration of p27. *EMBO J* 1999;18:5321–5333.

12. Wang G, Miskimins R, Miskimins WK. The cyclin-dependent kinase inhibitor p27Kip1 is localized to the cytosol in Swiss/3T3 cells. *Oncogene* 1999;18:5204–5210.

13. Tomoda K, Kubota Y, Kato J. Degradation of the cyclin-dependent-kinase inhibitor p27Kip1 is instigated by Jab1. *Nature* 1999;398:160–165.

14. Smitherman M, Lee K, Swanger J, Kapur R, Clurman BE. Characterization and targeted disruption of murine nup50, a p27(Kip1)-interacting component of the nuclear pore complex [In Process Citation]. *Mol Cell Biol* 2000;20:5631–5642.

15. Soucek T, Yeung RS, Hengstschlager M. Inactivation of the cyclin-dependent kinase inhibitor p27 upon loss of the tuberous sclerosis complex gene-2. *Proc Natl Acad Sci USA* 1998;95:15653–15658.

16. Ponce-Castaneda MV, Lee MH, Latres E, Polyak K, Lacombe L, Montgomery K, et al. p27Kip1: chromosomal mapping to 12p12-12p13.1 and absence of mutations in human tumors. *Cancer Res* 1995;55:1211–1214.

17. Pietenpol JA, Bohlander SK, Sato Y, Papadopoulos N, Liu B, Friedman C, et al. Assignment of the human p27Kip1 gene to 12p13 and its analysis in leukemias. *Cancer Res* 1995;55:1206–1210.

18. Bullrich F, MacLachlan TK, Sang N, Druck T, Veronese ML, Allen SL, et al. Chromosomal mapping of members of the cdc2 family of protein kinases, cdk3, cdk6, PISSLRE, and PITALRE, and a cdk inhibitor, p27Kip1, to regions involved in human cancer. *Cancer Res* 1995;55:1199–1205.

19. Fero ML, Randel E, Gurley KE, Roberts JM, Kemp CJ. The murine gene p27Kip1 is haplo-insufficient for tumour suppression. *Nature* 1998;396:177–180.

20. Philipp J, Vo K, Gurley KE, Seidel K, Kemp CJ. Tumor suppression by p27Kip1 and p21Cip1 during chemically induced skin carcinogenesis. *Oncogene* 1999;18:4689–4698.

21. Park MS, Rosai J, Nguyen HT, Capodieci P, Cordon-Cardo C, Koff A. p27 and Rb are on overlapping pathways suppressing tumorigenesis in mice. *Proc Natl Acad Sci USA* 1999;96:6382–6387.

22. Elledge SJ, Harper JW. The role of protein stability in the cell cycle and cancer. *Biochim Biophys Acta* 1998;1377:M61–M70.

23. Pagano M, Tam SW, Theodoras AM, Beer-Romero P, Del Sal G, Chau V, et al. Role of the ubiquitin-proteasome pathway in regulating abundance of the cyclin-dependent kinase inhibitor p27. *Science* 1995;269:682–685.

24. Piva R, Cancelli I, Cavalla P, Bortolotto S, Dominguez J, Draetta GF, Schiffer D. Proteasome-dependent degradation of p27/kip1 in gliomas. *J Neuropathol Exp Neurol* 1999;58:691–696.

25. Agus DB, Cordon-Cardo C, Fox W, Drobnjak M, Koff A, Golde D W, Scher HI. Prostate cancer cell cycle regulators: response to androgen withdrawal and development of androgen independence. *J Natl Cancer Inst* 1999;91:1869–1876.

26. Loda M, Cukor B, Tam SW, Lavin P, Fiorentino M, Draetta GF, et al. Increased proteasome-dependent degradation of the cyclin-dependent kinase inhibitor p27 in aggressive colorectal carcinomas. *Nat Med* 1997;3:231–234.

27. Shamma A, Doki Y, Tsujinaka T, Shiozaki H, Inoue M, Yano M, et al. Loss of p27(KIP1) expression predicts poor prognosis in patients with esophageal squamous cell carcinoma. *Oncology* 2000;58:152–158.
28. Cavalla P, Piva R, Bortolotto S, Grosso R, Cancelli I, Chio A, Schiffer D. p27/kip1 expression in oligodendrogliomas and its possible prognostic role. *Acta Neuropathol (Berl)* 1999;98: 629–634.
29. Palmqvist R, Stenling R, Landberg G. Prognostic significance of p27(Kip1) expression in colorectal cancer: a clinico-pathological characterization. *J Pathol* 1999;188:18–23.
30. Agrawal D, Hauser P, McPherson F, Dong F, Garcia A, Pledger WJ. Repression of p27kip1 synthesis by platelet-derived growth factor in BALB/c 3T3 cells. *Mol Cell Biol* 1996;16: 4327–4336.
31. Millard SS, Yan JS, Nguyen H, Pagano M, Kiyokawa H, and Koff A. Enhanced ribosomal association of p27(Kip1) mRNA is a mechanism contributing to accumulation during growth arrest. *J Biol Chem* 1997;272:7093–7098.
32. Millard SS, Vidal A, Markus M, Koff A. A U-Rich Element in the 5' untranslated region is necessary for the translation of p27 mRNA. *Mol Cell Biol* 2000;20:5947–5959.
33. Hanahan D, Weinberg RA. The hallmarks of cancer. *Cell* 2000;100:57–70.
34. Reed SI. Control of the G1/S transition. *Cancer Surv* 1997;29:7–23.
35. Montagnoli A, Fiore F, Eytan E, Carrano AC, Draetta GF, Hershko A, Pagano M. Ubiquitination of p27 is regulated by Cdk-dependent phosphorylation and trimeric complex formation. *Genes Dev* 1999;13:1181–1189.
36. Morisaki H, Fujimoto A, Ando A, Nagata Y, Ikeda K, Nakanishi M. Cell cycle-dependent phosphorylation of p27 cyclin-dependent kinase (Cdk) inhibitor by cyclin E/Cdk2. *Biochem Biophys Res Commun* 1997;240:386–390.
37. Mueller A, Odze R, Jenkins TD, Shahsesfaei A, Nakagawa H, Inomoto T, Rustgi AK. A transgenic mouse model with cyclin D1 overexpression results in cell cycle, epidermal growth factor receptor, and p53 abnormalities. *Cancer Res* 1997;57:5542–5549.
38. Nguyen H, Gitig DM, Koff A. Cell-free degradation of p27(kip1), a G1 cyclin-dependent kinase inhibitor, is dependent on CDK2 activity and the proteasome. *Mol Cell Biol* 1999;19:1190–1201.
39. Sheaff RJ, Groudine M, Gordon M, Roberts JM, Clurman BE. Cyclin E-CDK2 is a regulator of p27Kip1. *Genes Dev* 1997;11:1464–1478.
40. Vlach J, Hennecke S, Amati B. Phosphorylation-dependent degradation of the cyclin-dependent kinase inhibitor p27. *EMBO J* 1997;16:5334–5344.
41. Nigg EA, Blangy A, Lane HA. Dynamic changes in nuclear architecture during mitosis: on the role of protein phosphorylation in spindle assembly and chromosome segregation. *Exp Cell Res* 1996;229:174–180.
42. Harbour JW, Luo RX, Dei Santi A, Postigo AA, Dean DC. Cdk phosphorylation triggers sequential intramolecular interactions that progressively block Rb functions as cells move through G1. *Cell* 1999;98:859–869.
43. Cheng M, Sexl V, Sherr CJ, Roussel MF. Assembly of cyclin D-dependent kinase and titration of p27Kip1 regulated by mitogen-activated protein kinase kinase (MEK1). *Proc Natl Acad Sci USA* 1998;95:1091–1096.
44. Roussel MF, Theodoras AM, Pagano M, Sherr CJ. Rescue of defective mitogenic signaling by D-type cyclins. *Proc Natl Acad Sci USA* 1995;92:6837–6841.
45. Matsushime H, Quelle DE, Shurtleff SA, Shibuya M, Sherr CJ, Kato JY. D-type cyclin-dependent kinase activity in mammalian cells. *Mol Cell Biol* 1994;14:2066–2076.
46. Reynisdottir I, Polyak K, Iavarone A, Massague J. Kip/Cip and Ink4 Cdk inhibitors cooperate to induce cell cycle arrest in response to TGF-beta. *Genes Dev* 1995;9:1831–1845.
47. Kiyokawa H., Koff A. Roles of cyclin-dependent kinase inhibitors: lessons from knock-out mice. *Curr Topics Microbiol Immunol* 1997;227:105–120.

48. Cheng M, Olivier P, Diehl JA, Fero M, Roussel MF, Roberts JM, Sherr CJ. The p21(Cip1) and p27(Kip1) CDK 'inhibitors' are essential activators of cyclin D-dependent kinases in murine fibroblasts. *EMBO J* 1999;18:1571–1583.
49. Zhang H, Hannon GJ, Beach D. p21-containing cyclin kinases exist in both active and inactive states. *Genes Dev* 1994;8:1750–1758.
50. Cross FR. Cell cycle arrest caused by CLN gene deficiency in Saccharomyces cerevisiae resembles START-I arrest and is independent of the mating-pheromone signalling pathway. *Mol Cell Biol* 1990;10:6482–6490.
51. Richardson HE, Wittenberg C, Cross F, Reed SI. An essential G1 function for cyclin-like proteins in yeast. *Cell* 1989;59:1127–1133.
52. Kato JY, Sherr CJ. Inhibition of granulocyte differentiation by G1 cyclins D2 and D3 but not D1. *Proc Natl Acad Sci USA* 1993;90:11513–11517.
53. Skapek SX, Rhee J, Spicer DB, Lassar AB. Inhibition of myogenic differentiation in proliferating myoblasts by cyclin D1-dependent kinase. *Science* 1995;267:1022–1024.
54. Halevy O, Novitch BG, Spicer DB, Skapek SX, Rhee J, Hannon GJ, et al. Correlation of terminal cell cycle arrest of skeletal muscle with induction of p21 by MyoD. *Science* 1995;267:1018–1021.
55. Liu M, Lee MH, Cohen M, Bommakanti M, Freedman LP. Transcriptional activation of the Cdk inhibitor p21 by vitamin D3 leads to the induced differentiation of the myelomonocytic cell line U937. *Genes Dev* 1996;10:142–153.
56. Tikoo R, Osterhout DJ, Casaccia-Bonnefil P, Seth P, Koff A, Chao MV. Ectopic expression of p27Kip1 in oligodendrocyte progenitor cells results in cell-cycle growth arrest. *J Neurobiol* 1998;36:431–440.
57. Bortner DM, Rosenberg MP. Induction of mammary gland hyperplasia and carcinomas in transgenic mice expressing human cyclin E. *Mol Cell Biol* 1997;17:453–459.
58. Bortner DM, Rosenberg MP. Overexpression of cyclin A in the mammary glands of transgenic mice results in the induction of nuclear abnormalities and increased apoptosis. *Cell Growth Differ* 1995;6:1579–1589.
59. Gomez Lahoz E, Liegeois NJ, Zhang P, Engelman JA, Horner J, Silverman A, et al. Cyclin D- and E-dependent kinases and the p57(KIP2) inhibitor: cooperative interactions in vivo. *Mol Cell Biol* 1999;19:353–363.
60. Jenkins TD, Mueller A, Odze R, Shahsafaei A, Zukerberg LR, Kent R, et al. Cyclin D1 overexpression combined with N-nitrosomethylbenzylamine increases dysplasia and cellular proliferation in murine esophageal squamous epithelium. *Oncogene* 1999;18:59–66.
61. Karsunky H, Geisen C, Schmidt T, Haas K, Zevnik B, Gau E, Moroy T. Oncogenic potential of cyclin E in T-cell lymphomagenesis in transgenic mice: evidence for cooperation between cyclin E and Ras but not Myc. *Oncogene* 1999;18:7816–7824.
62. Klug DB, Crouch E, Carter C, Coghlan L, Conti CJ, Richie ER. Transgenic expression of cyclin D1 in thymic epithelial precursors promotes epithelial and T cell development. *J Immunol* 2000;164:1881–1888.
63. Lovec H, Grzeschiczek A, Kowalski MB, Moroy T. Cyclin D1/bcl-1 cooperates with myc genes in the generation of B-cell lymphoma in transgenic mice. *EMBO J* 1994a;13:3487–3495.
64. Lovec H, Sewing A, Lucibello FC, Muller R, Moroy T. Oncogenic activity of cyclin D1 revealed through cooperation with Ha-ras: link between cell cycle control and malignant transformation. *Oncogene* 1994b;9:323–326.
65. Ma ZQ, Chua SS, DeMayo FJ, Tsai SY. Induction of mammary gland hyperplasia in transgenic mice over-expressing human Cdc25B. *Oncogene* 1999;18:4564–4576.
66. Muller D, Bouchard C, Rudolph B, Steiner P, Stuckmann I, Saffrich R, et al. Cdk2-dependent phosphorylation of p27 facilitates its Myc-induced release from cyclin E/cdk2 complexes. *Oncogene* 1997;15:2561–2576.
67. Nakagawa H, Wang TC, Zukerberg L, Odze R, Togawa K, May GH, et al. The targeting of the cyclin D1 oncogene by an Epstein-Barr virus promoter in transgenic mice causes dysplasia in the tongue, esophagus and forestomach. *Oncogene* 1997;14:1185–1190.

68. Pierce AM, Fisher SM, Conti CJ, Johnson DG. Deregulated expression of E2F1 induces hyperplasia and cooperates with ras in skin tumor development. *Oncogene* 1998a;16:1267–1276.
69. Pierce AM, Gimenez-Conti IB, Schneider-Broussard R, Martinez LA, Conti CJ, Johnson DG. Increased E2F1 activity induces skin tumors in mice heterozygous and nullizygous for p53. *Proc Natl Acad Sci USA* 1998b;95:8858–8863.
70. Pierce AM, Schneider-Broussard R, Gimenez-Conti IB, Russell JL, Conti CJ, and Johnson DG. E2F1 has both oncogenic and tumor-suppressive properties in a transgenic model. *Mol Cell Biol* 1999;19:6408–6414.
71. Robles AI, Larcher F, Whalin RB, Murillas R, Richie E, Gimenez-Conti IB, et al. Expression of cyclin D1 in epithelial tissues of transgenic mice results in epidermal hyperproliferation and severe thymic hyperplasia. *Proc Natl Acad Sci USA* 1996;93:7634–7638.
72. Rodriguez-Puebla ML, LaCava M, Conti CJ. Cyclin D1 overexpression in mouse epidermis increases cyclin-dependent kinase activity and cell proliferation in vivo but does not affect skin tumor development. *Cell Growth Differ* 1999;10:467–472.
73. Stepanova L, Finegold M, DeMayo F, Schmidt EV, Harper JW. The oncoprotein kinase chaperone CDC37 functions as an oncogene in mice and collaborates with both c-myc and cyclin D1 in transformation of multiple tissues. *Mol Cell Biol* 2000;20:4462–4473.
74. Wang D, Russell JL, Johnson DG. E2F4 and E2F1 have similar proliferative properties but different apoptotic and oncogenic properties in vivo. *Mol Cell Biol* 2000;20:3417–3424.
75. Wang TC, Cardiff RD, Zukerberg L, Lees E, Arnold A, Schmidt EV. Mammary hyperplasia and carcinoma in MMTV-cyclin D1 transgenic mice. *Nature* 1994;369:669–671.
76. Vidal A, Koff A. Cell-cycle inhibitors: three families united by a common cause. *Gene* 2000;247:1–15.
77. Rane SG, Dubus P, Mettus RV, Galbreath EJ, Boden G, Reddy EP, Barbacid M. Loss of Cdk4 expression causes insulin-deficient diabetes and Cdk4 activation results in beta-islet cell hyperplasia. *Nat Genet* 1999;22:44–52.
78. Tsutsui T, Hesabi B, Moons DS, Pandolfi PP, Hansel KS, Koff A, Kiyokawa H. Targeted disruption of CDK4 delays cell cycle entry with enhanced p27(Kip1) activity. *Mol Cell Biol* 1999;19:7011–7019.
79. Franklin DS, Godfrey VL, Lee H, Kovalev GI, Schoonhoven R, Chen-Kiang S, et al. CDK inhibitors p18(INK4c) and p27(Kip1) mediate two separate pathways to collaboratively suppress pituitary tumorigenesis. *Genes Dev* 1998;12:2899–2911.
80. Resnitzky D, Reed SI. Different roles for cyclins D1 and E in regulation of the G1-to-S transition. *Mol Cell Biol* 1995;15:3463–3469.
81. Geng Y, Whoriskey W, Park MY, Bronson RT, Medema RH, Li T, et al. Rescue of cyclin D1 deficiency by knockin cyclin E. *Cell* 1999;97:767–777.
82. Adachi M, Torigoe T, Takayama S, Imai K. BAG-1 and Bcl-2 in IL-2 signaling. *Leuk Lymphoma* 1998;30:483–491.
83. Besmer P. The kit ligand encoded at the murine Steel locus: a pleiotropic growth and differentiation factor. *Curr Opin Cell Biol* 1991;3:939–946.
84. Downward J. Mechanisms and consequences of activation of protein kinase B/Akt. *Curr Opin Cell Biol* 1998a;10:262–267.
85a. Downward J. Ras signalling and apoptosis. *Curr Opin Genet Dev* 1998b;8:49–54.
85b. Collado M, Medema RH, Garcia-Cao I, Dubuisson ML, Barradas M, Glassford J, et al. Inhibition of the phosphoinositide 3-kinase pathway induces a senescence-like arrest mediated by p27Kip1. *J Biol Chem* 2000;275:21960–21968.
86a. Attardi LD, Jacks T. The role of p53 in tumour suppression: lessons from mouse models. *Cell Mol Life Sci* 1999;55:48–63.
86b. Serrano M, Lin AW, McCurrach ME, Beach D, Lowe SW. Oncogenic ras provokes premature cell senescence associated with accumulation of p53 and p16INK4a. *Cell* 1997;88:593–602.
87. Attardi LD, Lowe SW, Brugarolas J, Jacks T. Transcriptional activation by p53, but not induction of the p21 gene, is essential for oncogene-mediated apoptosis. *EMBO J* 1996;15:3702–3712.

87. Vogt M, Haggblom C, Yeargin, J, Christiansen-Weber T, Haas M. Independent induction of senescence by p16INK4a and p21CIP1 in spontaneously immortalized human fibroblasts. *Cell Growth Differ* 1998;9:139–146.

88. Weber JD, Taylor LJ, Roussel MF, Sherr CJ, Bar-Sagi D. Nucleolar Arf sequesters Mdm2 and activates p53. *Nat Cell Biol* 1999;1:20–26.

88. Brugarolas J, Moberg K, Boyd SD, Taya Y, Jacks T, Lees JA. Inhibition of cyclin-dependent kinase 2 by p21 is necessary for retinoblastoma protein-mediated G1 arrest after gamma-irradiation. *Proc Natl Acad Sci USA* 1999;96:1002–1007.

89. Guillouf C, Grana X, Selvakumaran M, De Luca A, Giordano A, Hoffman B, Liebermann DA. Dissection of the genetic programs of p53-mediated G1 growth arrest and apoptosis: blocking p53-induced apoptosis unmasks G1 arrest. *Blood* 1995;85:2691–2698.

90. Brugarolas J, Chandrasekaran C, Gordon JI, Beach D, Jacks T, Hannon GJ. Radiation-induced cell cycle arrest compromised by p21 deficiency. *Nature* 1995;377:552–557.

91. McCurrach ME, Connor TM, Knudson CM, Korsmeyer SJ, Lowe SW. bax-deficiency promotes drug resistance and oncogenic transformation by attenuating p53-dependent apoptosis. *Proc Natl Acad Sci USA* 1997;94:2345–2349.

92. Aladjem MI, Spike BT, Rodewald LW, Hope TJ, Klemm M, Jaenisch R, Wahl GM. ES cells do not activate p53-dependent stress responses and undergo p53-independent apoptosis in response to DNA damage. *Curr Biol* 1998;8:145–155.

93. Corbet SW, Clarke AR, Gledhill S, Wyllie AH. P53-dependent and -independent links between DNA-damage, apoptosis and mutation frequency in ES cells. Oncogene 1999; 18: 1537–1544.

94. Strasser A, Harris AW, Jacks T, Cory S. DNA damage can induce apoptosis in proliferating lymphoid cells via p53-independent mechanisms inhibitable by Bcl-2 [see comments]. *Cell* 1994;79:329–339.

95. Wyllie FS, Haughton MF, Bond JA, Rowson JM, Jones CJ, Wynford-Thomas D. S phase cell-cycle arrest following DNA damage is independent of the p53/p21(WAF1) signalling pathway. *Oncogene* 1996;12:1077–1182.

96. Bodrug SE, Warner BJ, Bath ML, Lindeman GJ, Harris AW, Adams JM. Cyclin D1 transgene impedes lymphocyte maturation and collaborates in lymphomagenesis with the myc gene. *EMBO J* 1994;13:2124–2130.

97. Missero C, Di Cunto F, Kiyokawa H, Koff A, Dotto GP. The absence of p21Cip1/WAF1 alters keratinocyte growth and differentiation and promotes ras-tumor progression. *Genes Dev* 1996;10:3065–3075.

98. Quelle DE, Zindy F, Ashmun RA, Sherr CJ. Alternative reading frames of the INK4a tumor suppressor gene encode two unrelated proteins capable of inducing cell cycle arrest. *Cell* 1995;83:993–1000.

99. Quelle DE, Cheng M, Ashmun RA, Sherr CJ. Cancer-associated mutations at the INK4a locus cancel cell cycle arrest by p16INK4a but not by the alternative reading frame protein p19ARF. *Proc Natl Acad Sci USA* 1997;94:669–673.

100. Eischen CM, Weber JD, Roussel MF, Sherr CJ, Cleveland JL. Disruption of the ARF-Mdm2-p53 tumor suppressor pathway in Myc-induced lymphomagenesis. *Genes Dev* 1999;13:2658–2669.

101. Kamijo T, Weber JD, Zambetti G, Zindy F, Roussel MF, Sherr CJ. Functional and physical interactions of the ARF tumor suppressor with p53 and Mdm2. *Proc Natl Acad Sci USA* 1998;95:8292–8297.

102. Tao W, Levine AJ. Nucleocytoplasmic shuttling of oncoprotein Hdm2 is required for Hdm2-mediated degradation of p53. *Proc Natl Acad Sci USA* 1999;96:3077–3080.

103. Tao W, Levine AJ. P19(ARF) stabilizes p53 by blocking nucleo-cytoplasmic shuttling of Mdm2. *Proc Natl Acad Sci USA* 1999;96:6937–6941.

104. Zindy F, Eischen CM, Randle DH, Kamijo T, Cleveland JL, Sherr CJ, Roussel MF. Myc signaling via the ARF tumor suppressor regulates p53-dependent apoptosis and immortalization. *Genes Dev* 1998;12:2424–2433.

105. Kamijo T, van de Kamp E, Chong MJ, Zindy F, Diehl JA, Sherr CJ, McKinnon PJ. Loss of the ARF tumor suppressor reverses premature replicative arrest but not radiation hypersensitivity arising from disabled atm function. *Cancer Res* 1999a;59:2464–2469.
106. Kamijo T, Bodner S, van de Kamp E, Randle DH, Sherr CJ. Tumor spectrum in ARF-deficient mice. *Cancer Res* 1999b;59:2217–2222.
107. Kamijo T, Zindy F, Roussel MF, Quelle DE, Downing JR, Ashmun RA, et al. Tumor suppression at the mouse INK4a locus mediated by the alternative reading frame product p19ARF. *Cell* 1997;91:649–659.
108. Sherr CJ. Tumor surveillance via the ARF-p53 pathway. *Genes Dev* 1998;12:2984–2991.
109. Sherr CJ, Weber JD. The ARF/p53 pathway. *Curr Opin Genet Dev* 2000;10:94–99.
110. Kiyokawa H, Kineman RD, Manova-Todorova KO, Soares VC, Hoffman ES, Ono M, et al. Enhanced growth of mice lacking the cyclin-dependent kinase inhibitor function of p27(Kip1). *Cell* 1996;85:721–732.
111. Fero ML, Rivkin M, Tasch M, Porter P, Carow CE, Firpo E, et al. A syndrome of multiorgan hyperplasia with features of gigantism, tumorigenesis, and female sterility in p27(Kip1)-deficient mice. *Cell* 1996;85:733–744.
112. Nakayama K, Ishida N, Shirane M, Inomata A, Inoue T, Shishido N, et al. Mice lacking p27(Kip1) display increased body size, multiple organ hyperplasia, retinal dysplasia, and pituitary tumors. *Cell* 1996;85:707–720.
113. Latres E, Malumbres M, Sotillo R, Martin J, Ortega S, Martin-Caballero J, et al. Limited overlapping roles of P15(INK4b) and P18(INK4c) cell cycle inhibitors in proliferation and tumorigenesis. *EMBO J* 2000;19:3496–3506.
114. Chen P, Segil N. p27(Kip1) links cell proliferation to morphogenesis in the developing organ of Corti. *Development* 1999;126:1581–1590.
115. Lowenheim H, Furness DN, Kil J, Zinn C, Gultig K, Fero ML, et al. Gene disruption of p27(Kip1) allows cell proliferation in the postnatal and adult organ of corti. *Proc Natl Acad Sci USA* 1999;96:4084–4088.
116. Tong W, Kiyokawa H, Soos TJ, Park MS, Soares VC, Manova K, et al. The absence of p27Kip1, an inhibitor of G1 cyclin-dependent kinases, uncouples differentiation and growth arrest during the granulosa- >luteal transition. *Cell Growth Differ* 1998;9:787–794.
117. Casaccia-Bonnefil P, Hardy RJ, Teng KK, Levine JM, Koff A, Chao MV. Loss of p27Kip1 function results in increased proliferative capacity of oligodendrocyte progenitors but unaltered timing of differentiation. *Development* 1999;126:4027–4037.
118. Casaccia-Bonnefil P, Tikoo R, Kiyokawa H, Friedrich V Jr, Chao MV, Koff A. Oligodendrocyte precursor differentiation is perturbed in the absence of the cyclin-dependent kinase inhibitor p27Kip1. *Genes Dev* 1997;11:2335–2346.
119. Durand B, Fero ML, Roberts JM, Raff MC. p27Kip1 alters the response of cells to mitogen and is part of a cell-intrinsic timer that arrests the cell cycle and initiates differentiation. *Curr Biol* 1998;8:431–440.
120. Drissi, H., Hushka, D., Aslam, F., Nguyen, Q., Buffone, E., Koff, A., et al. The cell cycle regulator p27kip1 contributes to growth and differentiation of osteoblasts. *Cancer Res* 1999;59:3705–3711.
121. Cordon-Cardo C, Koff A, Drobnjak M, Capodieci P, Osman I, Millard SS, et al. Distinct altered patterns of p27KIP1 gene expression in benign prostatic hyperplasia and prostatic carcinoma. *J Natl Cancer Inst* 1998;90:1284–1291.
122. Clarke AR, Maandag ER, van Roon M, van der Lugt NM, van der Valk M, Hooper ML, et al. Requirement for a functional Rb-1 gene in murine development. *Nature* 1992;359:328–330.
123. Jacks T, Fazeli A, Schmitt EM, Bronson RT, Goodell MA, Weinberg RA. Effects of an Rb mutation in the mouse. *Nature* 1992;359:295–300.
124. Lee EY, Chang CY, Hu N, Wang, YC, Lai CC, Herrup K, et al. Mice deficient for Rb are nonviable and show defects in neurogenesis and haematopoiesis. *Nature* 1992;359:288–294.

125. Nikitin A, Lee WH. Early loss of the retinoblastoma gene is associated with impaired growth inhibitory innervation during melanotroph carcinogenesis in Rb+/– mice. *Genes Dev* 1996;10:1870–1879.
126. Yamasaki L, Bronson R, Williams BO, Dyson NJ, Harlow E, Jacks T. Loss of E2F-1 reduces tumorigenesis and extends the lifespan of Rb1(+/–) mice. *Nat Genet* 1998;18:360–364.
127. Williams BO, Remington L, Albert DM, Mukai S, Bronson RT, Jacks T. Cooperative tumorigenic effects of germline mutations in Rb and p53. *Nat Genet* 1994;7:480–484.
128. Brugarolas J, Bronson RT, Jacks T. p21 is a critical CDK2 regulator essential for proliferation control in Rb-deficient cells. *J Cell Biol* 1998;141:503–514.

3 Cell Cycle Control of Transcription at the G1/S Phase Transition

André J. van Wijnen, PhD,
Gary S. Stein, PhD, Janet L. Stein, PhD,
and Jane B. Lian, PhD

CONTENTS

1. INTRODUCTION

Competency for proliferation and cell cycle progression are functionally linked to the activities of regulatory factors that modulate the cell division cycle in response to the multi-directional signals of cell type specific signaling cascades. The parameters that mediate growth control are complex and interdependent, and whether cells grow or cease division reflects the integration of a broad spectrum of positive and negative growth regulatory signals that operate within distinct biological contexts. Equally important from a clinical perspective, fidelity of cell cycle regulatory mechanisms is compromised in transformed and tumor cells and in nonmalignant disorders, and reflects deregulation of cell growth or abrogation of cell death.

The conceptual foundation for understanding mammalian cell cycle control was provided by the documentation *(1)* that proliferation of eukaryotic cells, analogous to that of bacteria, requires discrete periods of DNA replication (S-phase) and mitotic division (M) with a postsynthetic, premitotic period designated G_2 and a postmitotic, presynthetic period designated G_1 (Fig. 1). Cell fusion and nuclear transplant experiments (reviewed in refs. *2,3*) revealed that

From: *Cancer Drug Discovery and Development:*
Cell Cycle Inhibitors in Cancer Therapy: Current Strategies
Edited by: A. Giordano and K. J. Soprano © Humana Press Inc., Totowa, NJ

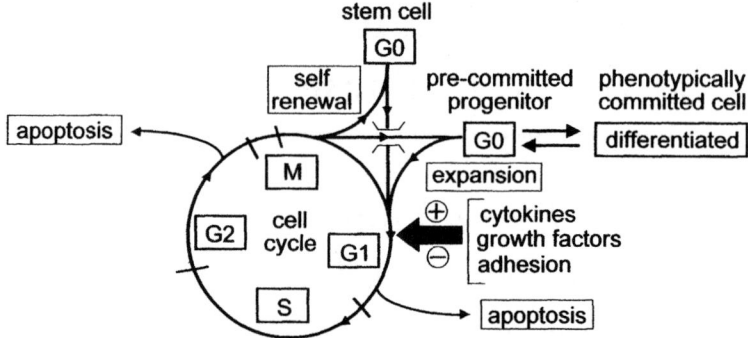

Fig 1. Control of cell proliferation. Cell cycle progression through the G_1, S, G_2, and M phases of the cell cycle is controlled in part by extracellular cues (e.g., growth factors, cytokines, and cell adhesion), as well as by a series of checkpoints (not indicated) that regulate multiple cell cycle transitions (e.g., G_1/S and G_2/M) and that involve surveillance mechanisms controlling apoptosis. The diagram also indicates the options of uncommitted stem cells and precommitted progenitor cells for clonal expansion prior to phenotype commitment and differentiation.

the regulation of DNA replication, which reflects the cellular commitment to duplicate the genome in anticipation of mitotic division, involves both positive and negative cell stage-specific factors.

Transcriptional control of gene expression during S phase in the cell cycle is required for rendering cells capable of replicating DNA and, subsequently, for packaging nascent DNA into chromatin, which permits chromosomal segregation at mitosis. Upon growth factor stimulation there are a series of checkpoints during the G_1 and S phases of the cell cycle where specific genes are activated or suppressed. These checkpoints in late G_1 and in early S phase include surveillance mechanisms that monitor growth factors concentrations, nutrient status and the integrity of the genome, and influence the regulatory activities of cell cycle stage-specific factors. In normal cells, editing mechanism that rectify DNA damage or restore the fidelity of the transcriptional machinery, influence the decision to resume progression through the cell cycle or to default to apoptotic pathways.

Promoters of genes and cognate factors together represent physiologically responsive transducers of growth regulatory signals within the nucleus by forming macromolecular complexes involving sequence-specific protein-DNA and protein-protein interactions. Formation of these macromolecular complexes may be facilitated by specific localization of genes with the nuclear space, subnuclear targeting of gene regulatory factors, local concentration of transcriptional regulators at specific nuclear domains, and *in situ* association with co-regulatory factors capable of modifying chromatin organization *(4)*. Furthermore, the gene-specific integration of cell signals requires remodeling of chromatin, which is

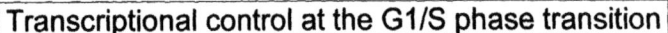

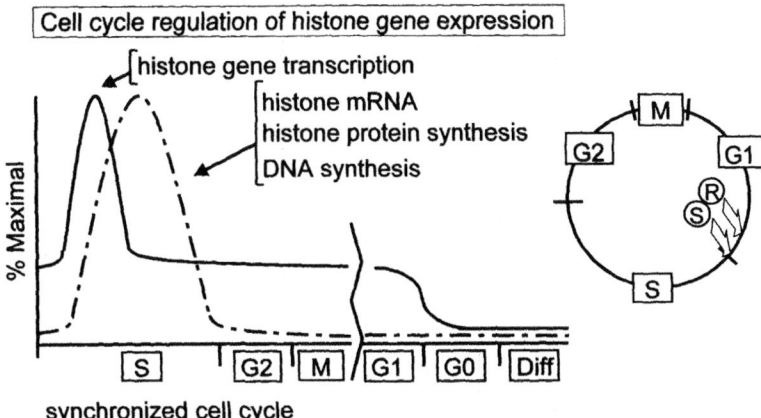

Fig. 2. Cell cycle regulation of histone gene expression. Histone gene regulation represents a paradigm for transcriptional control at the G_1/S phase transition. Cells synchronized at the G_1/S phase boundary progress through the S, G_2, M, and G_1 phases as indicated (horizontal axis). Accumulation of histone mRNA and histone proteins biosynthesis that parallel the rate of DNA synthesis (all depicted together by the dashed line; percentage of maximal value depicted on the vertical axis). The rapid accumulation of histone mRNAs during early S-phase is supported by a significant enhancement of histone gene transcription (solid line) immediately following entry into S-phase. The transcriptional upregulation of histone gene transcription at the G_1/S phase transition is mediated by an E2F-independent mechanism.

under control of SWI/SNF proteins and histone modifying enzymes, to render cis-acting promoter elements accessible to trans-acting regulatory proteins *(5)*. Current evidence suggests that aberrations in any of these steps mediating control of gene expression may deregulate cell growth regulatory pathways.

Transcriptional control is a dominant component of growth-related gene regulation, but post-transcriptional mechanisms are also operative. For example, 3' end processing of primary transcripts, mRNA splicing, RNA export from the nucleus, translational control, and the location of ribosomes within the cell represent potential targets for modulating gene expression. Messenger RNA stability is relevant to cell cycle-dependent control of gene expression. Transcripts from constitutively transcribed genes have finite half-lives. Histone gene expression is a striking example of the combined utilization of control at the levels of transcription, messenger RNA processing, and transcript stability (Fig. 2). Transcriptional upregulation occurs at the onset of S phase. Cell cycle stage-specific changes in transcript processing and turnover reflects the tight coupling of histone gene expression with DNA replication. Histone messenger RNAs are stable throughout S phase and are rapidly as well as selectively degraded at the S/G_2 transition or immediately following inhibition of DNA synthesis.

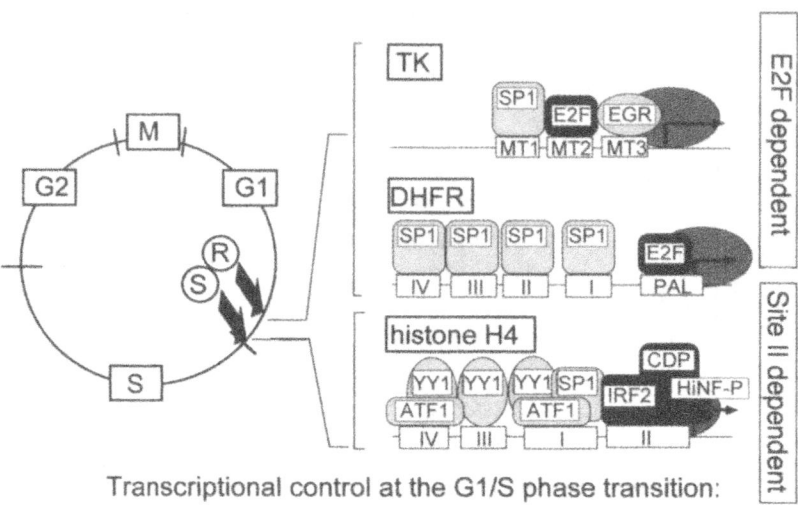

Fig. 3. Transcriptional control of genes regulated in late G_1 and the G_1/S phase transition. The promoters of the TK and DHFR genes integrate cell growth regulatory cues at the Restriction point and are regulated by E2F and SP1. Histone gene promoters are activated after cells have reached growth factor independence at the R-point, and are regulated by E2F-independent mechanisms.

2. TRANSCRIPTIONAL CONTROL DURING THE CELL CYCLE

Insight into transcriptional control at strategic points during the cell cycle has been provided by characterization of promoters and cognate factors, which regulate expression of genes associated with competency for proliferation, cell cycle progression, and mitotic division. The modular organization of these gene promoter elements offers a blueprint of responsiveness to a broad spectrum of physiological regulatory signals, which determine levels of transcription. The overlapping sequence organization of each promoter domain and the multipartite complexes that involve protein/DNA and protein/protein interactions facilitate the convergence of growth regulatory signals to accommodate cell cycle and growth control under diverse biological circumstances. Transcriptional modulation of gene expression is required throughout the cell cycle and is linked to a temporal sequence of events that is necessary for proliferation. However, for clarity of presentation we will confine our considerations to examples of transcriptional control which are operative during G_1 and at the onset of S phase (Fig. 3).

2.1. Transcriptional Activation and Suppression of Genes Involved in Nucleotide Metabolism at the Restriction Point Preceding the G_1/S Transition

During the G_1/S phase transition, three critical events associated with activities of cell cycle checkpoints occur which prepare the cell for the duplication of chromatin. First, genes encoding enzymes involved in nucleotide metabolism are activated to ensure that cellular deoxynucleotide triphosphate pools are adequate for the onset of DNA synthesis. Second, multiprotein complexes at DNA replication origins are assembled that regulate both the initiation of DNA synthesis and prevent re-initiation at the same origin. Third, histone proteins are synthesized *de novo* to accommodate the packaging of newly replicated DNA into nucleosomes. Transcriptional activation of gene expression at the G_1/S phase transition represents the initial rate-limiting step for cell cycle progression into S phase.

The restriction point prior to the G_1/S phase transition integrates a multiplicity of cell signaling pathways that monitor growth factor levels, nutrient status and cell/cell contact. This integration of positive and negative cell cycle regulatory cues culminates in the transcriptional upregulation of genes encoding enzymes and accessory factors that directly and indirectly control nucleotide metabolism and DNA synthesis (Fig. 3). Analysis of the thymidine kinase (TK) promoter and cognate promoter factors has revealed that maximal TK gene transcription involves at least three distinct cis-acting elements (MT1, MT2, and MT3) *(6–11)*. These elements interact with cell cycle-dependent (e.g., Yi1 and Yi2) and constitutive (e.g., SP1) DNA binding proteins. The Yi-complexes interacting with the MT2 motif are associated with p107, as well as cyclin- and cdk-related proteins *(7–11)*. The Yi-complexes are analogous to or identical with E2F related higher-order complexes containing cyclins, CDKs and pRB related proteins. Interestingly, cyclins A and E may represent the labile and rate-limiting restriction point proteins, which were originally postulated based on results from early studies on cell growth control *(12)*.

Each of the G_1/S phase genes is controlled by different arrays of cis-acting promoter elements and cognate factors. One unifying theme among many promoters of the R-point genes is the presence of E2F and SP1 consensus elements. Thus, one mechanism by which the cell achieves coordinate and temporal regulation of these genes at the G_1/S phase boundary is directly linked to the release of transcriptionally active E2F from inactive E2F/pRB complexes (Fig. 4). The disruption of E2F/pRB is mediated by CDK4/CDK6-dependent phosphorylation of pRB in response to growth factor stimulation and cell cycle entry. Hence, the E2F dependent activation of the R-point genes provides linkage between the onset of S phase and control of cell growth.

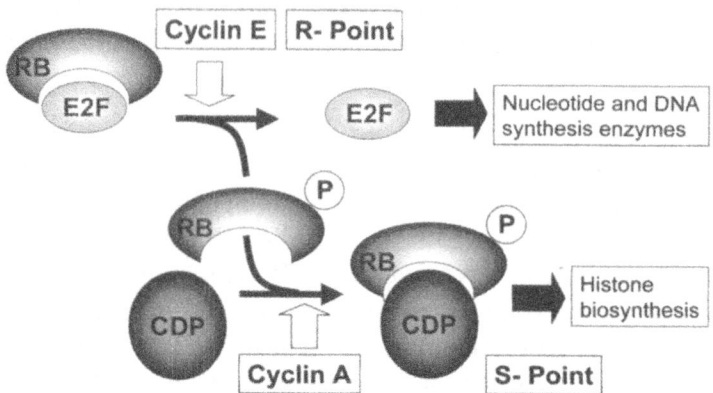

Fig. 4. Postulated functions of pRB during the cell cycle. The function of the pRB tumor suppressor protein as a transcriptional co-regulator may be transduced through E2F and non-E2F factors. E2F factors are activated at the R-point by Cyclin E/CDK2 mediated phosphorylation of pRB which disrupts the pRB/E2F interaction. Release of pRB from E2F is involved in transcriptional enhancement of genes (e.g., TK, DHFR) that regulate nucleotide metabolism. Hyperphosphorylation of pRB coincides with emergence of the histone gene transcription factor complex HiNF-D which contains the CDP-cut homeodomain protein in association with pRB and Cyclin A. The pRB/CDP-cut complex (i.e., HiNF-D) is involved in the regulation of histone gene transcription at the G_1/S phase transition when DNA synthesis has been initiated (designated S-point).

The E2F transcription factor represents a heterogenous class of heterodimers formed between one of five different E2F proteins (i.e., E2F-1 to E2F-5) and one of three distinct DP factors (DP-1 to DP-3). The various E2F factors may display preferences in promoter-specificity, differ in the regulation of their DNA binding activities during the cell cycle, and bind selectively to distinct pRB proteins *(13,14)*. The mechanism by which this multiplicity of E2F factors orchestrate transcriptional regulation of diverse sets of genes at the G_1/S phase transition is only beginning to be understood. Apart from the role of "free" E2F in activating genes at the G_1/S phase transition, promoter-bound complexes of E2F factors associated with pRB-related proteins, cyclin A and CDK2 have active roles in repression of gene expression during early S phase *(15)*.

E2F-responsive transcriptional modulation of R-point genes requires partici-pation of the SP1 family of transcription factors (e.g., SP1 and SP3). For example, the TK promoter contains one E2F site and one SP1 site and both are required for maximal transcriptional responsiveness at the G_1/S phase boundary *(16)*. This synergistic enhancement involves direct protein/protein interactions between E2F and SP1. Consistent with the critical role of SP1 in cell cycle control of gene expression, protein/protein interactions between SP1 and pRB can also occur, suggesting that pRB can modulate the activities of E2F and SP1 in concert.

Analogous to the TK promoter, the DHFR promoter is regulated by four SP1 elements, which together with E2F mediate transcriptional upregulation at the G_1/S phase transition *(17–24)*. Interestingly, SP3 selectively represses SP1 activation of the DHFR promoter, but not the TK or histone H4 promoter *(25,26)*. It appears that the cellular ratio of SP1 and SP3 levels may influence specific classes of cell cycle regulated genes, but the physiological function of this regulatory mechanism remains to be elucidated.

2.2. E2F Dependent Integration of Cell Growth Regulatory Signals at the Restriction Point Late in G1

Computer-assisted analysis of gene promoters for the presence of E2F consensus elements has identified many cell cycle related genes that are or may be potential targets for E2F transcription factors *(27)*. The set of known or putative E2F dependent target genes include cell cycle-related genes such as those encoding E2F transcription factors, cyclins (e.g., cycD1, cycA, cycB1), cyclin-dependent kinases (e.g., CDK1/cdc2) and phosphatases (cdc25C), inhibitors of cyclin-dependent kinases (e.g., p21), tumor suppressors (p53, and the retinoblastoma-related proteins RB1 and p107), and ARF; factors and enzymes involved in DNA replication, DNA repair, and nucleotide metabolism (e.g., DHFR, TK); transcription factors of the Myc, Myb, and AP-1 families, nucleolins, RNA polymerases, and genes encoding components of signal transduction pathways (plk) *(27)*. This broad spectrum of target genes includes genes that exhibit G_2-specific expression patterns indicating that E2F-mediated transcriptional regulation is not restricted to the G_1/S phase. Thus, E2F may perform a more ubiquitous gene regulatory role in proliferating cells analogous to that of other transcription factors involved in cell cycle control, including the CCAAT-box binding protein NF-Y, the GC-box binding protein Sp1, and the octamer binding factor Oct1.

E2F dependent regulation of genes during the cell cycle involves sequential interactions with distinct members of the E2F and pRB families as cells progress through G_1 following growth factor stimulation. This principle is exemplified by studies with the DHFR gene. The interaction of E2F proteins with two overlapping E2F sites in the DHFR gene is critical for the cell cycle-dependent repression and induction of DHFR gene expression in late G_1 *(24)*. One of the proteins involved in repression is the pRB related p130 protein. Growth factor stimulation reduces the levels of E2F-4/DP-1/p130 repressor complexes, and the inactivation of p130-mediated repression permits transcriptional enhancement by positively acting E2F complexes (i.e., E2F-4 and E2F-2 with DP-1) during late G_1. The recruitment of p130 by E2F-4 to repress genes in quiescent cells correlates with decreased acetylation *(28)*. Upon cell cycle entry, gene induction is reflected by binding of E2F-1, E2F-2, or E2F-3 to different promoters and occurs concomitant with acetylation of histones H3 and H4 at E2F-responsive promoters.

Certain histone genes, whose expression remains high throughout S-phase and into G_2 phase, also appear to have E2F binding sites. However, the great majority of DNA replication-dependent histone genes do not have E2F binding sites, and all cell cycle regulatory elements that have been identified in histone gene promoters lack E2F recognition motifs *(29–32)*. The dependence of DNA replication during S phase on the products of E2F dependent genes, and the reliance of histone genes on other gene regulatory factors, indicates that cell cycle control at the G_1/S phase transition is achieved by the integration of both E2F dependent and independent pathways.

2.3. Transcriptional Control by pRB Proteins Independent of E2F During the Cell Cycle

The retinoblastoma tumor suppressor protein (pRB) is a transcriptional co-regulator that mediates several cell cycle related functions. These functions are sequentially activated and inactivated by distinct CDK/cyclin complexes during the G_1- and S-phases *(33)*. Phosphorylation of pRB by CDK/cyclin complexes prevents pRB from suppressing transcription of cell cycle regulatory genes resulting in stimulation of cell cycle progression. The function of pRB as a co-regulator necessitates the action of a sequence-specific transcription factor capable of targeting pRB to appropriate genes. One principal class of partner proteins for pRB are the E2F transcription factors. Several genes that are up-regulated in G_1 by the E2F class of transcription factors can be repressed by pRB. The selectivity of pRB function is reflected by its contribution to the transcriptional downregulation of genes related to the G_1/S phase transition, including E2F-1, E2F-2, dihydrofolate reductase, thymidine kinase, c-myc, proliferating-cell nuclear antigen, p107, and p21/Cip1 genes *(34)*. However, pRB does not appear to regulate transcription of other related genes (e.g., E2F-3, E2F-4, E2F-5, DP-1, DP-2, or p16/Ink4). Apart from the formation of pRB/E2F repressor complexes on gene promoters, it is important to note that E2F independent mechanisms for mediating the transcriptional functions of pRB are also operative (Fig. 4).

DNA replication-dependent histone gene promoters lack E2F binding sites and interact with pRB proteins through a proliferation-specific multimeric complex (designated HiNF-D) containing the CDP/cut homeodomain transcription factor *(30)*. Consistent with this finding, pRB-family proteins can also interact with transcription factors containing paired-like homeodomains *(35,36)*. The HMG-box protein-1 (HBP-1) is also known to directly interact with pRB, and HBP-1 suppresses the gene encoding the Cdk inhibitor p21 (WAF1/CIP1) *(37)*. HBP-1 mediated transcriptional repression prevents the E2F dependent induction of p21 expression. Thus, the interplay between the activities of the pRB binding protein HBP1 and E2Fs on the p21 promoter may account for modulations in p21 gene expression. Recent finding suggests that the runt-related transcription factor RUNX2 (CBFA1/AML3/PEBP2alphaA) interacts with the retinoblastoma protein. The resulting complex appears to function as a transcriptional activator that controls cell growth and differentiation in osteoblasts *(38)*.

2.4. Transcriptional Control at the G1/S Phase Transition that is Functionally Coupled with Initiation of DNA Synthesis

Conditions that establish competency for the initiation of DNA synthesis in vertebrates are monitored in part by the origin recognition complex (ORC) *(39,40)*. This complex appears to contain sequence-specific proteins that mark the location of DNA replication origins. Prior to S-phase, the labile Cdc6p protein associates with ORC, which stages the subsequent binding of Mcm proteins ("licensing factors") to form large origin-bound prereplication complexes. The mechanism by which these complexes facilitate the onset of template directed synthesis of DNA remains to be established. However, activation of S phase dependent CDKs is required for the initiation of DNA replication, but this event is also thought to prevent assembly of new prereplication complexes *(40)*. This hypothesis provides a potential mechanism for stringent control of chromosomal duplication, which should occur only once during each somatic cell cycle. Thus, checkpoint controls at the onset of DNA synthesis serve to signal cellular competency for S-phase entry and maintenance of the normal diploid genotype upon mitosis.

Once DNA synthesis has been initiated, replicative activity is confined to specific locations within the nucleus, referred to as DNA replication foci. DNA replication foci represent subnuclear domains that are thought to be highly enriched in multi-subunit complexes ("DNA replication factories") containing enzymes involved in DNA synthesis, including DNA polymerases α and δ, PCNA, and DNA ligase *(39,41,42)*. The concentration of these factors at DNA replication foci that are associated with the nuclear matrix provides a solid-phase frame-work for understanding catalytic and regulatory components of DNA replication.

2.5. Coordinate Activation of Multiple DNA Replication-Dependent Histone Genes at the Onset of S Phase

The initiation of histone protein synthesis at the G_1/S phase transition is tightly coupled to the start and progression of DNA synthesis (Fig. 2). To prevent disorganization of nuclear architecture and chromosomal catastrophe during chromosome segregation at mitosis, it is critical that newly replicated DNA is packaged immediately into nucleosomes. Histones permit the precise packaging of 2 m of DNA into chromatin within each cell nucleus (diameter approx 10 μm). This functional and temporal coupling poses stringent constraints on multiple parameters of histone gene expression, because somatic cells do not have storage

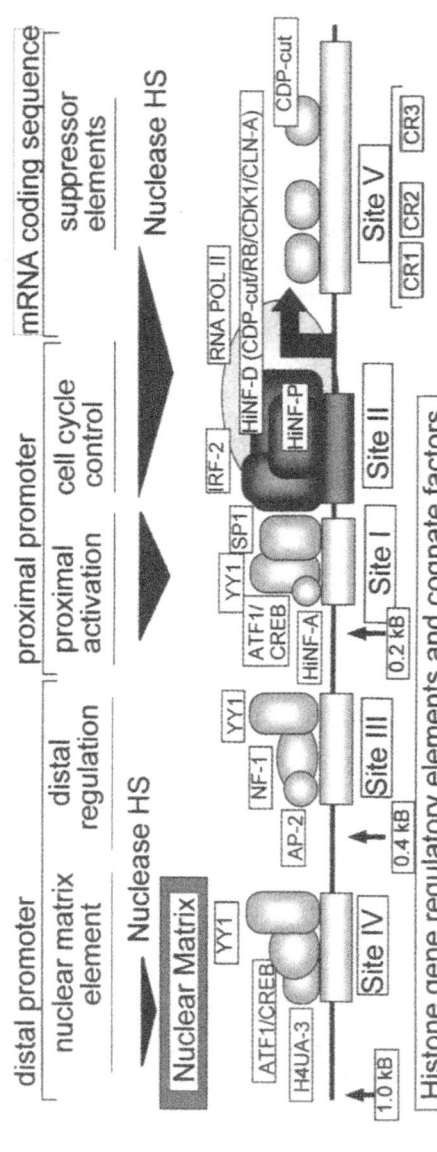

Fig. 5. Regulation of histone gene transcription at the G_1/S phase transition. The diagram depicts the promoter of a prototypical histone gene (referred to as H4/n, H4FN, H4.1, or F0108) located on human chromosome 1. The promoter contains a series of multipartite regulatory domains (Sites I, II, III, IV, and V) that interact with a series of factors. The Site II element mediates cell cycle control of transcription. Nuclease hypersensitive sites and nuclear matrix attachment regions are indicated above the diagram.

pools for histone protein or histone mRNAs. The vast number of histone polypeptides that must be synthesized and the limited time of S phase allotted for this process, necessitates a high histone protein synthesis rate. Mass production of each histone subtype occurs at an average rate of several thousand proteins per second throughout S-phase. Moreover, because each 0.2 kB of DNA is packaged by nucleosomal octamers composed of histone H2A, H2B, H3, and H4, the stoichiometric synthesis of each of the histone subtypes is essential for efficient DNA packaging. Consequently, histone gene regulatory factors integrate a series of cell-signaling pathways that monitor the onset of S phase and coordinate the expression of 50–100 distinct histone genes.

The first rate-limiting factor of histone gene expression is the enhancement of a low transcription rate that persists throughout the cell cycle (Fig. 2) *(43)*. Histone H4 gene transcription has been extensively studied, and a series of cis-acting elements and cognate factors have been identified by our laboratory (Fig. 5) *(26,30,44–49)*. We first showed that genomic occupancy of histone gene promoter elements occurs throughout the cell cycle *(50)*, which was subsequently also shown for the R-point gene DHFR *(20)* by others. The constitutive occupancy of promoter regulatory elements is consistent with the concept that protein/protein interactions, post-translational modifications and alterations in chromatin structure are important factors in modulating transcription of histone genes and other genes expressed during S phase *(51–54)*. Similar to the R-point genes, the presence of SP1 binding sites is critical for maximum activation of histone genes (Fig. 5). However, unlike the R-point genes, the majority of histone genes does not contain E2F elements. Rather, a sophisticated and E2F independent transcriptional mechanism has evolved for coordinate activation of histone genes.

As with E2F responsive genes, E2F independent transcriptional control mechanisms must account for G_1/S phase-dependent enhancement of transcription, as well as attenuation of gene transcription at later stages of S phase (Fig. 5). The key cell cycle element for histone H4 genes is a highly conserved promoter domain designated Site II, which encompasses binding sites for IRF2, the homeodomain-related "CCAAT Displacement Protein" CDP/cut, and the TATA binding complex TFIID *(44,45,47,55–59)*. IRF2 is required for maximal activation of histone gene transcription, and appears to function at the G_1/S phase boundary in a manner analogous to "free" E2F by enhancing cell cycle-dependent transcription rates by about threefold *(44)*. Phosphorylation of IRF2 in vivo occurs primarily on serine residues, which may be mediated by several ubiquitous kinases including Casein Kinase II, Protein Kinase A (PKA), and Protein Kinase C (PKC) *(60)*. Interestingly, IRF2 activity does not appear to be directly linked to phosphorylation by mitogen-activated protein (MAP) kinases or CDKs.

Involvement of the CDP/cut homeodomain protein in cell cycle control was initially established by the finding that this factor is a component of the HiN

F-D complex *(30)*. In the multi-subunit HiNF-D complex, the CDP/cut protein is associated with pRB, cyclin A, and CDK1/cdc2 *(45,61,62)*. HiNF-D may have a bifunctional role in H4 gene transcription. For example, binding of the HiNF-D complex to the H4 promoter is essential for maximal H4 gene promoter activity in cells nullizygous for IRF2. However, overexpression of the CDP/cut DNA binding subunit of HiNF-D results in repression of H4 promoter activity *(30)*. CDP/cut in association with pRB, CDK1/cdc2, and cyclin A may perform a function very similar to that of the multiplicity of higher-order E2F complexes (Fig. 3). These CDP complexes bound to cyclins, CDKs, and pRB related proteins attenuate the enhanced levels of histone gene transcription during mid S phase when physiological demand for histone mRNAs begins to diminish.

Similar to the R-point genes, histone gene promoters have auxiliary elements (e.g., Site I) that support transcriptional activation during the cell cycle. For example, histone H4 genes contain binding sites for YY1 and SP1. The interaction of SP1 with Site I modulates the efficiency of H4 gene transcription by an order of magnitude *(26)*. The binding of YY1 to multiple sites in the histone H4 promoter may facilitate gene/nuclear matrix interactions *(63;* unpublished data). In addition, it has been shown that YY1 associates with histone deacetylase rpd3. The possibility arises that post-translational modifications of histone proteins when bound as nucleosomes to the H4 promoter, may parallel the modifications in chromatin structure that accompany modulations of histone H4 gene expression *(51,64)*.

Stoichiometric synthesis of histone mRNAs and proteins requires coordinate control of histone gene expression at several gene regulatory levels. At the transcriptional level, coordinate activation of the five histone gene classes at the G_1/S phase transition may be mediated by CDP/cut, which has been shown to interact with the promoters of all major histone gene subtypes. The association of CDP/cut with pRB, cyclin A, and CDK1/cdc2 as components of the HiNF-D complexes interacting with DNA replication-dependent histone genes, provides direct functional linkage between transcriptional coordination of histone gene expression and cyclin/CDK signaling mechanisms that mediate cell cycle progression.

A second link involving between cyclin/CDK complexes and histone gene expression is provided by the NPAT (nuclear protein, ataxia-telangiectasia locus) protein, which is a substrate for cyclin E/CDK2 complexes. NPAT co-localizes during S phase with the two major DNA replication-dependent histone clusters on chromosomes 1 and 6 *(65,66)*. NPAT is capable of modulating histone gene transcription and this stimulation appears to be enhanced by the activity of cyclin E-Cdk2 *(65)*. Because NPAT does not appear to bind DNA directly, the mechanism by which NPAT regulates histone gene transcription is not clear at present. It is conceivable that NPAT may form protein/protein interactions in histone H4 gene promoters with any of the three Site II binding proteins, including HiN

F-M/IRF-2, HiNF-P/H4TF-2, or HiNF-D (CDP-cut/pRB/CDK1/cyclin A containing complex). Furthermore, whether NPAT can directly mediate the enhancement of histone gene transcription through known cell cycle regulatory sequences in synchronized cells progressing towards the G_1/S phase transition remains to be established. The role of NPAT may be analogous to that of BZAP45, a 45 kD protein that stimulates histone gene transcription through cell cycle regulatory sequences, but is not capable by itself of binding to DNA directly *(67)*.

The secondary levels at which histone gene expression is coordinated occur by post-transcriptional mechanisms, including transcript elongation and 3' end processing, which produce mature histone mRNAs. Histone mRNAs do not have poly A tails, but instead contain a unique histone specific hairpin-loop structure. Histone 3' end processing is mediated by U7 snRNP complexes *(68,69)*, and accessory proteins that recognize histone mRNA 3' ends are being characterized. It has been postulated that histone mRNA 3' end processing is a key step in histone gene expression *(68–70)*, but the regulatory events that connect activation of this process to cell cycle progression remain to be established. However, because all histone mRNAs have highly similar structural elements at the 3' end, the recognition of these structures by regulatory factors *(71,72)* may represent an important mechanism by which mature histone mRNAs are produced, transported to specific cytoplasmic locations, translated, and degraded.

2.6. Selective Downregulation of Histone Gene Expression Upon Cessation of DNA Replication at the S/G2 Transition

When cells approach the S/G_2 transition, most of the genome has been replicated, and the demand for histone proteins to package newly replicated DNA diminishes (Fig. 1). Cells must ensure that histones do not accumulate in excess as these highly basic proteins would likely interfere with cellular and particularly nucleic acid metabolism. Therefore, histone mRNAs are selectively degraded during late S phase in concert with the completion of DNA synthesis. Molecular mechanisms have been elucidated that account for post-transcriptional control of histone gene expression during S phase by modulating mRNA stability. The histone mRNA-specific stem-loop structure plays a key role in regulating histone mRNA turn-over. This stem-loop motif is present in all mRNAs encoding the live cell cycle-regulated histone subtypes. Therefore, this structure is considered pivotal in maintaining the stoichiometric balance of the five histone classes and coupling with DNA replication. Selective degradation of histone mRNA when DNA synthesis is halted is mediated by a 3' exonuclease, and requires active translation of histone mRNA bound to polyribosomes *(68,69,73,74)*. Interestingly, mRNA destabilization does not occur when histone mRNA is targeted to membrane-bound ribosomes rather than to ribosomes associated with the nonmembranous cytoskeleton. Thus, histone mRNA degradation is a dynamic process that requires macromolecular complexes at specific subcellular locations.

It has been shown that histone proteins mediate histone mRNA degradation *(75)* and that histone mRNA half-lives are modulated during the cell cycle *(76)*. Because histone mRNAs are most stable when free histone protein concentrations are minimal and highly unstable when histone proteins accumulate in excess, it appears that selective downregulation of histone gene expression is achieved by an autoregulatory mechanism.

ACKNOWLEDGMENTS

This work was supported by grants from the National Institutes of Health (P01 CA82834, R01 AR39588, R01 GM32010). The contents of this manuscript are solely the responsibility of the authors and do not necessarily represent the official views of the National Institutes of Health.

REFERENCES

1. Howard A, Pelc SR. Nuclear incorporation of 32p as demonstrated by autoradiography. *Exp Cell Res* 1951;2:178–187.
2. Prescott DM. *Reproduction of Eukaryotic Cells.* Academic Press, New York, 1976.
3. Heichman KA, Roberts JM. Rules to replicate by. *Cell* 1994;79:557–562.
4. Stein GS, Montecino M, van Wijnen AJ, Stein JL, Lian JB. Nuclear structure—gene expression interrelationships: implications for aberrant gene expression in cancer. *Cancer Res* 2000;60:2067–2076.
5. Workman JL, Kingston RE. Alteration of nucleosome structure as a mechanism of transcriptional regulation. *Annu Rev Biochem* 1998;67:545–579.
6. Fridovich-Keil JL, Markell PJ, Gudas JM, Pardee AB. DNA sequences required for serum-responsive regulation of expression from the mouse thymidine kinase promoter. *Cell Growth Differ* 1993;4:679–687.
7. Dou QP, Zhao S, Levin AH, Wang J, Helin K, Pardee AB. G1/S-regulated E2F-containing protein complexes bind to the mouse thymidine kinase gene promoter. *J Biol Chem* 1994;269:1306–1313.
8. Dou QP, Molnar G, Pardee AB. Cyclin D1/cdk2 kinase is present in a G1 phase-specific protein complex Yi1 that binds to the mouse thymidine kinase gene promoter. *Biochem Biophys Res Commun* 1994;205:1859–1868.
9. Dou QP, Pardee AB. Transcriptional activation of thymidine kinase, a marker for cell cycle control. *Prog Nucleic Acid Res Mol Biol* 1996;53:197–217.
10. Li LJ, Naeve GS, Lee AS. Temporal regulation of cyclin A-p107 and p33cdk2 complexes binding to a human thymidine kinase promoter element important for G1-S phase transcriptional regulation. *Proc Natl Acad Sci USA* 1993;90:3554–3558.
11. Good L, Chen J, Chen KY. Analysis of sequence-specific binding activity of cis-elements in human thymidine kinase gene promoter during G1/S phase transition. *J Cell Physiol* 1995;163:636–644.
12. Dou QP, Levin AH, Zhao S, Pardee AB. Cyclin E and cyclin A as candidates for the restriction point protein. *Cancer Res* 1993;53:1493–1497.
13. Meyers S, Hiebert SW. Indirect and direct disruption of transcriptional regulation in cancer: E2F and AML-1. *Crit Rev Eukary Gene Expr* 1995;5:365–383.
14. Chen PL, Riley DJ, Lee WH. The retinoblastoma protein as a fundamental mediator of growth and differentiation signals. *Crit Rev Eukaryot Gene Expr* 1995;5:79–95.

15. Krek W, Ewen ME, Shirodkar S, Arany Z, Kaelin WG, Jr., Livingston DM. Negative regulation of the growth-promoting transcription factor E2F-1 by a stably bound cyclin A-dependent protein kinase. *Cell* 1994;78:161–172.
16. Karlseder J, Rotheneder H, Wintersberger E. Interaction of Sp1 with the growth- and cell cycle-regulated transcription factor E2F. *Mol Cell Biol* 1996;16:1659–1667.
17. Wade M, Blake MC, Jambou RC, Helin K, Harlow E, Azizkhan JC. An inverted repeat motif stabilizes binding of E2F and enhances transcription of the dihydrofolate reductase gene. *J Biol Chem* 1995;270:9783–9791.
18. Good L, Dimri GP, Campisi J, Chen KY. Regulation of dihydrofolate reductase gene expression and E2F components in human diploid fibroblasts during growth and senescence. *J Cell Physiol* 1996;168:580–588.
19. Schulze A, Zerfass K, Spitkovsky D, Henglein B, Jansen-Durr P. Activation of the E2F transcription factor by cyclin D1 is blocked by p16INK4, the product of the putative tumor suppressor gene MTS1. *Oncogene* 1994;9:3475–3482.
20. Wells J, Held P, Illenye S, Heintz NH. Protein-DNA interactions at the major and minor promoters of the divergently transcribed dhfr and rep3 genes during the Chinese hamster ovary cell cycle. *Mol Cell Biol* 1996;16:634–647.
21. Azizkhan JC, Jensen DE, Pierce AJ, Wade M. Transcription from TATA-less promoters: dihydrofolate reductase as a model. *Crit Rev Eukaryot Gene Expr* 1993;3:229–254.
22. Schilling LJ, Farnham PJ. Transcriptional regulation of the dihydrofolate reductase/rep-3 locus. *Crit Rev Eukaryot Gene Expr* 1994;4:19–53.
23. Schilling LJ, Farnham PJ. The bidirectionally transcribed dihydrofolate reductase and rep-3a promoters are growth regulated by distinct mechanisms. *Cell Growth Differ* 1995;6:541–548.
24. Wells JM, Illenye S, Magae J, Wu CL, Heintz NH. Accumulation of E2F-4.DP-1 DNA binding complexes correlates with induction of *dhfr* gene expression during the G1 to S phase transition. *J Biol Chem* 1997;272:4483–4492.
25. Birnbaum MJ, van Wijnen AJ, Odgren PR, Last TJ, Suske G, Stein GS, Stein JL. Sp1 transactivation of cell cycle regulated promoters is selectively repressed by Sp3. *Biochemistry* 1995;34:16503–16508.
26. Birnbaum MJ, Wright KL, van Wijnen AJ, Ramsey-Ewing AL, Bourke MT, Last TJ, et al. Functional role for Sp1 in the transcriptional amplification of a cell cycle regulated histone H4 gene. *Biochemistry* 1995;34:7648–7658.
27. Kel AE, Kel-Margoulis OV, Farnham PJ, Bartley SM, Wingender E, Zhang MQ. Computer-assisted identification of cell cycle-related genes: new targets for E2F transcription factors. *J Mol Biol* 2001;309:99–120.
28. Takahashi Y, Rayman JB, Dynlacht BD. Analysis of promoter binding by the E2F and pRB families in vivo: distinct E2F proteins mediate activation and repression. *Genes Dev* 2000;14:804–816.
29. Stein GS, Lian JB, Stein JL, van Wijnen AJ, Montecino M. Transcriptional control of osteoblast growth and differentiation. *Physiol Rev* 1996;76:593–629.
30. van Wijnen AJ, van Gurp MF, de Ridder MC, Tufarelli C, Last TJ, Birnbaum M, et al. CDP/ cut is the DNA-binding subunit of histone gene transcription factor HiNF-D: a mechanism for gene regulation at the G_1/S phase cell cycle transition point independent of transcription factor E2F. *Proc Natl Acad Sci USA* 1996;93:11516–11521.
31. Heintz N. The regulation of histone gene expression during the cell cycle. *Biochim Biophys Acta* 1991;1088:327–339.
32. Osley MA. The regulation of histone synthesis in the cell cycle. *Annu Rev Biochem* 1991;60:827–861.
33. Adams PD. Regulation of the retinoblastoma tumor suppressor protein by cyclin/cdks. *Biochim Biophys Acta* 2001;1471:M123–M133.

34. Buchmann AM, Swaminathan S, Thimmapaya B. Regulation of cellular genes in a chromosomal context by the retinoblastoma tumor suppressor protein. *Mol Cell Biol* 1998;18:4565–4576.
35. Eberhard D, Busslinger M. The partial homeodomain of the transcription factor Pax-5 (BSAP) is an interaction motif for the retinoblastoma and TATA-binding proteins. *Cancer Res* 1999;59:1716s–1724s.
36. Wiggan O, Taniguchi-Sidle A, Hamel PA. Interaction of the pRB-family proteins with factors containing paired-like homeodomains. *Oncogene* 1998;16:227–236.
37. Gartel AL, Goufman E, Tevosian SG, Shih H, Yee AS, Tyner AL. Activation and repression of p21(WAF1/CIP1) transcription by RB binding proteins. *Oncogene* 1998;17:3463–3469.
38. Thomas DM, Carty SA, Piscopo DM, Lee JS, Wang WF, Forrester WC, Hinds PW. The retinoblastoma protein acts as a transcriptional coactivator required for osteogenic differentiation. *Molec Cell* 2001;8:303–316.
39. Hickey RJ, Malkas LH. Mammalian cell DNA replication. *Crit Rev Eukaryot Gene Expr* 1997;7:125–157.
40. Stillman B. Cell cycle control of DNA replication. *Science* 1996;274:1659–1664.
41. Leonhardt H, Rahn HP, Cardoso MC. Intranuclear targeting of DNA replication factors. *J Cell Biochem Suppl* 1998;30–31:243–249.
42. Leonhardt H, Cardoso MC. Targeting and association of proteins with functional domains in the nucleus: the insoluble solution. *Int Rev Cytol* 1995;162B:303–335.
43. Plumb M, Stein J, Stein G. Coordinate regulation of multiple histone mRNAs during the cell cycle in HeLa cells. *Nucleic Acids Res* 1983;11:2391–2410.
44. Vaughan PS, Aziz F, van Wijnen AJ, Wu S, Harada H, Taniguchi T, et al. Activation of a cell-cycle-regulated histone gene by the oncogenic transcription factor IRF-2. *Nature* 1995; 377:362–365.
45. van Wijnen AJ, Aziz F, Grana X, De Luca A, Desai RK, Jaarsveld K, et al. Transcription of histone H4, H3, and H1 cell cycle genes: promoter factor HiNF-D contains CDC2, cyclin A, and an RB-related protein. *Proc Natl Acad Sci USA* 1994;91:12882–12886.
46. Guo B, Stein JL, van Wijnen AJ, Stein GS. ATF1 and CREB trans-activate a cell cycle regulated histone H4 gene at a distal nuclear matrix associated promoter element. *Biochemistry* 1997;36:14447–14455.
47. Aziz F, van Wijnen AJ, Vaughan PS, Wu S, Shakoori AR, Lian JB, et al. The integrated activities of IRF-2 (HiNF-M) CDP/cut (HiNF-D) and H4TF-2 (HiNF-P) regulate transcription of a cell cycle controlled human histone H4 gene: mechanistic differences between distinct H4 genes. *Mol Biol Rep* 1998;25:1–12.
48. Aziz F, van Wijnen AJ, Stein JL, Stein GS. HiNF-D (CDP-*cut*/CDC2/cyclin A/pRB-complex) influences the timing of IRF-2 dependent cell cycle activation of human histone H4 gene transcription at the G1/S phase transition. *J Cell Physiol* 1998;177:453–464.
49. Stein GS, Stein JL, van Wijnen AJ, Lian JB. Transcriptional control of cell cycle progression: the histone gene is a paradigm for the G1/S phase and proliferation/differentiation transitions. *Cell Biol Int* 1996;20:41–49.
50. Green L, Whittle W, Dell'Orco R, Ostrer H, Stein G, Stein J. Human histone gene organization. Identification of a histone gene polymorphism prevalent in a black population. *Exp Cell Res* 1996;164:507–515.
51. Chrysogelos S, Riley DE, Stein G, Stein J. A human histone H4 gene exhibits cell cycle-dependent changes in chromatin structure that correlate with its expression. *Proc Natl Acad Sci USA* 1985;82:7535–7539.
52. Moreno ML, Chrysogelos SA, Stein GS, Stein JL. Reversible changes in the nucleosomal organization of a human H4 histone gene during the cell cycle. *Biochemistry* 1986;25:5364–5370.
53. Pemov A, Bavykin S, Hamlin JL. Proximal and long-range alterations in chromatin structure surrounding the Chinese hamster dihydrofolate reductase promoter. *Biochemistry* 1995; 34:2381–2392.

54. Ljungman M. Effect of differential gene expression on the chromatin structure of the DHFR gene domain in vivo. *Biochim Biophys Acta* 1996;1307:171–177.

55. Vaughan PS, van der Meijden CMJ, Aziz F, Harada H, Taniguchi T, van Wijnen AJ, Stein JL, Stein GS. Cell cycle regulation of histone H4 gene transcription requires the oncogenic factor IRF-2. *J Biol Chem* 1998;273:194–199.

56. Xie R, van Wijnen AJ, van Der MC, Luong MX, Stein JL, Stein GS. The cell cycle control element of histone H4 gene transcription is maximally responsive to interferon regulatory factor pairs IRF-1/IRF-3 and IRF-1/IRF-7. *J Biol Chem* 2001;276:18624–18632.

57. van der Meijden CMJ, Vaughan PS, Staal A, Albig W, Doenecke D, Stein JL, et al. Selective expression of specific histone H4 genes reflects distinctions in transcription factor interactions with divergent H4 promoter elements. *Biochim Biophys Acta* 1998;1442:82–100.

58. Staal A, Enserink JM, Stein JL, Stein GS, van Wijnen AJ. Molecular characterization of Celtix-1, a bromodomain protein interacting with the transcription factor interferon regulatory factor 2. *J Cell Physiol* 2000;185:269–279.

59. Stein GS, Stein JL, van Wijnen AJ, Lian JB. Histone gene transcription: a model for responsiveness to an integrated series of regulatory signals mediating cell cycle control and proliferation/differentiation interrelationships. *J Cell Biochem* 1994;54:393–404.

60. Birnbaum MJ, van Zundert B, Vaughan PS, Whitmarsh AJ, van Wijnen AJ, Davis RJ, Stein GS, Stein JL. Phosphorylation of the oncogenic transcription factor interferon regulatory factor 2 (IRF2) *in vitro* and *in vivo*. *J Cell Biochem* 1997;66:175–183.

61. van Wijnen AJ, Cooper C, Odgren P, Aziz F, De Luca A, Shakoori RA, et al. Cell cycle-dependent modifications in activities of pRb-related tumor suppressors and proliferation-specific CDP/cut homeodomain factors in murine hematopoietic progenitor cells. *J Cell Biochem* 1997;66:512–523.

62. Shakoori AR, van Wijnen AJ, Cooper C, Aziz F, Birnbaum M, Reddy GP, et al. Cytokine induction of proliferation and expression of CDC2 and cyclin A in FDC-P1 myeloid hematopoietic progenitor cells: regulation of ubiquitous and cell cycle-dependent histone gene transcription factors. *J Cell Biochem* 1995;59:291–302.

63. Guo B, Odgren PR, van Wijnen AJ, Last TJ, Nickerson J, Penman S, et al. The nuclear matrix protein NMP-1 is the transcription factor YY1. *Proc Natl Acad Sci USA* 1995;92:10526–10530.

64. Chrysogelos S, Pauli U, Stein G, Stein J. Fine mapping of the chromatin structure of a cell cycle-regulated human H4 histone gene. *J Biol Chem* 1989;264:1232–1237.

65. Zhao J, Kennedy BK, Lawrence BD, Barbie DA, Matera AG, Fletcher JA, Harlow E. NPAT links cyclin E-Cdk2 to the regulation of replication-dependent histone gene transcription. *Genes Dev* 2000;14:2283–2297.

66. Ma T, Van Tine BA, Wei Y, Garrett MD, Nelson D, Adams PD, et al. Cell cycle-regulated phosphorylation of p220(NPAT) by cyclin E/Cdk2 in Cajal bodies promotes histone gene transcription. *Genes Dev* 2000;14:2298–2313.

67. Mitra P, Vaughan PS, Stein JL, Stein GS, van Wijnen AJ. Purification and functional analysis of a novel embryonically expressed protein BZAP45 stimulating cell cycle regulated histone H4 gene transcription. *Biochemistry* 2002;40:10,693–10,699.

68. Marzluff WF, Pandey NB. Multiple regulatory steps control histone mRNA concentrations. *Trends Biochem Sci* 1988;13:49–52.

69. Schumperli D. Multilevel regulation of replication-dependent histone genes. *Trends Genet* 1988;4:187–191.

70. Harris ME, Bohni R, Schneiderman MH, Ramamurthy L, Schumperli D, Marzluff WF. Regulation of histone mRNA in the unperturbed cell cycle: evidence suggesting control at two posttranscriptional steps. *Mol Cell Biol* 1991;11:2416–2424.

71. Wang ZF, Whitfield ML, Ingledue TC3, Dominski Z, Marzluff WF. The protein that binds the 3' end of histone mRNA: a novel RNA-binding protein required for histone pre-mRNA processing. *Genes Dev* 1996;10:3028–3040.

72. Martin F, Schaller A, Eglite S, Schumperli D, Muller B. The gene for histone RNA hairpin binding protein is located on human chromosome 4 and encodes a novel type of RNA binding protein. *EMBO J* 1997;16:769–778.
73. Stein GS, Stein JL. Is human histone gene expression autogenously regulated? *Mol Cell Biochem* 1984;64:105–110.
74. Zambetti G, Stein J, Stein G. Targeting of a chimeric human histone fusion mRNA to membrane-bound polysomes in HeLa cells. *Proc Natl Acad Sci USA* 1987;84:2683–2687.
75. Peltz SW, Ross J. Autogenous regulation of histone mRNA decay by histone proteins in a cell-free system 1. *Mol Cell Biol* 1987;7:4345–4356.
76. Morris TD, Weber LA, Hickey E, Stein GS, Stein JL. Changes in the stability of a human H3 histone mRNA during the HeLa cell cycle. *Mol Cell Biol* 1991;11:544–553.

4 Tumor-Suppressor Genes as Diagnostic Tools

Lorenzo Leoncini, MD, PhD,
Cristiana Bellan, MD, PhD,
Caterina Cinti, PhD,
and Antonio Giordano, MD, PhD

CONTENTS

1. INTRODUCTION

Neoplastic transformation is a multistep process, involving the clonal accumulation of genetic lesions that affect proto-oncogenes or tumor-suppressor genes. The products of these later play a fundamental role in signal transduction pathways, by controlling cell cycle program, differentiation, or even cell death. There is now increasing evidence that progression of the normal cell cycle is the result of a balanced interaction among multiple regulators such as the oncosuppressor gene products and cell-cycle associated proteins. Therefore it is not surprising that fundamental alteration of oncosuppressor genes may result in an unregulated cell cycle and eventual neoplastic transformation (Table 1). As such, one might define cancer as a genetic disease of the cell cycle. An understanding of the regulatory control of the cell cycle will be needed to understand some of the most common genetic abnormalities of tumors.

From: *Cancer Drug Discovery and Development:*
Cell Cycle Inhibitors in Cancer Therapy: Current Strategies
Edited by: A. Giordano and K. J. Soprano © Humana Press Inc., Totowa, NJ

Table 1
Tumor-Suppressor Genes in Human Cancers

Gene	Function	Mutation	Familial form	Major tumor types
p53	Trans., Cycle	Point mut., del	Li-Fraumeni	Multiple types
RB	Cycle	Point mut., del	Retinoblastoma	Multiple types
RB2	Cycle	Point mut., del		Multiple types
BRCA 1,2	DNA repair	Del., Dup., Point mut	Familial breast and ovarian cancer	Breast and ovarian cancers
APC	Cytosk.	Point mut., del	FAP	Colorectal tumors
DCC	Surface	Del., Point mut.	None	Colorectal, others
MTS1	Cycle	Del., Point mut.	Melanoma	Multiple types
WT1	Trans.	Point mut., del	Denys-Drash	Wilm's tumor
VHL	?	Point mut., del	von Hippel-Lindau	Renal cell carcinoma
NF1	GAP	Del.,Point mut.	NF, type I	Peripheral neurofibromas
SCH	Cytosk.	Point mut., del	NF, type II	CNS schwannomas

2. TUMOR-SUPPRESSOR GENES AND CELL CYCLE CONTROL

The cell cycle can be seen as a serial recurrence of DNA synthesis (S phase) and mitosis (M phase), separated by the two intervening phases of cell growth (G_1 and G_2 phases). The entry of a cell into S phase is tightly controlled near the end of G_1 by key protein phosphorylation events, as the entry into M phase is controlled near the end of G_2 (1). The central decision-making machinery, known as the "cell cycle clock," which governs the cell's fate, is able to respond in normal situations to growth factor stimulation only during the first two-thirds of the G_1 phase. At the end of this period (restriction [R] point), the cells will continue the cycle, reenter the quiescent G_0 phase, attain a postmitotic differentiated state, or die (2). The phosphorylation of various proteins, involved in cell cycle control, is carried out by a family of enzymes (serine/threonine kinases), the different members of which have specific roles during certain parts of the cycle, and are termed cyclin-dependent kinases (CDK). The activity of the kinases involved is dependent on their binding to cyclin proteins, so named because they classically appear and disappear at characteristic times during the cell cycle.

2.1. CDKs

Nine CDKs have been identified so far (CDK1 to CDK9), although not all of them are involved directly in the cell cycle. They show remarkable structural similarities, with a 75% sequence homology. However, they possess unique binding sites to enable them to bind specifically to their activating cyclins (3,4).

2.2. Cyclins

Currently, 14 cyclins have been identified (cyclin A to cyclin J, some of which have been subdivided—for example, there are three D type cyclins: D_1, D_2, and D_3), although the functions of all of them have not been determined *(5)*. Common to the structure of all members of this family is the cyclin box, which is a series of 100 amino acids *(6)*. Some cyclins also have similar sequences of amino acids at their N-terminal region, called the destruction box, which brings about their own degradation *(7)*. The concentrations of different cyclins oscillate throughout the cell cycle. When the concentration is high, the cyclin can bind to the CDK, but when the activated CDK/cyclin complex is no longer required, the cyclin is destroyed and the concentration subsequently drops *(8)*.

Cyclins alone do not fully activate CDKs, as the latter also requires phosphorylation and dephosphorylation of the same specific amino acid residues to become fully functional. This is, in part, carried out by the CDK activating kinase (CAK), which is composed of cyclin H and CDK7 *(9,10)*. Thus, only when CDK has been activated by its partner cyclin and also by CAK and other similar functional proteins, can it carry out its role within the cell cycle. The cyclin A/Cdk4 complex, the cyclin E/Cdk2 complex, and the cyclin D/Cdk4 complexes appear to control entry into S phase *(11)*. The cyclin B/Cdk2 complex controls entry into M phase. Other cyclins and CDK proteins are known, and are thought to follow this basic functional scheme.

2.3. CKIs

Two families of Cyclin Kinase Inhibitors (CKIs) introduce an additional level of complexity for kinase activity control. Of most interest are p16, p19/ARF from the INK4 family, and p21 and p27 from the Cip1 family *(12,13)*. CKIs act as mediators of various signaling pathways resulting in the arrest of the cell cycle. The Cip 1 family consists of p21, p27, and p57. p21 was the first CKI to be identified; unfortunately it was described independently by several different workers and consequently been given a number of different names. Thus, p21 is also know as wild-type p53 activated fragment 1 (WAF1), CDK2 interacting protein 1 (CIP1), senescent derived inhibitor 1 (SDI1), and melanoma differentiation associated gene (mda-6). p21 is the prototype of universal inhibitors of CDK enzyme activity. It is capable of inactivating CDK activity when expressed at high levels and of inducing cell cycle arrest. p27 and p57 are also known as kinase inhibiting protein 1 (KIP1) and 2 (KIP2), respectively. These inhibitors tend to have wide ranging roles and can potentially inhibit a number of different CDKs. In particular, the inhibition of CDK-dependent activity by p27 targets all the cyclins/CDK complexes present during G_1/S phase progression, and overexpression of p27 is enough to induce G_1 arrest in many cells, independently from the function of the cyclin/CDK substrate. p27 accumulates in a variety of

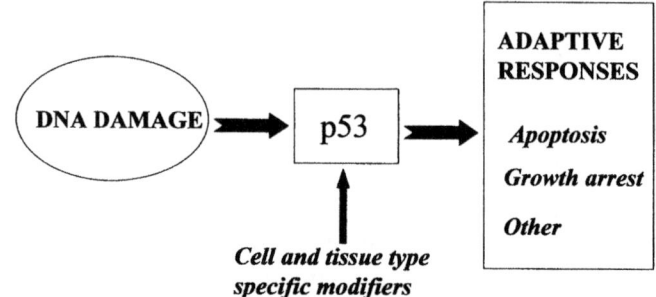

Fig. 1. The p53 pathway. p53 induces either growth arrest or apoptosis.

quiescent cells and disappears in response to mitogens as cells approach the G/S boundary *(14)*.

The role of INK4 family in cell cycle control will be discussed more in detail in the paragraph on the MTS1 gene.

2.4. p53, RB, MTS1, and the Cell Cycle

The prototype tumor-suppressor genes are p53 and RB. The involvement of these tumor-suppressor genes in cancer is widespread and often the genes show great specificity for particular tumor types. Recent studies have emphasized the very wide variety of functions exhibited among this class of cancer-associated genes. These studies produced some detailed models for the biochemical basis of tumor suppression *(1,5)*. A main target for the action of these genes is the cell cycle.

The most common alteration found in these genes is represented by deletion or point mutation. In addition, inactivation of tumor-suppressor genes may result from interaction with viral oncoproteins. In fact, viral agents are capable of integration into the host's genetic material and may interfere with the regulation of normal cell growth and proliferation by interacting with the function of tumor-suppressor genes such as the p53 and pRb families *(15,16)*.

2.4.1. P53 FAMILY GENES

The p53 gene is located on chromosome 17p13.1, know to be frequently lost in human cancers. p53 was discovered as a nuclear protein bound by the large T (tumor) antigen of the transforming virus SV40. p53 is a DNA-binding protein that stimulates transcription of a number of genes, including GADD45, Mdm2, p21, IGF-BP3, Bax, and cyclin G. Perturbations to cellular metabolism that stabilize the normally unstable wild-type protein induce either growth arrest or apoptosis (Fig. 1). In healthy cells an important function of p53 is to cause progression through cell cycle to cease when damage to the cellular genome is detected. This activity has been referred to as checkpoint control, which may be defined as a surveillance mechanism that blocks cell cycle transition. Subsequent to DNA damage, there is also an increase in the stability of the p53 protein, probably the result of phosphorylation. p53 may be phosphorylated by a variety of kinases, including PKC, casein kinase II, CDK1, DNA-dependent protein kinase, ERK, JNK, and PKA, although which of these are most relevant physiologically remains to be determined *(17)*.

In the normal cell, murine double minute 2 (Mdm2) negatively regulates p53 by forming a complex with it and eliciting its degradation in an ubiquitin-dependent, proteosome-mediated manner *(18)*. Thus, p53 stimulates the expression of a gene whose product shortens its own (p53s) lifetime. p53 modified by certain mutations, or by stress-induced modifications, is resistant to Mdm2-provoked degradation, thereby accumulating to increased levels. Additionally, phosphorylation of Mdm2 by the DNA-dependent PK impairs its binding to p53.

Different conformational forms of p53 may be phosphorylated via different signaling pathways, giving rise to versions of the tumor suppressor protein with different activities *(19)*. p53 induced p21 expression results in an inhibition of CDK4 (complexed with cyclin D), CDK2 8 (complexed with either cyclin A or cyclin E), and CDK1 (complexed with cyclin B), thus effectively blocking progression into and through S phase.

If the genome is severely damaged, or if abnormal oncogene-mediated signaling is detected, p53 induces an apoptotic response, possibly by stimulating Bax gene expression and thus decreasing the Bcl2/Bax ratio *(20)*.

Deacetylation of p53 also modulates its effect on cell growth and apoptosis The mechanism by which acetylated p53 is maintained in vivo remains unclear. Recently, it has been shown that the deacetylation of p53 is mediated by an histone deacetylase-1 (HDAC1)-containing complex. A p53 target protein in the deacetylase complexes (designated PID; but identical to metastasis-associated protein 2 (MTA2)) has been identified as a component of the NuRD complex. PID specifically interacts with p53 both in vitro and in vivo, and its expression significantly reduces the steady-state levels of acetylated p53. PID expression strongly represses p53-dependent transcriptional activation, and, notably, it modulates p53-mediated cell growth arrest and apoptosis. These results show that deacetylation and functional interactions by the PID/MTA2-associated NuRD complex may represent an important pathway to regulate p53 function *(21)*.

It is in these various capacities, particularly that of inducing cell death, that p53 exerts its control over the development of a malignancy. Early surveys of the structure and expression of the tumor suppressor gene p53 suggested that inactivating mutations might be a common denominator in the vast majority of human cancers. Indeed, it was initially suggested that p53 mutation (or the associated elevation of cellular p53 protein levels) might even be a molecular diagnostic marker of the malignant state *per se*. Subsequently, analyses of large series of individual tumor types have, however, revealed a much complex story.

It is now known that some cancers uniformly show a very low rate of mutation of p53. Others use indirect means to inactivate p53, notably gene amplification and, hence, overexpression of the functional inhibitor Mdm2. Yet, in some common epithelial cancer types, p53 mutation is often observed, but only in a subset of cases. Furthermore, there is now a consensus that these mutant p53 cases have a significantly poorer prognosis, making them of clinical as well as biological interest *(22)*.

To date, the existence of such a mutant p53 subgroup has been explained conventionally on the "play of chance," i.e., that these are cancers that just happened to acquire a p53 mutation, whereupon the resulting subclone gained a persistent growth advantage *(17)*.

Recently, a fundamentally different hypothesis has been proposed. According to this hypothesis, the liability of a given tumor to exhibit p53 mutation is predetermined by the nature of its cell of origin and, more specifically, depends on the extent to which wild-type p53 forms a rate-limiting step in the control of proliferative life span in that cell. The life span-regulatory role of p53 varies dramatically between epithelial cells of the same "lineage," depending on their initial differentiation state. The existence of phenotypically distinct mutant or wild-type p53 subgroups within a given cancer type can therefore be reinterpreted as the result, not of random differences in acquired genetic events acting on a common cell, but rather of an underlying difference in the phenotype of the cell of origin, which subsequently dictates both the tumor phenotype and the "choice" of somatic genetic events *(23)*.

A novel member of the p53 family is p73 gene at chromosome 1q36.3, on which frequent defects are seen at the locus in many tumors including neuroblastoma. Besides structural similarities, the fact that p73 functions in the regulation of the cell cycle and apoptosis prompts the expansion of the research field concerning p53-associated tumor progression *(24)*.

2.4.2. RB Family Genes

The RB/p105 gene maps to 13q14 chromosome, on which deletions or constitutional heterozygous mutations have been found in several human neoplasias *(25,26)*. The retinoblastoma (RB) gene codes for a 105 kDa protein, which is involved in numerous areas of cellular control at different times during the cell cycle. pRB/p105 is essential in initiating cell cycle arrest, in multiple differentiation processes during development and in aspects of apoptosis *(27,28)*. The retinoblastoma protein is further involved in cell cycle control by regulating the restriction point transition, where it acts as a gatekeeper *(29)*. The protein has been proven to be essential for growth arrest in the case of DNA damage and in acting as an antiapoptotic agent *(30,31)*. pRB/p105 itself is the target of caspases and is rapidly inactivated once the apoptotic stimulus becomes overwhelming *(28,32)*.

RB2/p130 gene, which maps to 16p12.2 chromosome, codes for a 130kDa protein, which seems to be more restricted in its function of controlling gene expression in cells that are not in the proliferative cell cycle *(33)*. This protein is stabilized and activated as soon as the cell withdraws from the cell cycle during cell cycle arrest and cellular differentiation. pRB2/p130 is powerful in arresting cell culture models if ectopically expressed *(34,35)*.

The p107 gene maps to a chromosome region (20q11.2) not frequently found to be altered in human neoplasias *(36)*. p107 codes for a 107 kDa protein that is most prominently present during G_1 and S phase and disappears in arrested and differentiated cells. The actual role of this family member is the least understood and future studies will have to define its role in the control of cellular expression.

The retinoblastoma family members, pRb/p105, pRb2/p130, and p107, are structurally and biochemically similar proteins and, as a consequence, they carry out similar functional tasks. The retinoblastoma family proteins share large regions of homology, especially in a bipartite region that makes up the "pocket domain or pocket region." In this region, pRb2/p130 and p107 are much more closely related to each other with about 50% amino acid identity, than they are to pRb/p105 (30–35% identity). The conserved pocket region, which confers a peculiar steric conformation to retinoblastoma family members, is responsible for many of the protein–protein interactions and characterizes the functional activity of these proteins in the homeostasis of cell cycle *(37,38)*. A number of common target proteins have been found to interact with the pocket region, including members of the E2F family of transcription factors, oncoproteins from several DNA tumor viruses, the D-type cyclins, and the histone deacetylase *(29,39)*. It is interesting to note that even though all three members share high homologies and overlapping features and activities, it is safe to state that each protein has a unique function and plays a unique, nonredundant role *(35)*. However, there might be scenarios where they become redundant as the mutational loss of one member is functionally compensated for by that of another. In fact, it seems that the Rb family of proteins do not each have fixed functions *(32,40,41)*. This notion conforms to the existence on nuclear Rb family products of multifunctional domains, which permit complex interactions with the cellular transcription apparatuses *(42)*.

The regulation of all three members of the retinoblastoma family of proteins is complex and unique for each single member. Regulation of all three genes occurs at the transcriptional as well as at the post-translational level *(43,44)*. pRB/p105, pRB2/p130, and p107 are similar in sequence and protein structure homology but differ in the timely expression pattern detected in different tissues. pRB/p105 is abundant at all times with slight variations in expression levels but significant differences in its phosphorylation status, whereas p107 expression is lost in cells withdrawn from the cell cycle but high throughout the proliferative cell cycle. pRB2/p130, described as the protein defining G_0, is detectable at high levels in nonproliferating cells.

According to the pattern of its phosphorylation and phosphorylation-dependent growth suppressive properties, pRb might function as the guardian of the G_1/S phase transition at the R-point gate. Before G_1 phase progression is initiated by mitogen stimulation, pRb is underphosphorylated, a form known to be active in repressing cell cycle progression. As the cells progress into G_1/S phase, pRb becomes phosphorylated, which causes the inactivation of its growth inhibitory function. pRb then maintains this hyperphosphorylated configuration throughout the remainder of the cell cycle, becoming underphosphorylated once again upon emergence from M *(29)*. The sites of phosphorylation of pRb/p105 are targeted by cyclin/CDKs specifically induced during different stages of G_1/S phase progression. Thus, cyclin/CDK-mediated phosphorylation of pRb is likely to be the mechanism by which the growth suppressive function of pRb is turned off during the G_1/S phase transition and the following phases of the cell cycle. pRb exerts its antiproliferative function by regulating a number of downstream effectors *(45)*. The best characterized pRb targets are the members of the E2F/ DP family of transcription factors, generically referred to as E2F. Five E2F species (E2F-5) and three DP family members (DP1-3) have been identified and characterized *(46)*. E2F and DP members heterodimerize in various combinations to bind to a consensus sequence (E2F site) present in the promoter of genes required for progression from G_1 to S, including c-myc, N-myc, B-myb, cdc2, DHFR, thymidine synthetase, thymidine kinase, and DNA polymerase α *(47)*. Extensive studies have shown that E2F/DP free heterodimers are active in promoting the transcription of downstream genes and that the interaction with unphosphorylated pRb represses activation of E2F-responsive genes. pRb preferentially binds to a subset of E2F members, E2F1-3, via the "pocket region" *(15, 28, 29)*. The pRb-bound E2F species does not account for all E2F activity during the cell cycle. In fact, the most predominant E2F species in quiescent cells are E2F4 and E2F5 *(48)*. At this stage of the cell cycle, E2F4 is found in a complex with a pRb-related protein, pRb2/p130. p107/E2F complexes and pRb2/p130/ E2F complexes possess a common function, for which pRB/E2F complexes are either insufficient or which they are incapable of performing, that is needed for p16-induced cell cycle arrest (Fig. 2) *(49)*.

Based on the experimental data, a model for pRb2/p130 and p107 control during cell proliferation has been previously proposed. In quiescent G_0 cells, the nuclear E2F-pRb2/p130 complex is responsible for the active repression of a number of cellular promoters, including those of E2F1, E2F2, and p107. After its release into the cell cycle, pRb2/p130 is phosphorylated by G^1 cyclin-CDKs and subsequently degraded through a proteosome-dependent mechanism. pRb2 protein level thus drops dramatically to almost undetectable levels, resulting in

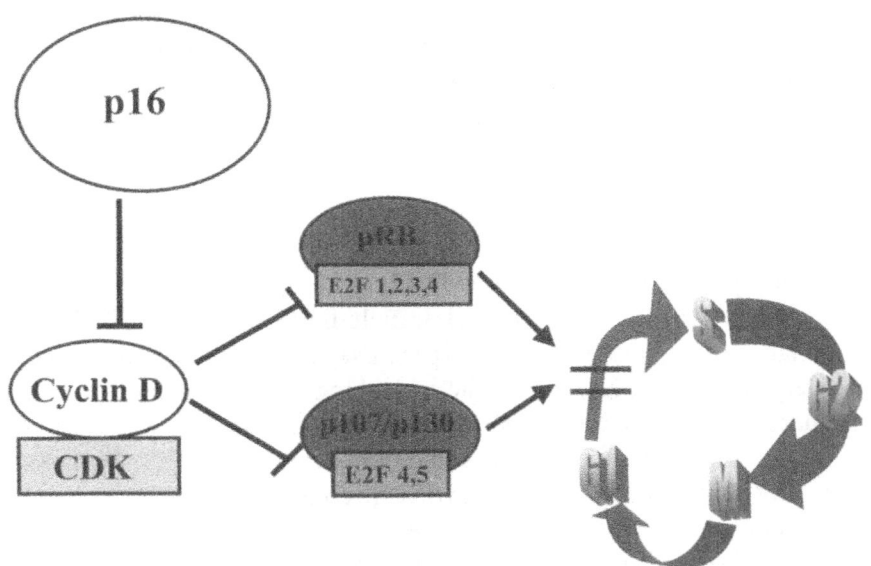

Fig. 2. p16[INK4]–induced arrest requires pRB/E2F complex, p107/E2F complex, and p130/E2F.

the derepression of a variety of genes, including p107. The accumulated p107 protein then is able to interact with E2F4 and E2F5, which have been released from pRb2/p130 and associate with cyclin A/cdk2 *(50,51)*.

By inhibiting the enzymatic kinase potential of cyclin D1/CDK4, cyclinE/ CDK2, and cyclinA/CDK2, an accumulation of hypophosphorylated forms of pRB/p105 and pRB2/p130 and p107 are detectable. This subsequently affects transcription from promoters containing sites for E2F transcription factors for example. In such a scenario, cell cycle progression toward the S phase is blocked and the cell gains time to prepare itself for tasks to come or perform DNA repair. Overexpression of pRB2/p130 and p107 arrests cells not only by their binding to E2F but also affects the kinase activity of CDKs. The spacer region of pRB2/ p130 and the N-terminus of p107 bind and thereby inhibit the kinase activity of cyclin/CDK2 complexes *(52,53)*.

Whereas RB complies with all the requirements in order to be considered a tumor suppressor gene, the role of RB2/p130 and p107 as oncosuppressor genes is still controversial *(29,54)*. However, there has recently been increased evidence in favor of the oncosuppressive activity of RB2/p130. Different mechanisms of its inactivation have been demonstrated to play a role in various human neoplasia. Several mutations in the RB2/p130 gene have been found, resulting in modification of the primary protein structure, which strongly impairs the gene's function *(55)*. Besides mutations of the gene, interaction with viral oncoproteins is another important mechanism of inactivation of RB2/p130, as oncoviral disruption of E2F/DP complexes reinduce site-dependent transcription and cell cycle progression. However, due to the high GC content in the promoter region, one might speculate whether methylation of the gene could be an issue in tumor samples and cell lines where low or null levels of pRB2/p130 protein or mRNA have been described. Future studies are necessary to verify such assumptions.

2.4.3. MTS1

The multiple tumor suppressor (MTS1) gene, located on chromosome 9p, encodes for the INK4 family molecules, including $p16^{INK4A}$, $p15^{INK4B}$, $p14^{ARF}$ (the human homologue of $p19^{ARF}$), and p18. They function as inhibitors of cyclin-dependent kinases (CDKs) and are the critical regulators of progression from G_1 to S-phase. Point mutations, heterozygous and homozygous losses of MTS1, have been found in a variety of sporadic tumor types. $p16^{INK4A}$ with $p14^{INK4B}$ specifically binds to CDK4 and CDK6 that are competing with the cyclin D_1, and prevents phosphorylation of the Rb protein. $p16^{INK4A}$ thus may act normally to preserve unphosphorylated Rb, the form thought to inhibit cellular entry into S phase. The ability of CKI p16 to arrest cells has been linked to the activity of pRB/p105 but recent studies have demonstrated that the p16-induced arrest is not mediated exclusively by pRb, but depends on the nonredundant functions of at least two pRB-family members, pRB2/p130 or p107 *(49)*. The regulatory control of the G_1-S boundary appears to be a major determinant of cellular proliferation. Presumably, a lack of MTS1 would cause dysregulation of this G_1-S control point. The importance of CKIs is underscored by the fact that components like CKI p16 and p27 have been described to be functionally lost in a high percentage of human neoplasias originating from various tissues *(13,14)*. The loss of p16 can be caused by mutation or by hyper-methylation of its promoter, and elevated cyclinE/CDK2 activity eliminates p27 via phosphorylation, which causes subsequent ubiquitin-dependent degradation *(56,57)*.

3. OTHER TUMOR-SUPPRESSOR GENES: APD, DCC, WT1, VHL, NF1, SCH, AND PTEN

3.1. APC

The Adenomatous poliposis coli (APC) gene product binds to the cytoskeletal proteins α- and β-catenin, but otherwise its biochemical function is essentially unknown. Mutations usually cause a truncated protein, which provides the basis of a number of simple assays for these mutations. Germline mutations of the APC gene are the cause of Familial Adenomatous Poliposys (FAP). Somatic mutations of APC are nearly ubiquitous in sporadic colorectal adenomas and carcinomas *(58–61)*.

3.2. BRCA1 and BRCA2

The BRCA 1 gene was discovered by genetic linkage analysis of cancer pedigrees with families having a history of both breast and ovarian cancer on the chromosome 17q21.3 (62). Subsequent analysis of families with a history of breast cancer not linked to BRCA1 led to the discovery of another breast cancer susceptibility gene, BRCA2, on chromosome 13q12-13. In accordance with the Knudson's model, both BRCA 1 and BRCA2 are regarded as classical tumor suppressor genes.

Although the biological functions of the BRCA1 and BRCA2 proteins remain unclear, several functional domains in these proteins have been identified. The BRCA1 and BRCA2 proteins have been shown to share numerous similarities. They contain putative transcriptional activation domains and interact with each other, suggesting that they may function in the same pathway. Their association with human RAD51, which mediates homologous DNA repair and strand exchange, implies that both BRCA1 and BRCA2 are components of a multiprotein repair complex (63).

3.3. DCC

DCC (*deleted in colorectal carcinoma*) is the candidate tumor suppressor gene located at the site deletions of 18q, which are now known to occur in 80% of colorectal carcinomas as well as in a variety of other human neoplasms. DCC is a cell-surface protein of the immunoglobulin superfamily type, perhaps involved in cell-cell interactions. Failure in contact inhibition and other types of cell surface interactions are often seen among neoplastic cells. The DCC gene is more than a megabase in length, making it one of the largest genes known. This immense size has provided practical problems for the study of gene function. No familial disease is known to be associated with abnormalities of DCC (64).

3.4. WT1

The WT1 gene codes for a DNA-binding protein that may act to repress transcription at specific sites. It is involved in a rare germline susceptibility to Wilm's tumor (Denys-Drash syndrome), and somatic mutations occur in some sporadic Wilm's tumors. A second major tumor suppressor gene for Wilm's tumor has also been localized; it is affected in Beckwith-Widemann syndrome, a syndrome of abnormal development that includes multiple bilateral Wilm's tumors (65).

3.5. VHL

VHL is mutated in the germline of patients having Von Hippel-Lindau syndrome. Somatic point mutations and deletions of this gene occur in sporadic renal cell carcinomas as well. VHL is on chromosome 3p. Deletions of 3p occur in a wide variety of tumor types, and at least three tumor-suppressor genes are thought to lie on this chromosomal arm. Thus, the possible participation of VHL in other neoplasms has not been defined *(66).*

3.6. NF1 and SCH

Germline mutations of NF1, encoding a GTPase-activating protein, are the cause of neurofibromatosis type I, also called peripheral neurofibromatosis. NF1 may interact with RAS to control its signaling activity. SCH is responsible for the central nervous system schwannomas of neurofibromatosis type II. Its product has homology with proteins at the plasma membrane-cytoskeleton interface, a putative site of tumor-suppressive action perhaps similar to that suggested for APC product *(67).*

3.7. PTEN

PTEN (phosphatase and tensin homolog deleted on chromosome 10q23) is a recently discovered tumor suppressor gene. In general terms, PTEN has been show to modulate, mostly as a inhibitor factor, two seemingly distinct cellular functions: cell growth/survival and cell migration/adhesion through its lipid and protein phosphatase activities, respectively. PTEN's ability to induce growth suppression appears to be mediated by at least two mechanisms: it promotes cell-cycle arrest at the G_1 phase and also increases apoptosis induced by multiple distinct stimuli. The first mechanisms seem to be via p27^{KIP1} cyclin-dependent kinase inhibitor. In fact, it has been shown that PTEN induces p27 expression and allows the formation of complexes with cyclin E. This, in turn, reduces specifically cyclin-dependent kinase 2 (CDK2) activity and, consequently, results in low phosphorylation of the pRb protein. Low pRb phosphorylation leads to arrest in cell cycle progression. Another potential mechanism of cell-cycle control by PTEN may be through inhibition of cyclin D accumulation. Further insights into the mechanisms of PTEN-induced apoptosis are still required to allow for a complete understanding of its functional role.

Germline PTEN mutations have been reported in patients affected with two tumor-predisposing syndromes, each having overlapping clinical features: Cowden disease and Bannayan-Riley-Ruvalcaba syndrome, which are two hamartoma syndromes with an increased risk of breast and thyroid tumors. PTEN has also been found to be defective in large number of sporadic human tumors *(68,69).*

4. TUMOR-SUPPRESSOR GENES IN ANIMAL MODELS

Despite the fact that the profile of discrete genetic alterations characterizing the development of a specific type of malignant neoplasm arising in a particular experimental animal model of multistage carcinogenesis may not be identical to that which may have been detected in a corresponding human cancer, it is nevertheless important to emphasize that such animal models have considerable value with respect to validating the oncogenic potential of such genetic alterations, as well as in defining more precisely how independent molecular events may relate to a specific stage of multistage carcinogenic process. Transgenic animal technology, in which foreign genes are stably introduced into the germline of mice primarily (and now into the germline of other rodent species, such as the rat), has proven to be of considerable value in assessing the oncogenic potential of inactivated tumor suppressor genes. A few specific examples demonstrating the usefulness of transgenic animals in the study of multistage tumorigenesis are briefly presented as follows: 1) transgenic mice homozygous for the null p53 allele (p53-deficient mice) have been shown to be prone to the spontaneous development of a variety of malignant neoplasms (malignant lymphoma being the most frequently occurring) by 6 mo of age, emphasizing the importance of p53 as a tumor suppressor gene; 2) deletion of pRB/p105 leads to death of affected embryos at d 13–15 and animals haploid for pRB/p105 are at a high risk of developing multiple tumors (70); 3) loss of either pRB2/p130 or p107 has no such effect on the survival rate of the offspring, nor does it increase the tumor incidence in adult mice (hetero- or homozygously deleted). In transgenic mouse models, deficiency for pRB2/p130 causes high levels of p107 proteins and cellular control does not seem to be affected despite the loss of one of the pocket proteins. Such a functional compensation is probably restricted to pRB2/p130 and p107, which are highly related and equally distant from pRB/p105. Only the loss of both pRB2/p130 and p107 causes death shortly after birth (71,72). The inactivation of pocket proteins in the germline has not led to mouse models comparable to human cancer. In order to get a more precise picture dealing with the loss of retinoblastoma proteins, future studies are necessary in which these genes are inactivated in a tissue-specific and development-dependent setting, as recently shown for pRB/p105 (73).

However, it is important to mention that another group of researchers detected lethal effects of loss of pRB2/p130 in a mouse strain with a different genetic background. This opens the question about the relevance of data generated in one mouse strain vs another inbred mouse strain (74).

Various issues could be learned from the analysis of mouse models; however, many questions remain open, such as in which tissues and when the tumors occur or their dependence on the genetic background of the mouse strain used. Sophisticated methods need to be developed and explored to disrupt these tissue- and development-specific genes and gain improved insight into their roles in guaranteeing cellular homeostasis. More recently, triple knock-out mouse embryonic fibroblasts (TKO MEFs) have been developed, suggesting the involvement of all three Rb-related proteins downstream of multiple cell cycle control pathways, and further highlighting the link between loss of cell cycle control and tumorigenesis (75).

5. TUMOR-SUPPRESSOR GENES IN HUMAN CANCERS

5.1. Tumors of Nervous System

Genetic alterations are frequently observed in high-grade adult astrocytomas occurring in either the p53/MDM2/p14ARF or Rb/CDK4/p16INK4a tumor suppressor pathways. Two major differences in the genetic pathway(s) leading to the formation of *de novo* high-grade astrocytomas in children compared to those of the adult have been reported. Preferential inactivation of the p53 tumor-suppressor pathway occurs in >95% of pediatric astrocytomas versus inactivation of the Rb tumor-suppressor pathway in <25% of the same tumors. In sporadic ependymoma, the most frequent genetic change is monosomy 22, suggesting the presence of an ependymoma tumor-suppressor gene on that chromosome *(76,77)*.

5.2. Retinoblastoma

Retinoblastoma is a rare childhood neoplasia first identified as an inherited disease. This neoplasm gave the Rb-family of cell cycle regulators its name because mutations of RB/p105 gene were first found on both alleles in cases of retinoblastoma *(78)*. Bilateral familial retinoblastomas show germline mutation in pRb/p105, and tumors develop when the second allele becomes lost or mutated, following the concept of the two-hit model for inactivation of tumor-suppressor genes proposed by Knudson *(79)*. However, tumor penetrance varies among carriers in different family pedigrees. These discrepancies may be due to differences in the severity of the defect in mutant RB1 alleles. Alternatively, they may suggests that other genes can affect the risk of retinoblastoma development. These data are supported by mouse studies of retinoblastoma showing that heterozigous mutation of pRb/p105 (pRb+/-) only is not sufficient to develop the tumor, while mice carrying pRb+/- and p107-/- develop retinal dysplasia, indicating that p107 is able to prevent this type of tumor in pRb+/- mice and therefore acts as a tumor suppressor *(80)*. Recently, mutations in the Rb-related Rb2/p130 gene have been found in eight out of ten cases of retinoblastomas *(81)*. In addition, two potential hot spots for mutations clustered in the pocket and carboxiterminal regions of the gene have been identified. These results conform to the experimental evidence that mutations other than those of RB1 gene are probably necessary for retinoblastoma development. Further investigation of the mechanisms by which children develop retinoblastoma will contribute to a better understanding of principles of neoplastic transformation.

5.3. Nasopharyngeal Carcinoma

Nasopharyngeal carcinoma (NPC) is an endemic cancer with a very high incidence in southeastern China (32% of all cancers) and in North Africa. Several research groups have reported p53 gene mutations, which occur preferentially in exon 5 and 8, suggesting its possible involvement in NPC development. No pRb/

p105 gene rearrangement has been found in this class of tumor. Claudio and coworkers have shown a drastic reduction in the expression level of pRb2/p130 in nasopharyngeal cell line (HONE-1) and in primary tumors, while the other retinoblastoma family members remained at a consistently elevated level. The altered expression of pRb2/p130 is due to mutations that occur in the COOH-terminal functional domain and impair the stability of this oncosuppressor protein. Reintroduction of wild-type pRb2/p130 in these tumor cell lines causes a dramatic reduction in colony formation *(35,82)*.

5.4. Thyroid Carcinoma

Thyroid cancer, normally, is a disease with a good prognosis, but about 30% of the tumors de-differentiate and may finally develop into highly malignant anaplastic thyroid carcinomas with a mean survival time of less than 8 mo. The study of thyroid tumor genetics is of great relevance in understanding tumor pathogenesis and facilitates prediction of tumor behavior, and decision management. The p53 tumor-suppressor gene seems to play a role only in the final de-differentiation process, in particular p53 appears to be involved in the process of transformation to the anaplastic phenotype *(83,84)*. Although the role of PTEN tumor-suppressor gene in thyroid carcinoma is still controversial, recent studies demonstrate that PTEN mutations in sporadic thyroid cancer are infrequent, it may act as a suppressor of thyroid cancerogenesis as the constitutive re-expression of PTEN into two different thyroid cell lines markedly inhibits cell growth *(85)*.

5.5. Malignant Mesothelioma

Cytogenetic changes in known and putative tumor-suppressor genes have been reported in a number of mesotheliomas, although it is possible that even the relatively low frequencies reported have been overestimated due to extensive inferences from results obtained with established mesothelioma cell lines rather than primary tumors *(86)*. Furthermore, the tumor-suppressor genes most commonly altered in other human malignancies, including p53 and Rb, are only rarely mutated in malignant mesothelioma *(87)*.

It has been recently demonstrated that asbestos fibers can affect cell cycle by blocking it in different phases depending on the type of asbestos fibers. Even though asbestos fibers revealed a G_2/M accumulation, chrisotile fibers produced a p53, p21-dependent G_0/G_1 accumulation whereas crocidolite fibers induced a non-p53-dependent delay in G_1/S transition *(88)*. These findings suggest an underlying abnormal cyclin expression that is worth of further investigation.

Several studies indicated that the incidence of mesotheliomas may not only correlate with the extensive asbestos exposure, but may also correlate with the unintentional inoculation of SV40 into the population, through SV40 contaminated polio vaccine. Recent results have shown that SV40 Tag is capable to interacting with Rb family proteins and p53 in human specimens, supporting the conclusion that SV40 could play a role in the pathogenesis of mesothelioma by impairing the function of Rb2 and p53 *(89–91)*.

5.6. Lung Cancer

Lung cancer is one of the leading causes of death by cancer in the world. Recent studies have indicated that several distinct chromosomal loci are altered, suggesting that sequential genetic alterations are necessary for initiation and progression of lung carcinogenesis. Molecular mechanisms altered in lung cancer include induced expression of oncogenes such as ras, myc, c-erbB and Bcl2, and loss of tumor-suppressor genes, such as p53, pRb/p105, pRb2/p130, and p16 *(92)*. It was found that p53 inactivation through mutations is the most frequent alteration in lung cancer (75%) *(93)*. Mutation or deletions of the pRb/p105 gene have been found frequently in small cell lung cancer (SCLC) (90%). In non-small lung cancer (NSCLC) there is absence or abnormal pRb/p105 mRNA in 10% of cell lines. Some authors have assigned a prognostic significance to the loss pRb/p105 alone or combined with the loss of ras or p53 in patients with NSCLC, while there seems to be no prognostic correlation with the expression of these molecules in squamous cell carcinoma. Most of pRb/p105-positive lung cancer cell lines are p16 negative.This would indicate that the pathogenesis of some lung cancers could occur due to the absence of p16 inhibitor, which functions to keep retinoblastoma proteins hypophosphorylated *(94–96)*. Immunohistochemical analysis of pRb/p105 and pRb2/p130 expression in patients with lung cancer has shown an inverse correlation between the histological grading of the tumor, the development of metastasis and the level of expression of these retinoblastoma proteins. Molecular analysis in primary lung cancer has revealed mutations in the retinoblastoma-related gene Rb2/p130 in 78.5% of patients, demonstrating the involvement of this gene in lung carcinogenesis. In addition, retroviral-mediated delivery of wild-type Rb2/p130 to the lung tumor cell line H23 inhibits tumorigenesis in vitro by dramatic growth arrest in colony formation, and in vivo by suppression of tumor formation in nude mice, suggesting that pRb2/p130 might be a good candidate for use in lung cancer therapy *(97)*.

5.7. Colorectal Cancer

Colorectal cancer is a major cause of morbidity and mortality among the different types of cancer. Significant progress has been made in understanding the molecular mechanisms that lead to it. Much knowledge has been obtained through study of genetic changes that occur in individuals with a familial predisposition to colorectal cancer, including familial adenomatous polyposis (FAP) and hereditary nonpolyposis colorectal cancer (HNPCC) syndromes. The gene with mutations that result in FAP has been identified as adenomatous polyposis coli (APC) *(98)*. Similarly, mutations in several genes that normally function in

DNA mismatch repair result in HNPCC. Colorectal cancer is the result of accumulated mutations in several additional oncogenes or tumor-suppressor genes; this information is necessary in order to formulate a genetic model for the disease. Recent studies have also identified a relatively prevalent polymorphism in the APC gene in Ashkenazi Jews that is associated with an increased risk for colorectal cancer. These studies present a paradigm based on the APC mutation for the screening of cancer susceptibility genes in the population at large *(99)*.

In addition mutations in the p53 gene have been implicated in the development of colorectal adenocarcinomas and have been associated with poor clinical outcome, although these data are still subject of controversy *(100)*.

5.8. Renal Tumors

The two main renal tumors, Wilm's tumor and renal cell carcinoma, are associated with distinct molecular genetic abnormalities. Probably more than any other group of tumors, they show a strong correlation between genetics and histopathology and serve as an illustration and experimental system for a diverse range of genetic mechanisms of disease *(101)*. These include mutation, loss of heterozygosity, deletion and contiguous gene syndromes, altered transcription and methylation, imprinting, and chromosomal loss.

Wilm's tumor (WT), a kidney malignancy found in children, occurs in hereditary and sporadic forms. Linkage analysis of families with a hereditary predisposition to WT and loss of heterozygosity (LOH) studies of hereditary and sporadic WT have led to the cloning of three WT susceptibility genes: WT1, WIT1, and WT2 *(102,103)*.

In WT, LOH at more than one locus suggests that multiple genetic events are required to give rise to a fully malignant phenotype, so that WT genesis may be complex. Cloning and characterization of additional WT-predisposing genes will lead to elucidation of interactions between different WT suppressor genes and their protein products. Identification of downstream target genes of WT suppressor genes is a very important step toward understanding how mutations of WT suppressor genes result in tumor formation, and should yield insight into tissue-specific carcinogenesis.

Two main studies on p53 mutations in WT have also been reported *(104)*. In WT, the high levels of p53 expression have been associated with sensitivity to chemotherapy, raising the possibility that chemosensitivity is dependent on a p53 dependent apoptosis.

Both sporadic and familial renal cell carcinomas have been reported to demonstrate chromosome 3p losses *(105)*. The most common cause of familial renal cell carcinoma is von Hippel Lindau syndrome, associated with abnormalities of 3p25-26. However, other familial forms of renal cell carcinoma are associated with abnormalities in other parts of chromosome 3p. The VHL gene maps in this region. Three studies have implicated somatic mutation of the VHL gene in sporadic renal cell carcinoma *(106)*. Mutations of the VHL gene were detected in a large number of sporadic renal cell carcinomas of the nonpapillary type. Mutations were not seen in other types of renal tumors or in nonrenal tumors associated with 3p losses. These data, along with the information gathered about VHL syndrome, suggest that the VHL gene is a relatively tissue-specific tumor suppressor gene, in accordance with Knudson's two hit model of tumorigenesis.

The existing data regarding renal tumors indicates that p53 alteration is rare, but when it does occur, it may be of biological significance. Mutations in p53 appear to be even less frequent in renal cell carcinoma, which could indicate that such mutations play a minor role in renal cell carcinoma progression *(107)*.

5.9. Prostate Cancer

The most commonly altered tumor suppressor gene in human cancers, p53, is involved in the late stages of prostate cancer progression. Molecular and immunohistochemical assays indicate that p53 alterations are associated with the progression of prostate cancer and loss of differentiation. These alterations are also associated with metastatic prostate tumors and androgen-insensitive tumors, suggesting that p53 alterations are late events *(108)*.

RB1 is one of the regions frequently deleted in prostate cancer *(109)*. Recent studies have demonstrated that restoring normal RB1 expression in the human prostate carcinoma cell line DU-145 suppresses tumorigenicity *(110)*. However, others have not found such a correlation *(111)*. The role of RB1 in prostate cancer therefore remains to be clarified.

A group from Johns Hopkins University Hospital has identified a metastasis-suppressor gene, called KAI1, in human prostate cancer. KAI1 belongs to a family of membrane glycoproteins and is thought to function in cell-cell interactions and cell migration *(112)*. This gene (located on chromosome 11p11.2) can suppress metastasis when introduced into rat prostate cancer cells. Expression of this gene was reduced in human cell lines derived from metastatic prostate tumors. The MMAC1/PTEN gene, recently identified and mapped to chromosome 10q23, is probably a tumor-suppressor gene for prostate cancer *(113)*.

5.10. Bladder Cancer

Studies on loss of heterozygosity using polymorphic markers have identified specific allelic deletions in many bladder cancers (BCs) that are not present in the DNA from normal tissues *(114)*. The retinoblastoma (RB) gene and the p53 gene play an important role in the progression of BC and possibly in its development. RB gene mutations are seen in approximately 30% of BCs. Inability to detect pRb immunohistochemically is associated with increased tumor grade and stage, especially muscle invasion.

Approximately 50% of muscle-invasive BCs show nuclear overexpression of p53, indicating the presence of a mutated protein. This is associated with increased stage and grade. Although it appears that altered p53 status is associated with a poorer prognosis, the practical clinical implications need to be further elucidated. Additionally, since deletions on chromosome 9 are found in more than 60% of BCs, there is strong evidence that at least two BC suppressor genes are present on that chromosome. In fact, deletions on chromosome 9 not only appear to occur in over 60% of BC across all grades and stages, but also are likely to be an initiating event. Indeed, at least one of the regions on the long arm of chromosome 9 (9q) is deleted primarily in low-grade superficial transitional cell carcinomas, which suggest a different molecular pathway in urothelial tumorigenesis than that which occurs with p53 or pRb inactivation *(115)*.

5.11. Breast and Gynecological Cancers

The etiology of breast cancer involves a complex interplay of genetic, hormonal, and probably dietary factors. Clustering of breast and ovarian cancers in families suggests an inherited susceptibility to these cancers *(116)*. Genetic linkage analysis of cancer pedigrees with families having a history of both breast and ovarian cancer led to the localization of the first breast cancer susceptibility gene on chromosome 17q21.3 *(61)*. This is the position of BRCA1 gene, but subsequent analysis of families with a history of breast cancer not linked to BRCA1 led to the discovery of another breast cancer susceptibility gene, BRCA2, on chromosome 13q12-13. Each gene product interacts with recombination/DNA repair proteins in pathways that participate in preserving intact chromosome structure. However, it is unclear to what extent such functions specifically suppress breast and ovarian cancer.

Similarly to the RB gene, both BRCA1 and BRCA2 are regarded as classic tumor-suppressor genes for two reasons. First, germline mutations in BRCA1 and/or BRCA2 are associated with tumor development and predispose the carriers to breast cancers. Second, loss of the wild-type allele is frequently observed in sporadic and familial breast tumors. These two events lead to inactivation of the tumor-suppressor function and loss of control of cell growth *(62)*.

Additional mutations of known tumor-suppressor genes have been reported in breast carcinoma. Mutations of the Rb gene, including deletions and duplications, were found in breast tumor cell lines and primary tumors *(117)*. Studies in primary breast tumors show LOH for the RB gene in approx 36% of the breast tumors examined *(118)*. But in all cases where loss of RB expression was observed, a number of tumor cells still expressed RB. This suggests that RB alteration is not an initiating event but a progressive event in breast cancer.

It is likely that mutation of RB promotes breast cancer progression. However, children inheriting one mutant RB allele rarely suffer from breast carcinomas; therefore, additional pathways may also augment mammary tumorigenesis; in fact, LOH of p53 is the most common mutation in breast cancer. Approximately 30% of p53 mutations in breast tumors are missense mutations, and many p53 mutations are single base changes that produce p53 variants with abnormally long half-lives. The reduction of ability to grow in soft agar and the reduction of tumorigenicity in nude mice that is caused by transfection or viral infection of wild-type p53 indicates that the quantity of wild-type p53 and mutant p53 is crucial in determining which form functions dominantly over the other *(119)*. The ability of p53 expression and RB expression to suppress tumorigenicity of breast cancer cells provides functional evidence that deletion or inactivational mutations of tumor-suppressor genes represent important steps in breast cancer genesis. Recent experimental data suggest the existence of subsets of breast cancers that, because of their phenotypic characteristics, could be derived from subpopulations of normal breast cells that probably use different control mechanisms of cell proliferation and neoplastic progression, p53 dependent in the cases with a stem cell phenotype and p53 independent in the cases with a luminal phenotype. In the latter an alteration of cell growth control is probably due to genetic lesions involving the Rb pathway *(120,121)*.

Mutations in the p53, RB2, BRCA1, DCC, and PTEN genes have been reported in gynecological neoplasias such as ovarian, cervical, and endometrial cancer. Human papillomaviruses are of major interest because specific types (HPV-16, -18, and several others) have been identified as causative agents in at least 90% of cancers of the cervix. Some studies summarized the available information regarding the implication of specific oncogenes, oncosuppressor genes, and HPV in the development of female genital malignancies *(122–125)*.

5.12. Bone and Soft-Tissue Sarcoma

Alterations in tumor-suppressor genes have been evaluated in normal cells and in tumor cells from sarcoma patients. p53 mutations in tumor cells have been reported in about 30% of bone and soft-tissue sarcomas *(126–128)*. Germline p53 mutations have been found in 10% patients with rhabdomyosarcoma *(129)*. LOH for 17p (the locus for p53) has been reported in 25% of chondrosarcomas, with high-grade tumors demonstrating a higher incidence of p53 allelic loss than low-grade lesions *(130)*.

In the single study published to date relating p53 gene mutation to outcome in soft-tissue sarcoma, immunohistochemistry was used to evaluate p53 and did not correlate well with sequencing of gene mutations *(131)*. This study reported that p53 mutations were correlated with both grade and outcome. However, in multivariate analysis, only grade remained a significant predictor of outcome. This finding suggests that mutations in p53 are found more frequently in higher-grade sarcomas. However, the effect of p53 status on clinical outcome in a group of pure high-grade sarcomas has not been investigated.

The coexistence of p53 and Rb abnormalities in the same sarcoma has been reported *(132)*. Approximately 50% of osteosarcomas fail to express Rb protein, and Rb abnormalities are associated with high-grade sarcomas and poor clinical outcome *(133,134)*. These patients carry an increased risk of cancer in all of the body's cells. This type of alteration in tumor-suppressor gene function is observed in the familial cancer syndromes and is associated with susceptibility to a variety of different cancers.

Although identification of the genotypic alterations evident in various sarcomas is crucial to understanding the origin of these lesions, this information has not, so far, helped clinicians to stratify sarcomas in relation to the risk of metastasis or local progression. To date, recognition of molecular alterations has correlated highly with the tumor grade and has provided no extra prognostic information. To further assess the effect of known genetic abnormalities on clinical outcome, it will be necessary to develop banks of tumors that permit evaluation of molecular characteristics in panels of homogeneous sarcoma type.

5.13. Malignant Lymphomas

The karyotypic picture of cytogenetically abnormal lymphomas is generally complex; tumors with a single clonal aberration are detected infrequently, more often than not, numerous chromosome aberrations are found concurrently. Several of the common translocations that occur in malignant lymphomas involve the TCR or Ig genes. These presumably occur as recombination errors at the time of antigen receptor gene rearrangement. As a consequence of many such translocations, an oncogene is placed under the influence of the enhancer region of the antigen receptor gene. The abnormally regulated oncogene may result in uncontrolled cell proliferation or in a failure of cells to undergo apoptosis.

A different mechanism of lymphomagenesis is that in which loss of genetic sequences takes place due to chromosome deletion. Consistently, loss of chromosome bands or regions may harbor tumor-suppressor genes, the inactivation of which promotes the neoplastic process by causing disturbances in cell growth control.

The 11q13 translocations and bcl-1 rearrangement are characteristic features of Mantle cell lymphomas (MCL). These alterations lead to a constant overexpression of cyclin D_1, which plays an important pathogenetic role, probably deregulating cell-cycle control by overcoming the suppressor effect of the retinoblastoma protein and p27^{Kip1}. Aggressive variants of MCL have additional genetic alterations, including inactivation of p53 and p16INK4a tumor-suppressor genes. Deletion of p16INK4a occurs in approximately one-half of MCLs and is a more relevant indicator of the proliferative features as compared to morphological criteria *(135)*.

Several studies have reported alteration of the p53 gene in non-Hodgkin lymphomas (NHL). Gaidano et al. described loss and inactivation of p53 in more than 30% of Burkitt's lymphomas (BL) *(136)*. Others have revealed mutations of the p53 gene and/or abnormal expression of the p53 protein in a substantial number of patients with diffuse and follicular lymphomas. In particular, alteration of p53 has been suggested to play a role in the transformation of follicular lymphoma into diffuse large B-cell lymphoma (DLBCL) *(137)*. Yet, RB1 and p53 pathways are both important in the development of *de novo* DLBCL. It is thus possible to identify several distinct molecular types of DLBCL, corroborating the hypothesis that the heterogeneity of the disease relies on its pathogenetic heterogeneity *(138)*. In addition, p27 expression in diffuse large B-cell lymphomas with adverse clinical significance has been reported. This suggests that the anomalous p27 protein may be rendered nonfunctional through interaction with other cell cycle regulator proteins. Evidence in favor of p27 sequestration by cyclin D_3 was provided by co-immunoprecipitation studies in a Burkitt's cell line (Raji) showing the existence of cyclin D_3/p27 complexes and the absence of CDK2/p27 complexes. These results can support the hypothesis that there are cyclin D_3/p27 complexes in a subset of aggressive B-cell lymphomas in which p27 lacks the inhibitory activity found when it is bound to cyclin E/CDK2 complexes *(139,140)*.

A recent study indicates that p14(ARF) alterations occur in a subset of aggressive NHLs, but they are always associated with p16INK4a aberrations. Concomitant disruption of p16INK4a and p14(ARF)/p53 regulatory pathways may thus have a cooperative effect in the progression of these tumors *(141)*.

Besides the previously reported mechanisms, pRb2/p130 and p107 seem to be involved in the pathogenesis of NHL. Genetic alterations disrupting the nuclear localization of the retinoblastoma-related gene RB2/p130 have recently been documented in BL cell lines as well as in primary tumors. These mutations may impair the ability of the respective gene product to function as a growth-suppressor nuclear protein, pRb2/p130 being exclusively cytoplasmic. The distinct pattern of pRb2/p130 and p107 in a large cohort of NHL suggests the possibility of different pathogenetic mechanisms within and among lymphoma subtypes *(55,142)*. This further supports the REAL classification recommendation to examine each disease entity with respect to possibly divergent molecular features, growth patterns, and clinical aggressiveness.

The possible involvement of the p53 tumor-suppressor gene in the pathogenesis of Hodgkin's lymphomas (HD) is still under investigation. Conclusive data on p53 mutations in HD are still lacking mainly due to technical problems. In fact, the neoplastic tumor cell clone in HD is represented by the large Hodgkin and Reed-Sternberg cells, which account for only a minority of all cells in the tumor tissue (often < 1%). To identify putative HRS cell-specific mutations, analysis of single HRS cells from frozen or paraffin tissue sections of HD biopsy specimens is mandatory. By this method mutations of p53 have not been found. The accumulation of p53 protein in the HRS cells, as usually observed by immunohistochemistry, might be a consequence of p53 binding proteins such as certain viral products or the mouse double-minute 2 oncogene (MDM2) gene product. Since the cells of normal lymphoid tissue do not contain immunohistochemically detectable amounts of p53 and/or MDM2 (with rare exceptions), the overexpression and asymmetric distribution of p53 and MDM2 in HRS cells point toward a severely disordered cell cycle in these cells. It is likely that a major event in the pathogenesis of HD is the blockage of the apoptotic pathway. EBV, as well as genes monitoring the human genome for damaged DNA, such as p53, might be involved in the postulated hindrance of the apoptotic pathway, leading to the genesis of classic HRS cells. This is a hypothesis that is in harmony with the morphologic and molecular biologic evidence for a disturbance of the cell cycle and mitotic process in classic HRS cells (143).

Recently, a working model of a stepwise malignant transformation in the molecular pathogenesis of multiple myeloma (MM) was proposed, involving the tumor-suppressor gene TP53 and retinoblastoma gene (RB1). Monoallelic deletions of RB1 appear to be a frequent and early event in the pathogenesis of MM, without obvious relevance for disease progression (144).

5.14. Melanomas

It has been difficult to identify tumor-suppressor genes in malignant melanoma, as these tumors show a complex pattern of chromosome loss; only one familial melanoma syndrome has been mapped to a chromosome region that shows frequent LOH in sporadic melanomas (145). Sporadic melanomas show frequent LOH at chromosome arms 6q, 9p, 10q, 11q, and 18q, which suggests that these regions may contain tumor-suppressor genes. The importance of the CDKN2A (p16) gene in the development of sporadic melanomas is still not clear. Although this gene is frequently inactivated in melanoma cell lines, mutations are uncommon in sporadic melanomas. This finding, and the failure to detect CDKN2A mutations in families that show linkage to chromosome 9p, has led to speculation that there may be another tumor-suppressor gene of importance in melanoma development on chromosome 9p (146). Recent studies of genes identified in other cancers that map to chromosome regions frequently deleted in melanoma cell lines, or that are associated with pigmentary abnormalities, have led to the identification of some new tumor-suppressor genes of importance in melanoma development. PTEN is frequently deleted or mutated in melanoma cell lines (147). Mutations in the Peutz-Jeghers gene that encodes for a protein kinase have been identified in a small number of sporadic melanomas. Peutz-Jeghers syndrome is characterized by development of lentigines of the lips and mucosa but is not known to be associated with an increased melanoma risk. The RB tumor-suppressor gene is frequently inactivated in uveal melanoma by phosphorylation of residues in the COOH-terminal region that regulate its activity, and one mechanism for this phosphorylation is the overexpression of cyclin D (148).

Mutations of MTS1 gene can be found in the germline of the patients with familial susceptibility to melanoma (13,14). p53 mutations are common in nonmelanoma skin cancer and in related premalignant lesions such as actinic keratosis and Bowen's disease. More recently, p53 mutations have been identified in small clones of keratinocytes in sun-exposed human skin, which suggests that inactivation of this protein is an early event in skin cancer development. This observation of p53 mutations in clones of keratinocytes many years before skin cancers develop is consistent with its proposed role as a caretaker type of tumor-suppressor gene. In normal skin, wild-type p53 levels increase following exposure to ultraviolet radiation, this is thought to be an important protective response and is clearly demonstrated by studies in mice which lack p53, so-called knock-out mice, which show a marked increase in the rate of skin cancer development following exposure to UVR *(149)*.

6. CONCLUSIONS

Pathologists play multiple roles in the management of patients affected by cancer. First they must provide diagnoses that are both accurate and reproducible. It is also essential, however, that the diagnosis made have clinical relevance, providing information that is fundamental to prognosis and treatment. The traditional way to classifying tumors is by histopathology; the staining and analysis of tissues samples. Now, the ability to analyze changes at the molecular levels of the transcripts and/or protein products for literally thousands of genes promises interesting possibilities as a research tool, but also for tissue diagnosis. It is now possible to apply the knowledge of cell cycle control to the practical diagnostic pathology and better understand by which mechanisms cell growth can become deregulated in human neoplasia. Although most of the proteins involved in cell cycle control have been identified in low organisms such as yeast and bacteria, they show a high homology in eukariotic cells and it is now possible to detect many of these proteins in tissue sections, as monoclonal and/or polyclonal antibodies against cell cycle-related proteins are commercially available. Improvements in therapeutic approaches might then be made possible through a better genetic understanding of tumor classification and tumor cell biology. Personalized therapy tailored for patients with specific genetic makeups may become possible in the near future. Specific genes or gene expression are found to be altered in particular cancers and in some associated preneoplastic lesions. This diversity in genetic alteration is dependent in part of the organ of origin of the malignant neoplasm, its histologic type, and degree of progression.

Biologic approaches can enhance diagnostic accuracy and play a crucial role in a more accurate definition of neoplastic processes. Well over 150 human disease genes have been cloned and a large number of alleles have been identified. However, when a potential disease locus has been identified by genome wide marker analysis, a way to scan the coding sequences of all genes in the region quickly to find disease-associated nucleotide alterations is needed. Hybridization between complementary nucleotide sequences is also critical in what is currently the most widely used technique in molecular biology: the polymerase chain reaction (PCR). The PCR permits the in vitro amplification of defined regions of DNA provided that sequences surrounding the region to be amplified are known. The PCR amplification is carried out in repeated cycles of DNA synthesis in which the DNA polymerase copies the template sequences by extending the 3' end of the primers hybridized to the two strands of the template. The PCR technique of single-strand conformational polymorphism (SSCP), one of the most widely used methods for detecting single base pair changes in genomic DNA, is based on the principle that two single-strand DNA molecules of identical length but unlike sequence will migrate differentially in a nondenaturing acrylamide gel. Although SSCP is a rapid and easy procedure, studies have shown that it probably only detects about 70% of possible mutations. Therefore other PCR-based methods have been developed to try to increase this efficiency. One such procedure is called solid-phase chemical cleavage (SpCCM), which detects cleavage products that result from chemical modification of mismatches. Two other PCR-based methods for detecting single nucleotide differences are base excision sequence scanning (BESS), which uses an enzymatic sequencing method to detect thymidine residues in PCR products, and artificial mismatch hybridization (AMH), a method that exploits heteroduplex stability assays to detect single base pair mismatches. Finally the sequencing of PCR products will allow a definitive answer to the presence of genomic alterations.

Moreover, the recently developed DNA microarray technique can provide detailed information of the expression patterns of thousands of genes in tumors. The DNA microarrays consist of two centimeter wide slivers of silicon or glass impregnated with thousands of immobilized fragments of DNA serving as probes for detecting complementary DNA/RNA sequences. These will allow the analysis of expression patterns of thousands of genes simultaneously. Instead of following the expression of only one or two genes at a time, entire molecular pathways can now be followed. The unique expression patterns of cancer specific genes can be profiled in various tumors that are resistant or sensitive to various chemotherapeutic agents and/or radiotherapy, generating data that can be used not only at the diagnostic and prognostic levels but also to design novel therapeutic agents. The microchip arrays will accelerate the progress of medical research to a level never before imagined, ushering in a new era of molecular diagnostics and therapeutics. Once the genetic alterations have been identified at the molecular level, it is then possible to investigate how genetic diversity becomes phenotypic diversity, and to detect by immunohistochemistry the proteins and gene products.

p53 is often overexpressed in tumor cells, as can be demonstrated by immunohistochemistry in tissue sections or by protein analysis of cell preparations. This phenomenon affects both the wild-type and the mutant forms. p53

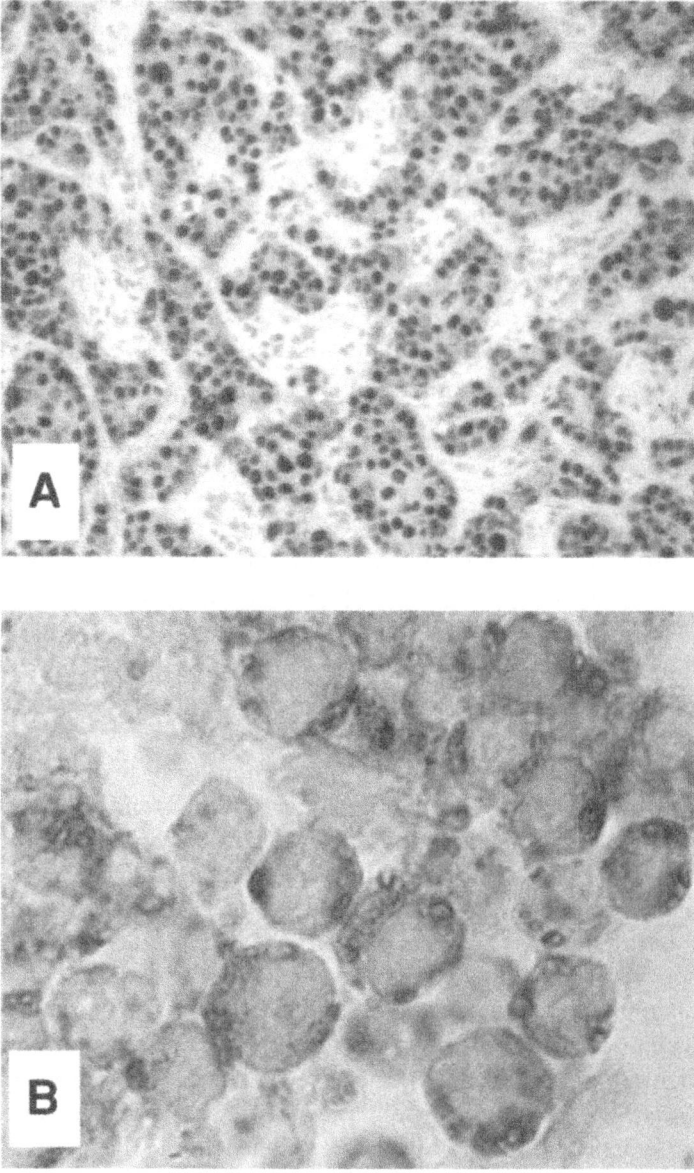

Fig. 3. (A) Immunohistochemical analysis of p53 in breast carcinomas. (B) Cytoplasmatic expression of pRb2/p130 by immunohistochemical analysis in Burkitt's lymphoma.

overexpression therefore is not always due to a mutation in the gene, but is more accurately seen as a property of many transformed cells. However, the use of immunostaining for p53 protein provides the highest estimate of abnormalities, even though this method will be expected to identify only miss-sense mutations and nontruncated proteins. Although without molecular analysis we cannot completely exclude false-negative or false-positive results, immunohistochemical analysis represents a rapid method to investigate p53 expression on tissue sections (Fig. 3A).

Mutations of RB and RB2 have been detected in many human tumors. The genetic alterations of RB and RB2 can result in the production of truncated or unstable protein whose function may be impaired; in this case, immunohistochemical analysis of RB or RB2/p130 gene products will reveal a negative or weak immunostaining. Still, mutations of RB2 nuclear localization signal results in the expression of the protein in the cytoplasm that can easily be detected by immunohistochemical analysis (Fig. 3B). Furthermore, an unusual expression of pRb2/p130 associated with high levels of proliferation-associated protein can suggest a mechanism of inactivation of pRb2/p130 by viral proteins as has been demonstrated in human mesothelioma and AIDS-related lymphomas.

An extensive knowledge of how underlying molecular mechanisms may be detected by immunohistochemistry on tissue sections, and is thus a powerful tool for pathologists in the assessment of prognosis and therapeutic approach.

REFERENCES

1. Lundberg AS, Weinberg RA. Control of cell cycle and apoptosis. *Eur J Cancer* 1999;35: 1886–1894.
2. Pardee AB. A restriction point for control of normal animal cell proliferation. *Proc Natl Acad Sci USA* 1974;71:1286–1290.
3. Morgan DO. Cyclin dependent kinases: engines, clocks and microprosessors. *Ann Rev Cell Dev Biol* 1997;13:261–291.
4. De Falco G, Giordano A. CDK9 (PITALRE): a multifunctional cdc2-related kinase. *J Cell Physiol* 1998;177:501–509.
5. Chellappan SP, Giordano A, Fisher PB. (1998) Role of cyclin dependent kinases and their inhibitors in cellular differentiation and development, in *Cyclin Dependent Kinase (CDK) Inhibitors*. Vagt PK, Reed SI, eds. Springer-Verlag, Berlin, pp. 57–103.
6. Lees EM, Harlow E. Sequences within the conserved cyclin box of human cyclin A are sufficient for binding to and inactivating of CDC2 kinase. *Mol Cell Biol* 1993;13:1194–1201.
7. Murray A. Cyclin ubiquitination: the destructive end of mitosis. *Cell* 1995;81:149–152.
8. King RW, Deshaies RJ, Peters JM, Kirshner MW. How proteolysis drives the cell cycle. *Science* 1996;274:1652–1659.
9. Solomon MJ, Lee T, Kirschner MW. Role of phosphorylation in p34^{CDC2} activation: identification of an activating kinase. *Mol Biol Cell* 1992;3:13–27.
10. Fischer RP, Morgan DO. A novel cyclin associates with MO 157CDK7 to form the CDK-activating kinase. *Cell* 1994;78:713–724.
11. Herzinger T, Leed SI. Cyclin D$_3$ in rate-limiting for G$_1$/S phase transition in fibroblasts. *J Biol Chem* 1998;273:14958–14961.

12. Mclachlan TK, Sang N, Giordano A. Cyclins, cyclin-dependent kinase and cdk inhibitors: implication in cell cycle control and cancer. *Crit Rev Eukaryot Gen. Expr* 1995;5:127–156.
13. Vidal A, Koff A. Cell-cycle inhibitors: tree families united by a common cause. *Gene* 2000;247:1–15.
14. Sgambato A, Cittadini A, Faraglia B, Weinstein, IB. Multiple functions of p27 (Kip 1) and its alterations in tumor cells: a review. *J Cell Physiol* 2000;183:18–27.
15. Nevins JR. E2F: a link between the Rb tumor suppressor protein and viral oncoproteins. *Science* 1992;258:424–429.
16. Flaitz CM, Hicks MJ. Molecular piracy: the viral link to carcinogenesis. *Oral Oncol* 1998;34:448–453.
17. Prives C, Hall PA. The p53 pathway. *J Pathol* 1999;187:112–126.
18. Haupt Y, Maya R, Kazaz A, Oren M. Mdm2 promotes the rapid degradation of p53. *Nature* 1997;387:296–299.
19. Hupp TR, Lane DP. Allosteric activation of latent p53 tetramers. *Curr Biol* 1994;4:865–875.
20. Miyashita T, Reed JC. Tumor suppressor p53 is a direct transcriptional activator of the human bax gene. *Cell* 1995;80:293–299.
21. Luo J, Su F, Chen D, Shildon A, Gu W. Deacetylation of p53 modulates its effect on cell growth and apoptosis. *Nature* 2000;408:377–381.
22. Harris CC, Hollestein M. Clinical implications of the p53 tumor-suppresor gene. *N Engl J Med* 1993;329:1318–1327.
23. Wyndoford-Thomas D, Blaydes J. The influence of cell context on the selection pressure for p53 mutation in human cancer. *Carcinogenesis* 1998;19:29–36.
24. Kaghad M, Bonnet H, Yang A. Monoallelicaly expressed gene related to p53 at 1p36, a region frequently deleted in neuroblastoma and other human cancers. *Cell* 1997;90:809–819.
25. Weinberg RA. Tumor suppressor genes. *Science* 1991;254:1138–1145.
26. Knudson AG. Retinoblastoma: clues to human oncogenesis. *Science* 1984;228:1028–1033.
27. Sidle A, Palaty C, Dirks P, Wiggan O, Kiess M, Gill RM, Wong AK, Hamal PA. Acitvity of the retinoblastoma family proteins, pRb, P107, and p30, during cellular proliferation and differentiation. *Crit Rev Biochem Mol* 1996;31:237–271.
28. Stiegler P, Kasten M, Giordano A. The RB family of cell cycle regulatory factors. *J Cell Biochem Suppl* 1998;31:30–36.
29. Weinberg RA. The retinoblastoma protein and cell cycle control. *Cell* 1995;81:323–330.
30. Harirngton EA, Bruce JL, Harlow E, Dyson N. pRb plays an essential role in cell cycle arrest induced by DNA damage. *Proc Natl Acad Sci USA* 1998;95:11945–11959.
31. Knudsen KE, Booth D, Naderi S, Sever-Chroneos Z, Fribour AF, Hunton IC, et al. RB-dependent S-phase response to DNA damage. *Mol Cell Biol* 2000;20:7751–7763.
32. Pucci B, Claudio PP, Masciullo V, Bellincampi L, Melino G, Giordano A. pRb2/p130 promotes radiation-induced apoptosis by Bcl-2 downregulation and p73 upregulation. (Submitted.)
33. Nevins JR. Toward an understanding of the functional complexity of the E2F and retinoblastoma families. *Cell Growth Differ* 1998;258:424–429.
34. Cludio PP, Howard CM, Baldi A, De Luca A, Fu Y, Condorelli G, et al. P130/pRb2 has growth suppressive properties similar to yet distinctive from those of retinoblastoma family members pRb and p107. *Cancer Res* 1994;54:5556–5560.
35. Claudio PP, De Luca A, Howard CM, Baldi A, Firpo EJ, Koff A, et al. Functional anlysis of pRb2/p130 interaction with cyclins. *Cancer Res* 1996;56:2003–2008.
36. Ewen ME, Xing EW, Larence JB, Livingston DM. Molecular cloning, chromosomal mapping, and expression of the cDNA for p107, a retinoblastoma gene product-related protein. *Cell* 1991;66:1155–1164.
37. Paggi, MG, Baldi A, Bonetto F, Giordano A. Retinoblastoma protein family in cell cycle and cancer. A reviewer. *J Cell Biochem* 1996;62:418–430.

38. Mayol X, Grana X, Baldi A, Sang N, Hu Q, Giordano A. Cloning of a new member of the retinoblastoma gene family (pRb2) which binds to E1A transforming domain. *Oncogene* 1993;8:2561–2566.
39. Lee JO, Russo AA, Pavletich NP. Structure of the retinoblastoma tumor-suppressor pocket domain bound to a peptide from HPV E7. *Nature* 1998;391:859–865.
40. Hass-Kogan DA, Kogan SC, Levi D, Dazin P, T'Ang A, Fung YK, Israel MA. Inhibition pf apoptosis by retinoblastoma gene product. *EMBO J* 1995;14:461–472.
41. Kasten M, Giordano A. pRb and Cdks in apoptosis and the cell cycle. *Cell Death Differ* 1998;5:132–140.
42. Kim YW, Otterson GA, Kratze RA, Coxon AB, Kaye FJ. Differential specificity for binding of the retinoblastoma binding protein 2 to RB, and TATA-binding protein. *Mol Cell Biol* 1994;14:7256–7264.
43. Smith EJ, Leone G, De Gregori J, Jakoi L, Nevins JR. The accumulation of an E2F-p130 transcriptional repressor distiguishes a G_0 cell state from a G_1 cell state. *Mol Cell Biol* 1996;16:6965–6976.
44. Smith EJ, Leone G, Nevins JR. Distinct mechanisms control the accumulation of the Rb-related p107 and p130 proteins during cell growth. *Cell Growth Differ* 1998;9:297–303.
45. Kouzarides T. Transcriptional control by the retinoblastoma protein. *Semin Cancer Biol* 1995;6:91–98.
46. La Thangue NB. E2F and the molecular mechanisms of the early cell-cycle control. *Biochem Soc Trans* 1996;24:54–59.
47. Adams PD, Kaelin WG Jr. Transcriptional control by E2F. *Semin Can Biol* 1995;6:99–108.
48. Moberg K, Starts MA, Lees JA. E2F4 switches from p130 to p107 and pRb in response to cell cycle reentry. *Mol Cell Biol* 1996;16:1436–1449.
49. Bruce JL, Hurfird RK Jr, Classon M, Koh J, Dyson N. Requirements for cell cycle arrest by p16INK4a. *Mol Cell* 2000;6:737–742.
50. Moberg K, Starts MA, Lees JA. E2F4 switches from p130 to p107 and prB in response to cell cyle reentry. *Mol Cell Biol* 1996;16:1436–1449.
51. Johnson DG. Regulation of E2F1 gene expression by p130 (Rb2) and D-type cyclin kinase activity. *Oncogene* 1995;11:1685–1692.
52. Johnson DG, Schneider-Broussard R. Role of E2F in cell cycle control and cancer. *Front Biosci* 1998;3:d447–d458.
53. Qian Y, Luckey C, Horton L, Esser M, Templeton DJ. Biological function of the retinoblastoma protein requires distinct domains for hyperphosphorylation and transcription factor binding. *Mol Cell Biol* 1992;12:5363–5372.
54. Paggi MG, Baldi A, Bonetto F, Giordano A. Retinoblastoma protein family in cell cycle and cancer: a review. *J Cell Biochem* 1996;62:418–430.
55. Cinti C, Leoncini L, Nyongo A, Ferrari F, Lazzi S, Bellan C, et al. Genetic alterations of the retinoblastoma-related gene Rb2/p130 identify different pathogenetic mechanisms in and among Burkitt's lymphoma subtypes. *Am J Pathol* 2000;156:751–760.
56. Slingerland J, Pagano M. Regulation of the cell cycle by the ubiquitin pathway. *Results Probl Cell Differ* 1998;22:133–147.
57. Slingerland J, Pagano M. Regulation of the cdk inhibitor p27 and its deregulation in cancer. *J Cell Physiol* 2000;183:10–17.
58. Mumetsu S, Souza B, Muller O, Albert I, Rubinfeld B, Polakos P. The APC gene product associateds with microtubules in vivo and promotes their assembly in vitro. *Cancer Res* 1994;54:3676–3681.
59. Groden J, Thlveris A, Samowitz W, Carlson M, Gelbert L, Alberstein H, et al. Identification and characterization of the familial adenomatous polyposis coli gene. *Cell* 1991;66:589–600.
60. Volgelstein B, Fearon ER, Kern SE, Hamilton SR, Preisinger AC, Nakamura Y, White R. Allelotype of colorectal carcinomas. *Science* 1989;244:207–211.

61. Kinzler KW, Nilbert MC, Volgelstein B, Braan TM, Lekid D, Smith KJ, et al. Identification of a gene located at chromosome 5q21 that is mutated in colorectal cancers. *Science* 1991;251:1366–1370.
62. Hall JM, Lee MK, Newman B, Marrow JE, Anderson LA, Huey B, King MC. Linkage of early onset familial breast cancer to chromosome 17q21. *Science* 1990;250:1684–1689.
63. Hofmann W, Schlag PM. BRCA1 and BRCA2- breast cancer susceptibility genes. *Cancer Res Clin Oncol* 2000;126:487–496.
64. Cho Y, Fearon ER. DCC: linking tumor suppressor genes and altered cell surface interactions in cancer? *Gen Dev* 1995;5:72–78.
65. Pritchard-Jones K, Fleming S, Davidson D, Bickmore W, Porteous D, Gosden C, et al. The candidate Wilm's tumour gene is involved in genitourinary development. *Nature* 1990; 346:194–197.
66. Whaley JM, Naglich J, Gelbert L, Lamiell JM, Green JS, Collins D, et al. Germline mutations in the von Hippel-Lindau tumor suppressor gene are similar to somatic von Hippel-Lindau aberrations in sporadic renal cell carcinoma. *Am J Hum Genet* 1994;55:1092–1102.
67. Gronostajski RM. Roles of the NFI/CTF gene family in transcription and development. *Gene* 2000;249:31–45.
68. Dahia PLM. PTEN, a unique tumor suppressor gene. *Endocr Rel Cancer* 2000;7:115–129.
69. Bonneau D, Longy M. Mutations of the human PTEN gene. *Hum Mut* 2000;16:109–122.
70. Jacks T, Fazeli A, Schmitt EM, Bronson RT, Goodel MA, Weinberg RA. Effects of an Rb mutation in the mouse. *Nature* 1992;359:295–300.
71. Cobrinik D, Lee MH, Hannon G, Mulligan G, Bronson RT, Dyson N, et al. Shared role of the pRb-related p130 and p107 proteins in limb development. *Genes Dev* 1996;10:1633–1644.
72. Mulligan G, Jacks T. The retinoblastoma gene family: cousins with overlapping interests. *Trends Genet* 1998;14:223–229.
73. Vooijs M, van der Valk M, te Riele H, Berns A. Flp-mediated tissue-specific inactivation of the retinoblastoma tumor suppressor gene in the mouse. *Oncogene* 1998;17:1–12.
74. LeCouter JE, Kablar B, Whyte PF, Ying C, Rudnicki MA. Strain-dependent embryonic lethality in mice lacking the retinoblastoma-related p130 gene. *Development* 1998;125: 4669–4679.
75. Sage J, Mulligan GJ, Attardi LD, Miller A, Chen S, Williams B, Theodorou E, Jacks T. Targeted disruption of the three RB-related genes leads to loss of G_1 control and immortalization. 2000. (Submitted.)
76. Tsuzuki T, Tsunada S, Sakaki T, Konishi N, Hiesa Y, Nakamura M. Alterations of retinoblastoma, p53, p16 (CDKN2), p15 genes in human astrocytomas. *Cancer* 1996;78:287–293.
77. Weiss WA. Genetics of brain tumors. *Curr Opin Pedriat* 2000;12:543–548.
78. Bignon YJ, Rio P. Retinoblastoma gene: with therapeutic use of its tumor suppressor properties be possible? *Bull Cancer* 1993;80:704–712.
79. Levine AJ. The tumor suppressor gene. *Annu Rev Biochem* 1993;62:623–651.
80. Lee MH, Williams BO, Mulligan G, Mukai S, Bronson RT, Dyson N, Harlow E. Targeted disruption of p107: functional overlap between p107 and Rb. *Genes Dev* 1996;16: 1621–1632.
81. Tosi GM, Cinti C, Claudio PP, Massaro-Giordano G, Filippone E, Ognibene A, et al. Alterations of the RB2/p130 gene in human retinoblastoma: implications for pathogenesis. (Submitted.)
82. Cluadio PP, Howard CM, Fu Y, Cinti C, Califano L, Micheli P, et al. Mutations in the retinoblastoma-related gene Rb2/p130 in primary nasopharingeal carcinoma. *Cancer Res* 2000;60:8–12.
83. Learoyd DL, Messina M, Zedenius J, Robinson BG. Molecular genetics of thyroid and surgical decision-making. *World J Surg* 2000;24:923–933.

84. Suarez HG. Molecular basis of ephitelial thyroid tumorigenesis. *C R Acad Sci III* 2000; 323:519–528.
85. Bruni P, Boccia A, Baldassarre G, Trapasso F, Santoro M, Chiappetta G, et al. PTEN expression is reduced in a subset of sporadic thyroid carcinomas: evidence that PTEN-growth suppressing activity in thyroid cancer cells mediated by p27kip1. *Oncogene* 2000;19:3146–3155.
86. Jaurand MC, Barrett JC (1994) Neoplastic transformation of masothelioma calls, in *The Mesothelial Cell and Mesothelioma*, Jaurand MC, Bignot J, eds. Marcel Dekker, New York, pp. 207–223.
87. Murthy SS, Testa JR. Asbestos, chromosomal deletions, and tumor suppressor gene alterations in human malignant mesothelioma. *J Cell Physiol* 1999;180:150–157.
88. Walker C, Everitt J, Barrett JC. Possible cellular and molecular mechanisms for asbestos carcinogenicity. *Am J Ind Med* 1992;21:253–273.
89. Procopio A, Strizzi L, Giuffrida A, Scarpa S, Giuliano M, Iezzi T, et al. Human malignant mesothelioma of the pleura: new perspectives for diagnosis and therapy. *Monaldi Arch Chest Dis* 1998;53:241–243.
90. Mutti L, De Luca A, Claudio PP, Convertino C, Carbone M, Giordano A. Simian virus 40-like DNA sequences and large-T antigen-retinoblastoma family protein pRb2/p130 interaction in human mesothelioma. *Dev Biol Stand* 1998;9:47–53.
91. De Luca A, Baldi A, Esposito V, Howard CM, Bagella L, Rizzo P, et al. The retinoblastoma gene family prb/p105, p107 pRb2/p130 and simian virus-40 large T-antigen in human mesothelioma. *Nat Med* 1997;3:913–916.
92. Sekido Y, Fong KM, Minna JD. Progress in understanding the molecular pathogenesis of human lung cancer. *Biochem Biophys Acta* 1998;1378:F21–F59.
93. Bennet WP, Hussain SP, Vahakangas KH, Khan MA, Shields PG, Harris CC. Molecular epidemiology of human cancer risk: gene-environment interactions and p53 mutation spectrum in human lung cancer. *J Pathol* 1999;187:8–18.
94. Shapiro GI, Edwards CD, Kobzik L, Godleski J, Richards W, Sugarbaker DJ. Reciprocal Rb inactivation and p16INK4 expression in primary lung cancer and cell lines. *Cancer Res* 1995;55:503–509.
95. Kinoshita, I., Dosaka-Akita, H., Mishina, T., Akie, K., Nishi, M., Hiroumi, H., et al. Altered p16INK4 and retinoblastoma protein status in non-small cell lung cancer: potential synergistic effect with altered p53 protein on proliferartive activity. *Cancer Res* 1996;56:5557–5562.
96. Baldi A, Esposito V, De Luca A, Howard CM, Mazzarella G, Baldi F, et al. Differential expression of retinoblastoma family members, pRb/p105, p107 and pRb2/p130 in lung cancer. *Clin Cancer Res* 1996;2:1239–1245.
97. Claudio PP, Howard CM, Pacilio C, Cinti C, Romano G, Minimo C, et al. Mutations in the retinoblastoma-related gene Rb2/p130 in lung tumors and suppression of tumor growth in vivo by retrovirus-mediated gene transfer. *Cancer Res* 2000;60:372–382.
98. Miyaki M, Konishi M, Kikuchi-Yanoshita R, Enomoto M, Igari T, Tanaka K, et al. Characterization of somatic mutation of the adenomatous polyposis coli gene in colorectal cancer. *Cancer Res* 1994;54:3011–3020.
99. Yang VW. The molecular genetics of colorectal cancer. *Curr Gastroenterol Rep* 1999;1: 449–454.
100. Fearon ER, Volgestein B. A genetic model for colorectal tumorigenesis. *Cell* 1990;61: 759–767.
101. Fleming S. The impact of genetics on the classification of renal carcinoma. *Histopathology* 1993;22:89–92.
102. Call KM, Glaser T, Ito Y, Bluckler AJ, Pelletier J, Haber PA, et al. Isolation and characterization of a zinc finger polypeptide gene at the human chromosome 11 Wilm's tumor locus. *Cell* 1990;60:509–520.

103. Gessler M, Poustka A, Cavenee W, Neve KL, Orkin SH, Brun S. Gap: Homozygous deletion in Wilms' tumor of a zinc finger gene identified by chromosome jumping. *Nature* 1990; 343:774–778.
104. Weber PG, Chen J, Nisen PD. Infrequency of ras, p53, WT1 or RB gene alterations in Wilms' tumors. *Cancer* 1993;72:3732–3738.
105. Erlandsson R, Boldog F, Sumegi J, Klein G. Do human renal cell carcinomas arise by a double loss mechanism? *Cancer Genet Cytogenet* 1988;36:197–203.
106. Gnarra JR, Lerman MI, Zbar B, Linehan WM. Genetics of renal-cell carcinoma and evidence for a critical role for von Hippel-Lindau in renal tumorigenesis. *Semin Oncol* 1995;22:3–8.
107. Fleming, S. Genetics of renal tumours. *Cancer Met Rev* 1997;16:127–140.
108. Voeller HJ, Sugars LY, Pretlow J, Gelmann EP. P53 oncogene mutastions in human prostate cancer specimens. *J Urol* 1994;151:492–495.
109. Phillips SMA, Morton DG, Lee SJ, Wallace DMA, Neoptolemas JP. Loss of heterozigosity of the retinoblastoma and adenomatous polyposis susceptibility gene loci and in chromosomas 10p, 10q and 16q in human prostate cancer. *Br J Urol* 1994;73:390–395.
110. Bookstein R, Shew JY, Chen PL, Scully P, Lee WH. Suppression of tumoregenicity of human prostate carcinoma cells by replacing a mutated RB gene. *Science* 1990:247:712–715.
111. Tricoli JV, Gumerlock PH, Yao JL, Chi SG, D'Sauza SA, Nestok BR, de Vere WR. Alteration of the retinoblastoma gene in human prostate adenocarcinoma. *Genes Chromosom Cancer* 1996;15:108–114.
112. Dong JT, Lomb PW, Rinker-Schaeffer CW, Vukanovic J, Ichikawa T, Isaacs JT, Barrett JC. KAI1, a metastasis suppressor gene for prostate cancer on human chromosome 11p11.2. *Science* 1995;268:884–886.
113. Cairns P, Okami K, Halachmi S, Halachmi N, Esteller M, Herman JG, et al. Frequent inactivation of PTEN/MMAC 1 in primary prostate cancer. *Cancer Res* 1997;57:4997–5000.
114. Knowles MA. Molecular genetics of bladder cancer. *Br J Urol* 1995;1:57–66.
115. Jung I, Messing E. Molecular machanisms and pathways in bladder cancer development and progression. *Cancer Control* 2000;7:325–334.
116. Lynch H. Hereditary breast cancer. *Ann Med* 1991;23:475–477.
117. Cox LA, Chen G, Lee EYHP. Tumor suppressor gene and their role in breast cancer. *Breast Cancer Res Treat* 1994;32:19–38.
118. Devilee P, Van Vliet M, Bardoel A, Kievits T, Kuipers-Dijshoorn N, Pearson PL, Cornelisse CJ. Frequent somatic imbalance of marker alleles for chromosome 1 in human primary breast carcinoma. *Cancer Res* 1991;51:1020–1025.
119. Hartmann A, Blaszyk H, Kovach JS, Sommer SS. The molecular epidemiology of p53 gene mutations in human breast cancer. *Trends Genet* 1997;13:27–33.
120. De Jong JS, Van Diest PJ, Michaelis RJ, Van der Valk P, Meijer CJ, Baak JP. Correlation of cyclin D_1 and Rb gene expression with apoptosis in invasive breast cancer. *J Clin Pathol Mol Pathol* 1998;51:30–34.
121. Megha T, Ferrari F, Benvenuto A, Bellan C, Lalinga AV, Lazzi S, et al. P53 mutation in breast cancer. Correlation with cell kinetics and cell of origin. *J Clin Path* 2002;55(6):461–466.
122. Buller RE, Sood A, Fullenkamp C, Sorosky J, Powills K, Anderson B. The influence of the p53 codon 72 polymorphism in ovarian carcinogenesis and prognosis. *Cancer Gene Ther* 1997;4:239–245.
123. Storey A, Thomas M, Kalita A, Harwood C, Gardiol D, Mantovani F, et al. Role of p53 polymorphism in the development of human papilomavirus-associated cancer. *Nature* 1998;393:229–234.
124. Gayther SA, Russel PA, Harrington PA, Antoniou AC, Easton DF, Ponder BAJ. The contribution of germline BRCA1 and BRCA2 mutations to familial ovarian cancer: no evidence for other ovarian cancer-susceptibility genes. *Am J Hum Genet* 1999;65:1021–1029.

125. Susini T, Baldi F, Howard CM, Baldi A, Taddei G, Massi D, et al. Expression of the retinoblastoma related gene Rb2/p130 correlates with clinical outcome in endometrial cancer. *J Clin Oncol* 1998;16:1085–1093.

126. Toguchida J, Yamaguchi T, Dayton SH, Beauchamp RL, Herrera GE, Ishizaki K, et al. Prevalence and spectrum of germline mutations of the p53 gene among patients with sarcoma. *N Engl J Med* 1992;326:1301–1308.

127. McIntyre JF, Smith-Soreson B, Friend SH, Kassell J, Borresen AL, Yan YX, et al. Germline mutations of the p53 tumor suppressor gene in children with osteosarcoma. *J Clin Oncol* 1994;12:925–930.

128. Toguchida J, Yamaguchi T, Ritchie B, Beuachamp RL, Dayton SH, Herrera GE, et al. Mutation spectrum of the p53 gene in bone and soft tissue sarcomas. *Cancer Res* 1992;52:6194–6199.

129. Diller L, Sexsmith E, Gottlieb A, Li FP, Malkin D. Germline p53 mutations are frequently detected in young children with rhabdomyosarcoma. *J Clin Invest* 1995;95:1606–1611.

130. Yamaguchi T, Toguchida J, Wadayama B, Kanoe H, Nakayama T, Ishizaki K, et al. Loss of heterozygosity and tumor suppressor gene mutations in chondrosarcomas. *Anticancer Res* 1996;16:1009–1015.

131. Cordon-Cardo C, Latres E, Drobnjak M, Oliva MR, Pollak D, Woodruff J, et al. Molecular abnormalities of mdm2 and p53 genes in adult soft tissue sarcomas. *Cancer Res* 1994;54: 794–799.

132. Stratton MR, Moss S, Warren W, Patterson H, Clark J, Fisher C, et al. Mutations of the p53 gene in human soft tissue sarcoma: association with abnormalities of the RB1 gene. *Oncogene* 1990;5:1297–1301.

133. Wadayama B, Toguchida J, Shimizu T, Ishizaki K, Sasaki MS, Kotoura Y, Yamamuro T. Mutation spectrum of the retinoblastoma gene in osteosarcomas. *Cancer Res* 1994;54: 3042–3048.

134. Wunder JS, Czitrom AA, Kandel R, Andrulis IL. Analysis of alterations in the retinoblastoma gene and tumor grade in bone and soft tissue sarcomas. *J Natl Cancer Inst* 1991;83:194–200.

135. Yufu Y, Goto T, Choi I, Uike N, Kozuru M, Ohshima K, et al. A new multiple myeloma cell line, MEF-1, possesses cyclin D_1 overexpression and p53 mutation. *Cancer* 1999; 85:1750–1757.

136. Gaidano G, Ballerini P, Gong JZ, Inghirami G, Neri A, Newcomb EW, et al. p53 mutations in human lymphoid malignancies: association with Burkitt lymphoma and chronic lymphocytic leukemia. *Proc Natl Acad Sci USA* 1991;88:5413–5417.

137. Natkunam Y, Warnke RA, Zehnder JL, Jones CD, Milatovich-Cherry A, Cornbleet PJ. Blastic/blastoid transformation of follicular lymphoma: immunohistologic and molecular analysis of five cases. *Am J Surg Pathol* 2000;24:525–534.

138. Moller MB, Kania PW, Ino Y, Gerdes AM, Nielsen O, Louis DN, Skjodt K, Pedersen NT. Frequent disruption of the RB1 pathway in diffuse large B cell lymphoma: prognostic significance of E2F-1 and p16INK4A. *Leukemia* 2000;14:898–904.

139. Saez A, Sanchez E, Sanchez-Beato M, Cruz MA, Chacon I, Munoz E, et al. P27KIP1 is abnormally expressed in Diffuse Large B-cell Lymphomas and is associated with an adverse clinical outcome. *Br J Cancer* 1999;80:1427–1434.

140. Sanchez-Beato M, Camacho FI, Martinez-Montero JC, Saez AI, Villuendas R, Sanchez-Verde L, et al. Anomalous high p27/KIP1 expression in a subset of aggressive B-cell lymphomas is associated with cyclin D_3 overexpression. P27/KIP1-cyclin D_3 colocalization in tumor cells. *Blood* 1999;94:765–772.

141. Pinyol M, Hernandez L, Martinez A, Cobo F, Hernendez S, Bea S, et al. INK4a/ARF locus alterations in human non-Hodgkin's lymphomas mainly occur in tumors with wild-type p53 gene. *Am J Pathol* 2000;156:1987–1996.

142. Leoncini L, Bellan C, Cossu A, Claudio PP, Lazzi S, Cinti C, et al. Retinoblastoma-related p107 and pRb2/p130 proteins in malignant lymphomas: distinct mechanisms of cell growth control. *Clin Cancer Res* 1999;5:4065–4072.

143. Montesinos-Rongen M, Roers A, Kuppers R, Rajewsky K, Hansmann ML. Mutation of the p53 gene is not a typical feature of Hodgkin and Reed-Sternberg cells in Hodgkin's disease. *Blood.* 1999;94:1755–1760.

144. Drach J, Kaufmann H, Urbauer E, Schreiber S, Ackermann J, Huber H. The biology of multiple myeloma. *J Cancer Res Clin Oncol* 2000;126:441–447.

145. Goldberg EK, Glendening JM, Karanjawala Z, Sridhar A, Walker GJ, Hayward NK, et al. Localization of multiple melanoma tumor suppressor genes on chromosome 11 by use of homozigosity mapping-of-deletion analysis. *Am J Hum Genet* 2000;67:417–431.

146. Borg A, Sandberg T, Nilsson K, Johannsson O, Klinker M, Masback A, et al. High frequency of multiple melanomas and breast and pancreas carcinomas in CDKN2A mutation-positive melanoma families. *J Natl Cancer Inst* 2000;92:1260–1266.

147. Reifenberger J, Wolter M, Bostrom J, Buschges R, Schulte KW, Megahed M, et al. Allelic losses on chromosome arm 10q and mutation of the PTEN (MMAC1) tumor suppressor gene in primary and metastatic malignant melanomas. *Virchows Arch* 2000;436:487–493.

148. Brantkey, MA Jr., Harbour JW. Inactivation of retinoblastoma protein in uveal melanoma by phosphorylation of sites in the COOH-terminal region. *Cancer Res* 2000;60:4320–4322.

149. Cree IA. Cell cycle and melanoma—two different tumours from the same cell type. *J Pathol* 2000;191:112–114.

5 Regulation of Cell Cycle and Apoptosis

Lucio Miele, MD, PhD

CONTENTS

Μοῖραν δ᾽ οὔ τινά φημι πεφυγμένον ἔμμεναι ἀνδρῶν,
οὐ κακόν, οὐδὲ μὲν ἐσθλόν, ἐπὴν τα πρῶτα γένηται

"But Fate, I tell you, no man can ever escape,
Whether evil or noble, from the first moment of life."
(Iliad, Homer VI:488–489.)

From: *Cancer Drug Discovery and Development:*
Cell Cycle Inhibitors in Cancer Therapy: Current Strategies
Edited by: A. Giordano and K. J. Soprano © Humana Press Inc., Totowa, NJ

1. INTRODUCTION: CANCER AS A DISEASE OF
CELL FATE DETERMINATION

The ancient Greeks believed that every life was subject to the whims of Fate or Moira, an inscrutable force that not even the gods could defy. Fate was often represented as three separate deities, the Moirae, who presided over the destiny of each life. Clotho spun the thread of life on her spool, Lakhesis measured it out, and Atropos cut the thread when a life had to end.

Today, one of the greatest challenges for biology and medicine is deciphering how the fate of a cell is decided. In a healthy multicellular organism, each cell "knows" whether and when to replicate, how long it has lived, and when it is time to die. Elucidating the molecular logic that underlies these decisions is the ultimate key to understanding normal and pathological development and to treating diseases ranging from birth defects to autoimmune disorders to cancer.

The many neoplastic diseases we commonly refer to as "cancer" are the result of cumulative genetic damage that disables key steps in cell fate decision processes. Cancer cells acquire an "illegitimate" immortality by losing cell cycle controls that normally delay or arrest proliferation, longevity controls that limit the number of replications and apoptosis programs that trigger suicide in response to genotoxic stress. This in turn results in increased genetic instability and accumulation of further mutations. Under selective pressure from tissue microenvironment and therapeutic interventions, this process eventually selects cells that can survive in hypoxic environments, induce neovascularization, and invade distant tissues. This natural history is common to most human malignancies. However, the molecular mechanisms that ultimately lead to the malignant phenotype are numerous and diverse. Even cancers that are morphologically indistinguishable can carry different combinations of genetic lesions and potentially respond differently to specific treatments.

Over the past three decades we have accumulated a massive amount of information on individual components of the molecular machinery that controls cell fate. The pace of information gathering has been dramatically accelerated by the parallel revolutions in molecular biology and information technology that have led to high-throughput genomics and proteomics. In 1971, when the "war on cancer" was declared, scientists could do little more than looking through microscopes, culturing cells and analyzing enzymes and simple chemicals extracted from cells and tissues. Today, for the first time in history, we are in a position to examine the molecular machinery inside our cells as a whole, and we are beginning to build a coherent picture from the data accumulated in decades of hard work. Assembling the whole puzzle will be a monumental task. However, the main outlines of cell fate decision processes are sufficiently clear, and what we know so far is surprisingly reminiscent of those ancient Greek myths. Each cell contains a cyclical molecular mechanism that controls and orchestrates replication, "spinning the spool of life." Each normal cell has a limited lifespan, and contains a clock that measures out the thread of life through chromosomal telomeres. And each cell contains a mechanims for quite literally cutting the thread of life and killing itself when it is time to die. These mechanisms are separate and can be studied individually. However, in living cells they are inextricably intertwined into a global decision-making program that monitors and integrates information from many sources inside and outside the cell and activates alternate fates based on this integrated input.

Despite this apparently hopeless complexity, some generalizations are possible. It is becoming apparent that most if not all oncogenic mutations ultimately converge on relatively few key pathways controlling cell cycle and apoptosis. In this chapter, I will provide a general overview of these pathways and of the mechanisms that integrate them, focusing on the general principles that have emerged from the available evidence. A detailed discussion of these signaling networks would be well beyond the scope of this discussion and the reader will be referred to comprehensive review articles wherever necessary.

2. SPINNING THE SPOOL OF LIFE: CELL CYCLE CONTROL AND THE G_1 RESTRICTION POINT

The replication of a eukaryotic cell follows a tightly orchestrated program that in most cells can be divided into discrete stages: G_1, which precedes DNA replication; S, during which DNA is replicated and new histones and other DNA-associated proteins are synthesized; G_2, during which the cell "checks" for completeness and accuracy of DNA replication; and finally M, the process of mitotic division itself, during which sister chromatides are condensed, positioned by specialized cytoskeletal structures, and separated before the two daughter cells physically divide. Cells that are not actively proliferating are locked into a G_1-like status that is sometimes referred to as G_0. This state of cell cycle arrest is irreversible in senescent cells (see below). Cells that are rapidly proliferating, such as embryonic cells during the first few divisions of a fertilized egg, have almost nonexistent G_1 lags and proceed from one cell division to the next. To ensure accurate transmission of the genome to the next generation of cells, the cell cycle must be tightly regulated. Each step must begin only after the previous step is complete, and damaged or erroneously replicated DNA must be repaired. Not surprisingly, the cell cycle machinery contains several "checkpoints" that can delay or stop the process if errors or damage are detected. The most important decision-making takes place in G_1, before the cell commits to replicate its DNA. Mechanisms operating in G_1 monitor the cell's internal and external environment to decide whether to proceed with the replication program or wait. Signals from growth factors, the extracellular matrix (ECM), and contiguous cells are integrated with "alarm signals" generated by DNA damage and other intracellular

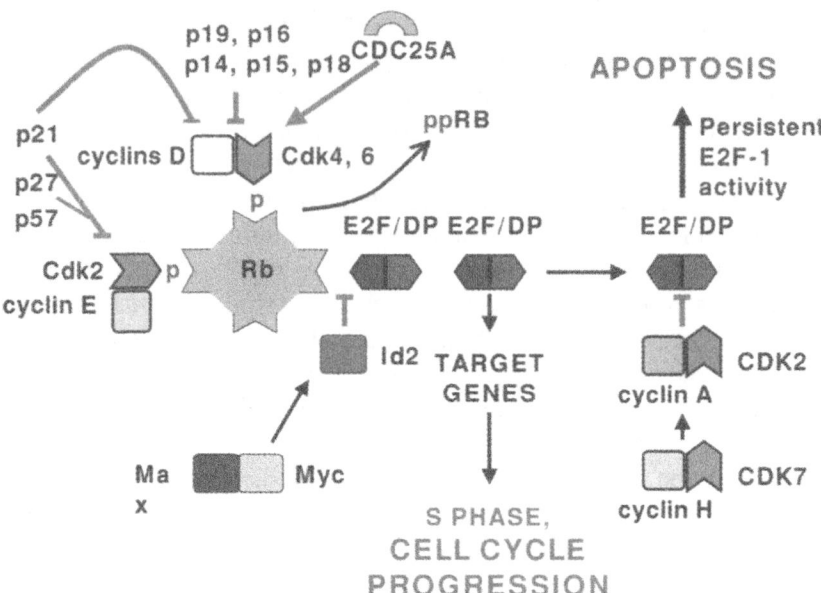

Fig. 1. Schematic representation of the G_1 restriction point. The activity of E2F transcription factors is controlled by their association with Rb and other pocket proteins. This association is inhibited by Id2, one of the mediators of Myc oncogenes. The complex of Rb and E2F represses transcription at E2F responsive elements, in part by recruiting histone acetyltransferase 1 (not shown). Sequential phosphorylation by cyclin D/CDK4 and 6 complexes and then by cyclin E/CDK2 complexes during late G_1 leads to inactivation of Rb which dissociates from E2F. E2F triggers entry into S-phase by transactivating a group of genes necessary for DNA replication. Cyclin A/CDK2 is activated by CAK, a complex of cyclin H and CDK7. Active cyclin A/CDK2 phosphorylates and inactivates E2F late during S phase (and also activates cyclin B/CDK1 during G_2, not shown). Persistent or unrestrained E2F activity beyond this point can lead to apoptosis by upregulating p19^{arf} and thus p53, and/or by inducing p73 (*see* below).

stress mediators to affect the decision to initiate DNA synthesis. These pathways converge on the so-called G_1 restriction point (Fig. 1).

The main components of the G_1 restriction point are the E2F family of transcription factors, the "pocket" proteins, Rb and its homologs p107 and p130, and the cyclin-dependent protein kinases (CDKs) that regulate their activities (*1–5*). E2F transcription factors are heterodimers comprised of one E2F subunit (E2F-1 through -6) and one DP subunit (DP-1or -2). A large body of evidence suggests that E2F, especially but not exclusively E2F-1, transactivate genes that are indispensable for progression from G_1 to S, such as DNA polymerase α, PCNA, thymidine kinase, cyclin E, and many others. Pocket proteins, of which Rb is the prototype, bind E2F heterodimers forming large complexes that also include chromatin remodeling molecules of the SWI/SNF family and histone deacetylases (HDAC) 1-3 *(2,5,6)*. Pocket proteins are characterized by a conserved "pocket" region, subdivided into subdomains A and B *(1)*. This region is the binding site for viral oncoproteins that inactivate Rb, such as SV40 large T, adenovirus E1A, and papillomavirus E7, as well as the primary interaction site with E2F.

The main effect of Rb binding to E2F is inhibition of E2F-dependent transcription, and thus, a delay in the G_1-S transition. CDKs active in G_1 sequentially phosphorylate Rb (first cyclin D/CDK4 or 6, then cyclin E/CDK2). Hyperphosphorylated Rb dissociates from E2F, thus relieving the inhibition and allowing G_1-S transition. During late S phase, cyclin A/cdk2 complexes inactivate E2F. In the simplistic scheme depicted in Fig. 1, Rb directly "blocks" E2F. More recent evidence suggests that Rb/E2F/HDAC complexes actively inhibit transcription at E2F-dependent promoters by acetylating histones and limiting promoter access through chromatin remodeling *(6)*. Other, HDAC-independent mechanisms of repression are also possible *(2,5)*. In addition to modulating E2F activity, Rb also interacts with other transcription factors, such as SP1, PU.1, Elf-1 and MyoD and regulates their activity, as well as with protein kinase c-Abl *(1)*. Rb-homologous pocket proteins p107 and p130 have partially overlapping functions with Rb. Both are capable of inactivating E2F factors, but appear to be more selective for E2F-4 and –5, while Rb binds E2F1-4. E2F4-p130 complexes are abundant in quiescent, differentiated cells where DNA synthesis is indefinitely repressed. A possible role for p107 and/or p130 in titrating cyclin E/CDK2 complexes, thus delaying Rb inactivation has been proposed *(5)*. In addition, p107 and p130 contain a p21-like sequence (see below) between pocket subdomains A and B, which contributes to their growth-arresting activity.

The rate of Rb inactivation by cyclin/CDK complexes controls the release of E2F transcriptional activity and thus the duration of G1 *(1,4)*. It appears that cyclin D/CDK4/6 phosphoryation of Rb derepresses the cyclin E gene, thereby allowing accumulation of cyclin E/CDK2 and complete inactivation of Rb. The activity of cyclin/CDK complexes is regulated in turn by several mechanisms. The intracellular levels of the various cyclin subunits oscillate during the cell cycle, and control the formation of active complexes. Phosphorylation at specific phosphoacceptor sites by cyclin-activating kinases (CAK), which themselves contain cyclin subunits, and dephosphorylation by CDC25 phosphatases at different sites are necessary for cdk activation. Additionally, two families of cdk inhibitors (CKI) modulate the activity of cyclin/cdk complexes. The family including p21$^{cip1/waf1}$, p27^{kip1}, and p57^{kip2} inhibits all known cdk complexes, while the ankyrin-repeat containing INK4 family, including p14, p15^{ink4b}, p16^{ink4a}, p18, and p19^{arf} are more specific for cdks 4 and 6. P16 and p19 are alternate products of the same locus.

Recent evidence *(7)* indicates that another key player in the mammalian G_1 restriction point is the inhibitory helix-loop-helix factor Id2. Id2 can bind Rb, preventing it from inactivating E2F, and thus promotes E2F activity. Importantly, Id2 is induced by oncogenes c-Myc and N-Myc and is necessary for their growth promoting activity.

In summary, the primary factor controlling G_1-S transition is the activity of E2F family transcription factors, especially E2F-1. E2F activity is downregulated by Rb and other pocket proteins. The balance between active and inactive E2F is controlled by sequential Rb phosphorylation by cyclin/CDK complexes and by Id2. Not surprisingly, mitogenic stimuli such as growth factors that activate the Ras signaling cascade often act by upregulating cyclin D_1 and other D-type cyclins (4), in turn leading to Rb phosphorylation by CDK4 and 6. Another gene that is generally upregulated by mitogenic stimuli is c-Myc, which in turn can cause Rb inactivation through a variety of mechanisms, including among others transactivation of Id2 (7) and of CDC25 CDK phosphatase (8).

The functional axis controlling the G_1 restriction point is deregulated in virtually all malignant cells (4). The importance of this mechanism is underscored by the fact that many DNA tumor viruses (e.g., human papillomaviruses, SV40, adenovirus) encode viral oncoproteins that inactivate Rb and are necessary for virus-induced transformation. In spontaneous human cancers, deregulation of the G_1 restriction point is caused by diverse mechanisms, such as cyclin D_1 overexpression, deletion, or epigenetic inactivation of key CKI such as p16, deletions and point mutations in Rb, autocrine production of growth factors, constitutive activation of growth factor receptors, and others.

In addition to the G_1 restriction point, additional checkpoints control cell cycle progression. Entry into mitosis from the G_2 phase requires the activation of cyclin B/CDK1 (previously known as cdc2). This complex accumulates at the end of S due to the action of cyclin A/CDK2, which phosphorylates and inactivates APC (anaphase-promoting complex), a ubiquitin ligase that drives cyclin B to degradation. The cyclin B/CDK1 complex is also negatively regulated by phosphoryation by Wee1 kinase and its homologues and positively regulated through dephosphorylation by phosphatase CDC25C. In turn, CDC25C is sequestered by 14.3.3σ. Checkpoint activation (for example by DNA damage) leads to arrest in G_2 by directly or indirectly blocking the activity of cyclin B/CDK1 (see below) (9–11). Active cyclin B/CDK1 enters the nucleus and phosphorylates histone H1, the nuclear envelope protein lamin and other substrates enabling the initiation of mitosis. Additional checkpoints operate during mitosis to ensure correct formation of the mitotic spindle and chromosomal alignment (12–14). Regulation of the APC plays a key role in mitotic checkpoints, as does the protein kinase BUBR1, which can inactivate the kinetocore motor CENP-E and APC in response to mitotic spindle damage (15,16). For the purpose of this chapter, it will suffice to say that elements of the G_1 restriction point have been implicated in regulating cell cycle steps beyond the G_1-S transition. Rb/E2F complexes, for example, downregulate the expression of cyclin A, and thus indirectly delaying the accumulation of cyclin B and entry into mitosis. Similarly, the broad spectrum CKI p21$^{cip1/waf1}$ through inhibition of various cyclin/CDK complexes can block the S-G2 transition and the G2-M transition. In addition, p21 can inhibit DNA synthesis directly by binding PCNA, a component of mammalian DNA polymerase delta required for processive "sliding" along template DNA.

3. MEASURING OUT THE THREAD: REPLICATIVE SENESCENCE AND TELOMERASE

It has been recognized for four decades that primary mammalian cells in culture can replicate a finite number of times before undergoing an irreversible cell cycle arrest called "replicative senescence." This limit to replication potential was named after its discoverer, L. Hayflick *(17–19)*. Neoplastic cells appear to have lost this internal "clock" and can divide indefinitely in culture, i.e., are theoretically immortal. Evidence accumulated in the last decade has elucidated some of the mechanisms responsible for replicative senescence. A key role in this process is played by specialized structures at the ends of eukaryotic chromosomes, the telomeres.

Eukaryotic chromosomes consist of exceedingly long, linear, double-stranded DNA molecules that are extensively supercoiled and folded by histones and other proteins into nucleosomal and higher-order chromatin structures. Each end of a chromosome is capped by structures, the telomeres, consisting of looped, single-stranded DNA containing a variable number of repetitive, G-rich hexanucleotide sequences, associated with specialized structural proteins TRF-1 and -2 *(20,21)*. The main functions of telomeres appear to be protecting the ends of chromosomes from forming illegitimate end-to-end fusions and from being recognized as double-stranded DNA breaks. Interestingly, certain DNA repair complexes appear to associate preferentially with the telomeres and are necessary for their function *(22)*. DNA replication in all living cells proceeds in 5'-3' direction and requires an RNA primer at the 5' end to which DNA polymerases attach the nascent new DNA. Primers are synthesized by DNA primases and are subsequently degraded and replaced with DNA by DNA polymerase α. The initiation of replication is preceded by the assembly of a primosome at origins of replication, which melts double-stranded DNA and synthesizes RNA primers. This poses a topological problem for replication of the very 3' end of a eukaryotic chromosome, where the assembly of a primosome and the synthesis of RNA primers are not possible. Thus, at each cell cycle some DNA at the 3' ends of both strands of the daughter DNA molecules is not replicated, resulting in shorter telomeres in the daughter cells (Fig. 2). It appears that when telomeres reach a critical length, this triggers the onset of replicative senescence *(17,18)*. In addition to telomere shortening, senescence can be induced by other

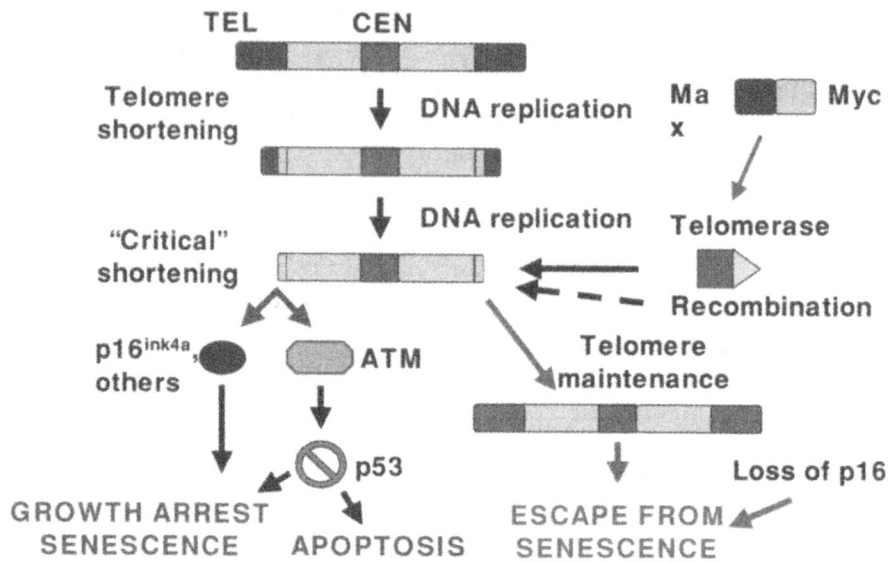

Fig. 2. Telomere maintenance and replicative senescence. The ends of eukaryotic chromosomes are capped by specialized structures called telomeres (TEL), whereas the centromere (CEN) is necessary for attachment to the mitotic spindle. In normal human cells, telomeres are shortened at each cell cycle. After a finite number of replications (the Hayflick limit), telomere length reaches a critical point that triggers a response similar to a DNA damage checkpoint. This response leads to upregulation of p16[ink4a] and other CKI, which trigger irreversible G_1 arrest and replicative senescence. Also, telomere shortening or damage to telomeric DNA can trigger a p53-dependent response through ATM, which in turn can lead either to reinforced cell cycle arrest via p21[cip1/waf1] or to apoptosis (*see* below). Activation of the Ras oncogene in otherwise normal cells triggers a similar response with p16[ink4a] and p19[arf] upregulation (not shown). Cells can escape senescence and become immortalized when they maintain telomere length through continuous replication. This is accomplished through induction of the expression of the catalytic subunit of telomerase (TERT) or through telomerase-independent mechanisms that may involve recombination. Induction of TERT is caused by activation of Myc oncogenes and by other, hitherto unclarified mechanisms. Another, complementary mechanism for escape from senescence is deletion or epigenetic inactivation of the ARF locus, that codes for both p16[ink4a] and p19[arf].

mechanisms. Ras activation, for example, can trigger senescence in cells with an intact G_1 restriction point. The mechanisms responsible for triggering senescence in response to critical telomere shortening or oncogene activation are still incompletely understood. However, it is fairly well established that the response to telomere shortening shares common features with a DNA damage response (*see* below): 1) it can result either in cell cycle arrest or in apoptosis, and 2) it is mediated at least in part by CKIs and p53. In a number of experimental models replicative senescence is associated with elevated levels of the CKI p16[ink4a] and/

or other CKI such as $p21^{cip1/waf1}$ and $p27^{kip1}$ (*18,23*). Activation of p53 via $p19^{arf}$ or other pathways (*see* below) can transactivate $21^{cip1/waf1}$ and participate in senescence inducion (*18,23–25*). Overexpression of ^{ink4b} can also trigger senescence (*26*). In Ras-induced senescence as well, the main mechanism seems to be the induction of CKIs $p16^{ink4a}$ and $p19^{arf}$, the latter resulting in p53 and $p21^{cip1/waf1}$ induction (*27*). Induction of the nuclear scaffold protein PML, which binds p53, also participates in Ras-induced senescence (*28*).

The main effect of these pathways is the maintainance of high levels of hypophosphorylated Rb, blocking the G_1-S transition. Thus, replicative senescence is achieved by enforcing a sustained block at the G_1 restriction point.

Senescent cells tend to be resistant to apoptosis, possibly because of their persistent G_1 arrest (*19,29*). However, as in the case of DNA damage checkpoints, signals that induce senescence can also trigger apoptosis depending on cellular context. Critical telomere shortening with loss of TRF-2 or accumulation of DNA damage at the telomeres can trigger either cell-cycle arrest or apoptosis, mainly via an ATM-p53-dependent pathway that is very similar to the DNA damage checkpoint (*see* below) (*30,31*). In a sense, telomeres may be thought of DNA damage sensors, that trigger either cell cycle arrest (senescence) or apoptosis when shortened and/or damaged (*31,32*).

Neoplastic cells bypass replicative senescence through a variety of mechanisms (Fig. 2). Telomere shortening can be prevented by inducing expression of the catalytic subunit (TERT) of the enzyme telomerase, an unusual reverse transcriptase that carries an endogenous RNA template and adds multiple units of a short repetitive sequence to the 3'end of chromosomal DNA (*18,33,34*). Inhibition of telomerase induces cell death in some human immortalized or transformed cells, making it a potential therapeutic target (*35,36*). Expression of telomerase is induced by oncogenes like c-Myc (*8,33*) and most likely by other mechanisms. In addition, telomerase-independent recombination events ("gene conversion") occuring during DNA replication can also prevent loss of telomere length (*37*). Deletion or epigenetic inactivation (through promoter methylation) of the ARF locus encoding both $p16^{ink4a}$ and $p19^{arf}$ is a common event in human malignancies (*4*). One consequence of functional loss of the ARF locus is inability to enforce replicative senescence and/or to induce a p53-dependent apoptosis in response to telomere shortening.

4. CUTTING THE THREAD OF LIFE: APOPTOSIS

Apoptosis (*38*) is an aptly chosen Greek word that literally means "dropping off." Initially defined in morphological terms as a series of hallmarks for certain types of cell death, this term is currently used to describe the process through which a eukaryotic cell self-destructs. This process, also known as programmed cell death or PCD, is essentially a controlled "implosion" through which a cell destroys molecules critical to life and generally cleaves its own genomic DNA while maintaining external integrity. Finally, an apoptotic cell exposes membrane markers that facilitate removal of its corpse by professional and nonprofessional phagocytes. In contrast, nonprogrammed, necrotic cell death induced by an overwhelming noxious agent can be compared to an uncontrolled "explosion," which is generally accompanied by loss of external integrity and spillage of cellular debris, including proteases, phospholipases, and other potentially damaging molecules. The latter process is thus more likely to cause damage to surrounding tissue and inflammation. The biology, biochemistry, and pharmacology of apoptosis have been recently reviewed in an oustanding series of articles (39–45).

In the life of a multicellular organism, apoptosis is used for many purposes. During development, it is used to remodel tissues and remove cells that are no longer needed, such as the salivary glands of insect larvae, the tail of tadpoles, or the interdigital webs in a primate embryo (43). During postnatal life, apoptosis is used to eliminate unnecessary or unwanted cells in the immune system (42) and it is the natural conclusion of the terminal differentiation process of continuously renewable cells in epithelial surfaces and in the hematopoietic system. A spectacular example of this is the human skin. Our bodies are surrounded by a covalently crosslinked layer of apoptotic keratinocytes, the stratum corneum of the epidermis. Epidermal keratinocytes cells undergo an orchestrated process of differentiation culminating in apoptosis (29). The integrity of this apoptotic cell layer maintains a barrier between our bodies and the external environment and is essential to life.

In contrast to physiological processes in which it is linked to differentiation, apoptosis is also used as an emergency self-destruction mechanism through which a cell that has sustained irreparable damage to its DNA or overwhelming metabolic stress commits suicide. The evolutionary importance of this damage-control apoptosis becomes apparent when considering that the primary task of any successfully surviving life form is the replication of its genome with as little error as possible. Allowing the uncontrolled replication of severely damaged DNA has potentially disastrous consequences for the life of individual cells and the survival of organisms and species.

"Emergency" apoptosis is of great interest to cancer researchers for two reasons: First, partial loss of this response contributes to the process of transformation, allowing neoplastic cells to proliferate under conditions that would trigger apoptosis in a normal cell, and to accumulate mutations in their genomes. This ability to survive despite genomic instability, combined with selective pressures from organism defenses and from therapy, is a major mechanism through which cancers select progressively more malignant cells and become resistant to therapy. Second, most nonsurgical strategies for the treatment of cancers aim to trigger a residual emergency apoptotic response in cancer cells, through radiation

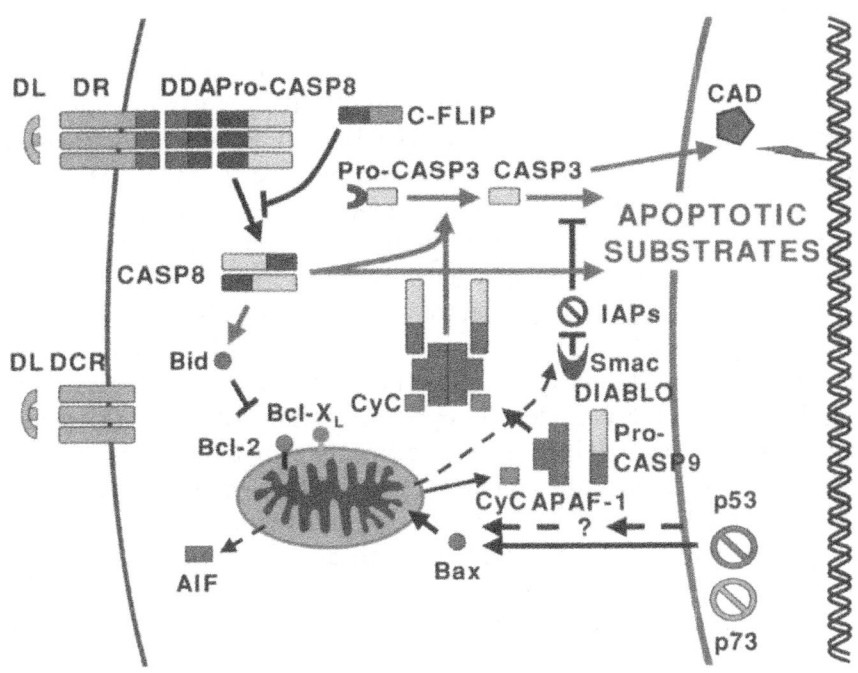

Fig. 3. Apoptotic cascades. Apoptosis can be triggered by several related death receptors (DR), such as Fas/CD95, the TNF receptor or DR5. These receptors are engaged by death ligands (DL) such as the Fas ligand, TNF-α, or TRAIL. Upon ligand engagement, death receptors self-associate and recruit death domain adaptors (DDA) through their death domains (DD, medium gray rectangles facing each other in both DR and DDA). Decoy receptors (DCR) lacking a death effector domain control death receptor activation by acting as a sink for death ligands at the cell surface. Death adaptors in turn recruit the proenzyme form of upstream caspases (CASP) such as caspase 8 or 10 through their Death Effector Domains (DED, dark gray rectangles within Pro-CASP8 and CASP8), leading to autocatalytic activation and generation of active caspases. Decoy inactive procaspases such as c-Flip can inhibit this process. Active upstream caspases can cleave apoptotic substrates directly, but function primarily through activation of downstream "effector" caspases such as caspase 3, and through cleavage and activation of pro-apoptotic BH family proteins such as Bid. Proteolytic steps are represented by light gray arrows. The mitochondria are a major control center for apoptosis, in most but not all cells. They act by releasing cytochrome c and other pro-apoptotic molecules including apoptosis inducing factor AIF from their intermembrane compartment into the cytoplasm. Cytochrome c associates with APAF-1 to form a complex that recruits procaspase 9 through its CARD domain (dark gray rectangle within Pro-CASP9 and CASP9), forming the apoptosome. This complex activates caspase 9, which in turn activates effector caspases. Once the effector caspases are activated, they cleave essential cellular components and activate CAD, a DNA-ase that causes extensive inter-nucleosomal cleavage of genomic DNA. The activity of caspases is inhibited by various inhibitors of apoptosis (IAPs), which in turn can be overwhelmed by anti-inhibitors such as Smac/DIABLO, also released from the mitochondria. BH family proteins act a the main rheostat controlling apoptosis. Anti-apoptotic family members such as Bcl-2 and Bcl-X $_L$ are associated

damage, chemical damage to DNA, elimination of survival signals, and other mechanisms. Even immunotherapy through T-cell vaccines or monoclonal antibodies (MAbs), and anti-angiogenic agents that limit nutrient supply to cancer cells, ultimately aim to induce or facilitate apoptosis in cancer cells.

A schematic representation of the basic machinery of apoptosis (39) is presented in Fig. 3. The key players are a family of cysteine-containing aspartyl proteases, the caspases. These can be divided into two families: signaling caspases, which transduce death receptor signals, and effector caspases, which are activated by the signaling caspases and mediate the "end-game" of apoptosis by destroying cellular targets. Caspases normally exist as proenzymes, with very low basal levels of activity. Under appropriate conditions, they can auto-activate by proteolytic cleavage and in turn activate downstream procaspases. Apoptosis can be induced by extracellular signals such as soluble or cell-associated "death ligands" (e.g., Fas ligand, TRAIL, TNF-α, etc.), or by intracellular mechanisms. Death ligands bind to one of several "death receptors" carrying an intracellular "death domain" (DD). Upon ligand binding, death receptors typically multimerize and recruit adaptor molecules to the membrane. These death adaptors (e.g., FADD, TRADD, RIP) contain death domains through which they associate with clustered death receptors and "death effector domains" (DED) that interact with homologous DED domains in pro-caspases. Thus, receptor engagement results in membrane recruitment of signaling procaspases such as caspase 8 or 10. The complex of death ligands, receptors, adapters, and signaling caspases is sometimes referred to as the DISC (death-inducing surface complex) (42). Within the context of the DISC, procaspases activate each other through proteolytic cleavage. Once activated, caspase 8 and other signaling caspases activate downstream effector caspases directly and also facilitate apoptosis by activating pro-apoptotic BH molecules (see below) such as Bid. Death ligand induced apoptosis is modulated by the levels of expression of the various death receptors and ligands, as well as by the expression of "decoy" death receptors lacking the DD domain. These decoy receptors act as a ligand sink, thus preventing the activation of death receptors. Similarly, the activation of procaspase 8 can be limited by c-FLIP, a catalytically inactive caspase homologue that acts intracellularly as a procaspase "decoy."

Fig. 3. *(Continued)* with mitochondrial membranes (and other intracellular membranes) and inhibit release of AIFs (and possibly also block the formation of the apoptosome directly). Pro-apoptotic family members such as Bax, Bid, or Bad, heterodimerize with anti-apoptotic members and prevent their function. The mechanism(s) of action of BH family proteins are still debated, and may involve controlling mitochondrial membrane permeability or the formation of a large protein channel in the mitochondrial membrane. One the main mechanisms of apoptosis induction by p53 is upregulation of Bax. The mechanisms of apoptosis induction by p73 are still unclear.

Intracellular signals such as DNA damage or severe metabolic imbalance can trigger apoptosis by inducing the release of proapoptotic molecules from the intermembrane compartment of mitochondria *(39,42)*. These include cytochrome c, a flavoprotein known as apoptosis-inducing factor (AIF) and procaspases 9, 2, and 3. Mitochondrial effectors activate the caspase cascade primarily though not exclusively via caspase 9, which in turn activates strictly "effector" caspases such caspase 3, 6, and 7. The best-characterized mechanims is mediated by cytochrome c. When released into the cytoplasm, cytochrome c complexes with an adaptor molecule, APAF-1, inducing self-association of APAF-1 and recruitment of procaspase 9 through its CARD domain (caspase activation and recruitment domain). This complex is sometimes called "apoptosome" and its formation leads to auto-activation of caspase 9, which in turn activates effector caspases such as caspase 3.

Once active, effector caspases cleave numerous intracellular targets including nuclear membrane component lamin, poly-ADP-ribose polymerase (a DNA damage marker), Rb, p21, cytoskeletal proteins gelsolin and fodrin, p21-activated kinase PAK, and many others, and activate a DNA-ase (caspase-activated DNA-ase or CAD) that catalyzes extensive internucleosomal cleavage of chromosomal DNA *(39)*. The latter is not an obligatory step in apoptosis but does occur in most "typical" apoptosis programs. The end result of this process is disappearance of the nuclear envelope, shrinkage (pyknosis) of the nucleus, and irreversible inactivation of genomic DNA. At the same time, caspase-dependent processes lead to membrane blebbing and surface exposure of phagocytosis targets such as phosphatidylserine. In some cells, sometimes referred to as "type I," the induction of apoptosis does not require mitochondrial signals because of highly effective DISC formation and activation of caspase 8, while in others, so-called "type II," very small amounts of DISC are formed and mitochondrial signals are necessary to amplify the death cascade *(42,46)*.

As we have seen for the cell cycle, the initiation and progress of the apoptotic program are regulated by the balance of multiple pro- and anti-apoptotic factors. The main group of apoptosis regulators is the growing family of Bcl-2 homologous proteins, characterized by the presence of BH (Bcl-2 homoloy) domains. This family includes anti-apoptotic proteins such as Bcl-2, Bcl-X_L and Mcl-1, and pro-apoptotic proteins such as Bax, Bad, Bak, or Bid). The anti-apoptotic members of the family contain 4 BH domains and tend to be permanently associated with mitochondrial membranes and other organelles *(39)*. The proapoptotic members tend to shuttle between cytoplasm and organelles, being directed to the mitochondria upon activation by cleavage or dephosphorylation. Members of the BH family can readily heterodimerize at the surface of mitochondria, forming pro- or anti-apoptotic complexes. Thus, the relative intracellular levels of active pro- and anti-apoptotic BH family proteins acts as a rheostat controlling the sensitivity of a cell to an apoptotic stimulus. The mechanism of apoptosis regulation by Bcl-2 family proteins is incompletely understood. It appears that anti-apoptotic complexes inhibit mitochondrial release of cytochrome c and other AIFs, while pro-apoptotic complexes facilitate such release. Pro-apoptotic BH complexes are thought to facilitate the formation of large, protein permeable pores or smaller ion channels through the mitochondrial membrane, thus allowing release of AIFs while anti-apoptotic BH proteins are suggested to inhibit this process. In addition, direct inhibition of APAF-1 apoptosome formation has been suggested for some anti-apoptotic family members.

In addition, a variety of endogenous caspase inhibitors referred to as inhibitors of apoptosis (IAPs) dampen the activation of effector caspases. These, in turn can be overwhelmed by anti-IAPs released by the mitochondria such as Smac/DIABLO.

In summary, apoptosis is controlled by an intricate network of opposing pro- and anti-apoptotic factors acting at multiple levels. The balance between pro- and anti-apoptotic signals at any given time determines the likelihood of activation of the self-destruction program. Every cell in a multicellular organism, it seems, stands constantly ready to self-destruct if the need arises. Using an analogy familiar to all computer users, one could say that every cell has an apoptotic program running "in the background," and it is ready to activate it if a "fatal error" occurs.

5. INTEGRATION OF CELL CYCLE AND APOPTOSIS PROGRAMS: A CHOICE BETWEEN TWO FATES

We have so far described in very general terms the cellular machineries that control cell cycle progression and apoptotic cell death. There is considerable evidence that these two mechanisms share components and are functionally integrated, providing the cell with the ability to chose between continued growth, growth arrest, and death by adjusting the levels and/or the activity of relatively few mediators. During the early years of oncogene discovery, it was recognized that the activation of specific oncogenes could signal cell proliferation or cell death depending on the cellular "context." The functional integration of the cell cycle and apoptosis machineries provides elegant explanations for many of these apparently puzzling observations.

It is possible to trigger apoptosis by simply activating the caspase cascade independently of cell cycle status and in fact, in anucleated cells (46). Activation of death receptors or severe metabolic stress leading to mitochondrial release of AIFs can occur without input from cell cycle components. However, in most nucleated cells there are several points of integration between the two programs. First, the detection of DNA damage or replication errors triggers a response that can result in either reversible cell cycle arrest followed by DNA repair or irre-

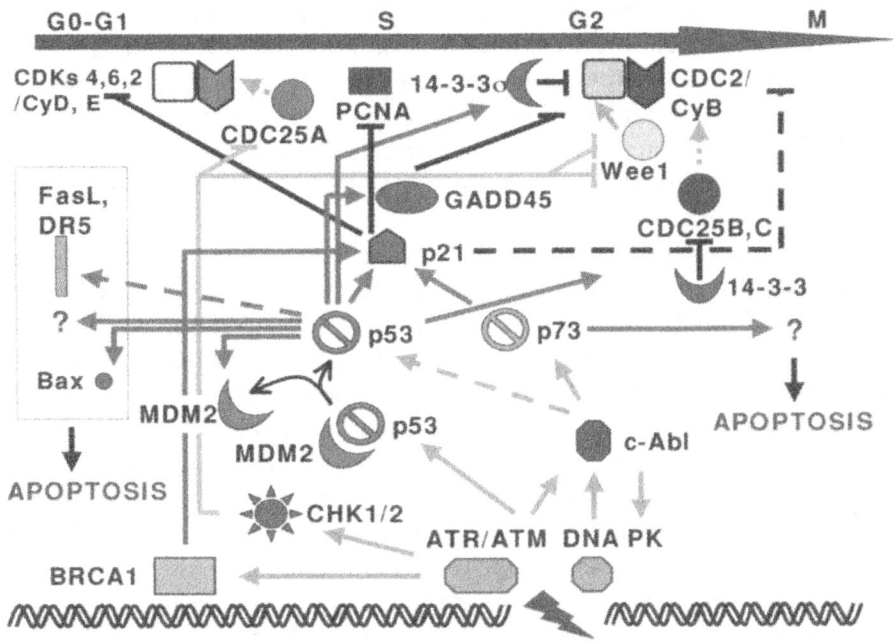

Fig. 4. The DNA damage response can result in cell cycle arrest or apoptosis. DNA damage (in this case, a double-strand break), is detected by sensors that are specialized protein kinases such as ATM, ATR, and DNA-PK. These set off a cascade of phosphorylation (light gray arrows), activating other protein kinases such as c-Abl and DNA damage response effectors such as BRCA-1 and CHK-1 and -2. Both directly and indirectly through other damage response effectors, DNA damage sensors induce cell cycle arrest. A key mediator of this effect is p53, with an accessory pathway mediated by p73. Post-translational modifications activate p53 and stabilize it, preventing its export from the nucleus and degradation by MDM2. Active p53 transactivates a number of mediator genes (dark gray arrows) including p21$^{cip1/waf1}$, GADD45, 14-3-3, and 14-3-3σ. These block cell cycle progression at several stages by directly inactivating (black crossed lines) various cyclin/CDK complexes and PCNA or by preventing CDK activation by CDC25 phosphatases (light gray dotted arrows). P21 is also induced directly by BRCA-1 and by p73. Damage detected during G_2 causes activation of protein kinase CHK-1, which phosphorylates and inactivates (light gray crossed lines) both Wee-1 (a CDK-1 activating kinase) and CDC25C (a CDK1-activating phosphatase), triggering G_2 arrest. Sustained p53 activation or p53 activation in the presence of a disabled G_1 restriction point triggers apoptosis via several mechanisms, including transactivation of death receptors and Bax. Recent data indicate that p73 can have similar effects. Dashed lines indicate effects whose mechanism is still unclear.

versible cell cycle arrest followed by apoptosis. Any irreparable damage detected during cell cycle progression (e.g., extensive DNA damage; failure to properly align sister chromatides, inappropriate initiation of mitosis) triggers emergency apoptosis *(40)*. Second, sustained or excessive activation of pathways that promote cell cycle progression, such as E2F-dependent transcription, triggers apoptosis rather than proliferation *(1–3,5)*. The CKI/CDK/Rb/E2F axis that controls the G_1 restriction point regulates apoptosis through several mechanisms, the most prominent of which involve p53 and/or its homologue p73. A highly simplified representation of the intricate interplay between cell cycle and apoptosis machinery is presented in Fig. 4. In the example presented, DNA damage is the emergency signal.

DNA damage occurs routinely in all living cells through a variety of mechanisms *(40)*. Deamination, oxidation, depurination, pyrimidine dimerization induced by UV light, single-strand breaks, and double-strand breaks have potentially disastrous consequences for cell viability and accuracy of genomic replication. Not surprisingly, cells have evolved numerous repair processes for DNA upkeep and maintenance. Base excision repair, nucleotide excision repair, and mismatch repair systems correct damage to individual nucleotides or errors introduced during replication. DNA ligases repair single-strand breaks. Double-strand breaks interrupt chromosome continuity and are potentially very dangerous for genomic integrity. These are repaired either by homologous recombination by borrowing a strand from the sister chromatid during DNA replication or by the less accurate nonhomologus end-joining. To attempt the repair of serious lesion, DNA replication must be prevented or arrested, and this is accomplished by the DNA damage response.

The presence of even a single a double-strand break in the whole genome is detected by specialized protein kinases such as ATM (ataxia-telangectasia mutated) and the related ATR (ataxia telangectasia Rad3 related) and DNA-PK (DNA-dependent protein kinases) *(40)*. These proteins bind directly to damaged DNA and set off a cascade of phosphorylation events that in turn trigger the expression of specific genes (Fig. 4). Damage detected during G_2 causes activation of protein kinase CHK-1, which phosphorylates and inactivates both Wee-1 (a CDK-1 activating kinase) and CDC25C (a CDK1-activating phosphatase) *(47)*. The net effect is G_2 arrest due to inactivation of cyclin B/CDK1.

A crucial effect triggered by most DNA damage sensors is activation of p53. In turn, p53 causes growth arrest or, if the damage is irreparable, apoptosis. The activation of the p53 pathway has been studied in detail, and it involves several components *(11)*. First, p53 is normally bound, exported from the nucleus, ubiquitinated, and degraded through the action of MDM2 (in human cells, HDM2). MDM2 is thought to catalyze the ubiquitination itself. Interestingly, p53 induces the expression of the MDM2 gene, thus limiting its own activity. In cells that have sustained DNA damage, p53 is stabilized through inhibition of MDM2 expression and through post-translational modification. Direct phosphorylation of p53 on Ser15 by ATM, ATR, or DNA-PK blocks its interaction with MDM2, thus leading to nuclear accumulation of p53. Other kinases that stabilize p53 include the proto-oncoprotein c-Abl (which is itself activated by

ATM in response to DNA damage) and the stress-activated kinase JNK (c-Jun-N-terminal kinase), a component of the Ras signaling network. Post-translational modifications also activate p53, making it capable to act as a transcription factor. These include phosphorylation in the N-terminal region by ATM, DNA PK, and JNK, and in the C-terminal region by casein kinase II, protein kinase C and CDKs. Phosphorylation by p38 MAP kinase stabilizes tetramer formation by p53. N-terminal phosphorylation enhances the binding of p53 to the transcriptional coactivator/histone acetyltransferase (HAT) p300. Both p300 and another HAT, PCAF, acetylate p53 on Lys residues in the C-terminal region. Finally, ATM-dependent dephosphorylation of Ser 376 enhances p53 binding to 14-3-3 proteins. This in turn increases the sequence-specific DNA binding of p53. Other proteins that interact with p53 and enhance its transcriptional activity include WT-1 (the gene mutated in Wilm's tumors), phosphorylated Rb, p19^{arf}, BRCA-1 (a gene frequently mutated in familial breast and ovarian cancers), and others *(11)*. Conversely, the transcriptional activity of p53 is inhibited by mot-1 (a heat-shock protein 70 family member), by the anti-apoptotic protein Bcl-2, by BRCA-2 (another gene frequently mutated in breast and ovarian cancers), and by the transcription factor c-Jun, a component of AP-1.

In addition to DNA damage, other forms of cell stress activate p53, including hypoxia, oxidative stress, a reduction in ribonucleotide triphosphate pool and other extracellular signals *(11)*. Conversely, survival signals such as IGF-1 (insulin-like growth factor 1), basic fibroblast growth factor (bFGF), and thyroid hormones antagonize p53 by upregulating MDM2.

The activity of p53 is finely modulated by such an intricate network for a very good reason: the choice between cell cycle arrest or apoptosis depends largely on the level and timing of p53 activity. In general, in nontransformed cells in which the G_1 restriction point is functional and damage is not irreparable, the effect of p53 activation by the DNA damage response is cell cycle arrest followed by DNA repair. However, if the G_1 restriction point is disabled, as is the case in most if not all transformed cells, or the damage is overwhelming, p53 activation triggers apoptosis.

Multiple mechanisms mediate growth arrest induced by p53 *(4,11,18)*. The most important one is transcriptional upregulation of the CKI p21$^{cip1/waf1}$. This pleiotropic inhibitor blocks the activity of cyclin/CDK complexes involved in the G_1-S transition, triggering Rb-mediated block of E2F-1, and in the G_2-M transition. Moreover, through its effect on PCNA, p21$^{cip1/waf1}$ inhibits DNA replication in S phase (*see* above). In addition to inducing p21$^{cip1/waf1}$, p53 directly inhibits CAK, the complex of cyclin H and CDK7 which activates the cyclin A/CDK2 complex necessary for G_1-S transition. G_2 block is induced by p53 through at least 2 mechanisms: upregulation of 14-3-3σ, which in turn sequesters the CDC25C phosphatase that is needed to activate the cyclin B/CDK1 complex that triggers the G_2-M transition, and upregulation of GADD45, which directly sequesters CDK1. These diverse mechanisms of growth arrest allow the cell to attempt repair of its DNA and eventually reenter the cell cycle. The effect of p53 is self-limited through the upregulation of MDM2, which sequesters p53.

Apoptosis induction by p53 is mediated by multiple mechanisms, some of which are dependent on transcriptional activation, while others are mediated by transcriptional repression or transcription-independent mechanisms (11). Transcription-dependent effects include upregulation of death receptors such as Fas/Apo1/CD95 and DR5, pro-apoptotic BH proteins such as Bax, of oxidoreductases that generate reactive oxygen radicals (ROS), and of anti-survival molecules such as IGF-BP3, which neutralizes IGF-1, an autocrine survival factor. Transrepression of survival molecules such as Bcl-2 and IGF-1 receptor also contributes to p53-induced apoptosis. Finally, direct effects of p53 on apoptosis cascade components, including activation of caspase 9, have been described.

Numerous factors influence the choice between growth arrest and apoptosis in response to p53 activation (11,40,48–50). The intensity of the stress signals, and thus the level and duration of p53 accumulation, can dictate whether a temporary growth arrest occurs, self-limited through induction of MDM2, or an apoptotic program is activated. One possible mechanism for this is the differential affinity of p53 for promoters in growth-arrest related genes, such as p21$^{cip1/waf1}$ and apoptosis genes, such as Bax. Low levels of p53 tend to preferentially activate p21$^{cip1/waf1}$ transcription, while higher levels activate Bax, which has a lower affinity p53 reponsive element in its promoter. The existing apoptotic threshold of the cell, dictated by the balance between pro- and anti-apoptotic molecules (see above) is paramount. For example, a number of growth factors protect cells from p53-induced apoptosis by activating the phosphoinositide 3-kinase (PI-3K) pathway (51), which leads to phosphorylation of the pro-apoptotic protein Bad through the downstream kinase Akt. Phosphorylated Bad is sequestered and inactivated by 14-3-3, thus tipping the balance in favor of anti-apoptotic BH family members such as Bcl-2 or Bcl-X_L (52). Another key pathway that modulates p53-induced apoptosis involves transcription factors of the NF-κB family. These factors are activated by numerous stress signals and in turn, regulate the expression of over 150 target genes, including a variety of anti- and pro-apoptotic proteins and cell cycle mediators (53–55). Whether NF-κB activation results in apoptosis or survival depends on the cellular context, but in most cases the effect is increased survival. Interestingly, NF-κB and p53 have been reported to antagonize each other's transcriptional effects (56), and inhibition of NF-κB by overexpression of wild-type p53 has been reported (57). On the other hand, induction of endogenous p53 has been shown to activate NF-κB and induce apoptosis in an NF-κB-*dependent* way (58). These findings have therapeutic implications in that NF-κB inhibitors are candidate anti-neoplastic agents, and their possible usefulness in p53-positive tumors depends on the functional relationship between NF-κB and p53.

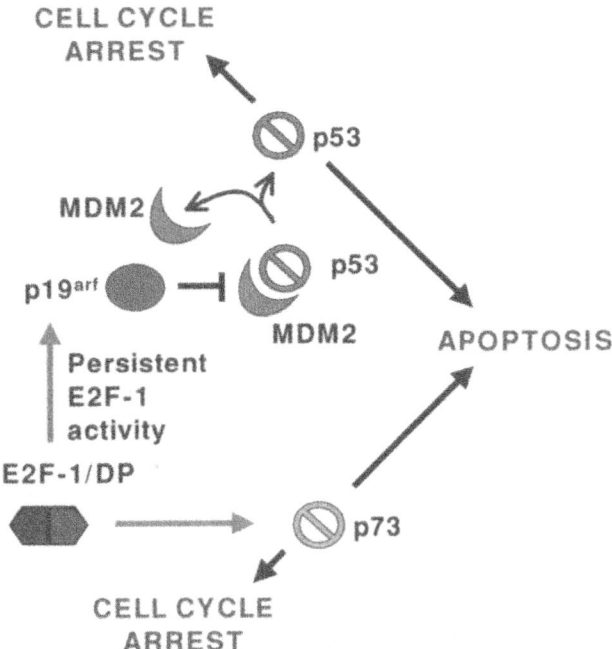

Fig. 5. E2F affects the choice between cell cycle arrest and apoptosis. Persistent activation of E2F in the presence of an active p53 or deregulated activation of E2F (by proliferative stimuli in the absence of survival signals) can lead to apoptosis. The best characterized pathway involves transactivation of p19^{arf}, which inactivates MDM2 and leads to nuclear accumulation of active p53. Depending on concomitant survival signals and the level of p53, this can result in apoptosis. Very recent evidence indicates that E2F can trigger apoptosis through p73 as well in a p53-independent way.

One key element of the cell cycle G_1 restriction point conditions the response to p53 (2–5). E2F-1 (and to a lesser extent, other E2F members) can lead to uncontrolled p53 activation by upregulating p19^{arf}, which in turn blocks MDM2 (Fig. 5). The end result is that p53 is not sequestered by MDM2 and accumulates in the nucleus. Thus, if the G_1 restriction point is functional, the growth arrest signals generated by p53 activation extinguish E2F activity through dephosphorylated Rb. On the other hand, if the G_1 restriction point is disabled (for example, by loss of Rb, functional loss of crucial CKIs, or overexpression of D-type cyclins), E2F activity is more difficult to block and growth arrest does not occur. Persistent E2F activity in the face of a growth arrest signal mediated by p53 lead to upregulation of p19^{arf} and thus to further accumulation of p53, which in turn activates the apoptotic program. This explains why many transformed cells are actually more sensitive to p53-induced apoptosis than their normal counterparts, which makes it possible to use DNA-damaging drugs and radiotherapy to preferentially induce apoptosis in cancers. Unfortunately, this also explains why loss or inactivation of p53 is the most common mutation event in human malignancies, and why recurrent cancer that have become resistant to treatment often result from selection of p53-null cells. Not suprisingly, oncogenic viruses have evolved mechanisms for inactivating simultaneously the G_1 restriction point and p53-induced apoptosis. SV40, human papillomaviruses (HPV) and Adenoviruses all produce proteins that inactivate Rb and p53. In some cases the same protein has both functions, such as SV40 large T, while in other cases two separate oncoproteins are needed, such as HPV E6 (which inactivates p53) and E7 (which inactivates Rb).

Despite its crucial role, p53 is not the only link between E2F and apoptosis. Like Rb, p53 has at least two homologues with partially overlapping functions, p63 and p73 *(59,60)*. It has been known for some time that apoptosis can be induced by E2F in a p53-independent way *(5)*. Very recent evidence has implicated the p53 homologue p73 in E2F-induced apoptosis *(61–63)*. Thus, p73 represents a "backup" or accessory mechanism through which apoptosis can be induced by unrestrained E2F activity. Additionally, E2F can repress the expression of antiapoptotic molecules such as TRAF-2 *(5)*.

In summary, a cell can respond to stress by either arresting the cell cycle and attempting to recover or by triggering apoptosis. Activation of p53 and/or its homologues can induce either response, depending on the overall balance of survival vs apoptosis pathways. The G_1 restriction point is crucial in determining the likelihood of apoptosis in response to stress. If the restriction point functions normally and E2F activity is suppressed by the CKI-Rb axis, cell cycle arrest is the preferred response to a stress that is not overwhelming. If the restriction point is disabled, unrestrained activation of E2F favors apoptosis through further activation of p53 and/or p53-independent mechanisms. The seemingly paradoxical observations that mitogenic signals including the activation of growth promoting oncogenes can lead to either growth or apoptosis depending on context can be largely explained by this cross-talk between the G_1-S transition machinery and the apoptotic machinery.

6. MULTIPLE PHYSIOLOGIC SIGNALS REGULATE CELL CYCLE AND APOPTOSIS

The picture presented so far indicates that each cell is constantly receiving and integrating internal and external signals that affect the overall balance between growth, survival, and death. These signals can be divided into two broad categories: "stress" signals that affect primarily cell survival, such as DNA damage, oxidative stress, nutrients, intracellular concentrations of ribonucleotide triphosphates, adhesion to the extracellular matrix and the like, and signals that modulate cell cycle and apoptosis in the context of a differentiation program, either during development or during postnatal life in self-renewing tissues. "Differentiation" programs, i.e., processes whereby a cell acquires a different or specialized phenotype, are inextricably linked to cell cycle and apoptosis. The "objective" of a differentiation program is to produce a population of cells with a certain phenotype, or more commonly multiple, parallel populations of cells with different phenotypes from common precursors (e.g., multiple blood cells from bone marrow stem cells, epidermis and hair follicles from epidermal stem cells etc.). Differentiating cells, such as embryonal neuroblasts, bone marrow hematopoietic cells, or skin keratinocytes, gradually alter their phenotypes over a number of cell cycles. Thus, differentiation programs must include signals that induce cell proliferation from relatively undifferentiated precursors, signals that guide the acquisition of different gene expression patterns in different daughter cells and quite often programs for orderly termination of cell life when the differentiation program is complete or when the differentiated cell has completed its function. Once the "differentiated" phenotype is attained, reversible or irreversible growth arrest generally occurs. In many cases, such as epidermal keratinocytes or mucosal epithelial cells, terminal differentiation is followed by timed apoptosis. The timing and direction of this process (i.e., at which point during differentiation must the cell exit from cell cycle, how long must apoptosis be inhibited, and which phenotype is ultimately going to be acquired by which cells) are crucial to the existance of all metazoa. Not surprisingly, altered differentiation signals feature prominently among the mechanisms of carcinogenesis and among candidate therapeutic targets.

The number of signals can affect the balance between cell cycle and apoptosis is vast, and any attempt at classifying them would inevitably be incomplete. The molecular information-processing machinery that responds to these signals is exceedingly complex and only partially understood. Each signal triggers a coordinated series of intermolecular interactions, post-translational modifications and transport mechanisms that ultimately transduce information to the genome and modulate gene-expression patterns. In turn, these gene-expression patterns adapt the composition of the cell and decide its ultimate fate. Our understanding of these processes is complicated by redundancy between individual signaling molecules and pathways, partially overlapping functions, extensive multifunctionality of key mediators, as well as cross-talk and feedback mechanisms that are dependent on time, the relative intracellular concentrations of the relevant mediators, and their cellular compartimentalization. The following description will briefly summarize the general aspects of the best-characterized mechanisms that transduce information to the genome, and focus on a few specific examples that are particularly relevant to cancer biology and/or especially novel.

In general terms, relatively few common mechanisms have been identified that transduce information to the genome *(64)*. Some of the signals connect directly to the nucleus through ligand-modulated transcriptional regulators that

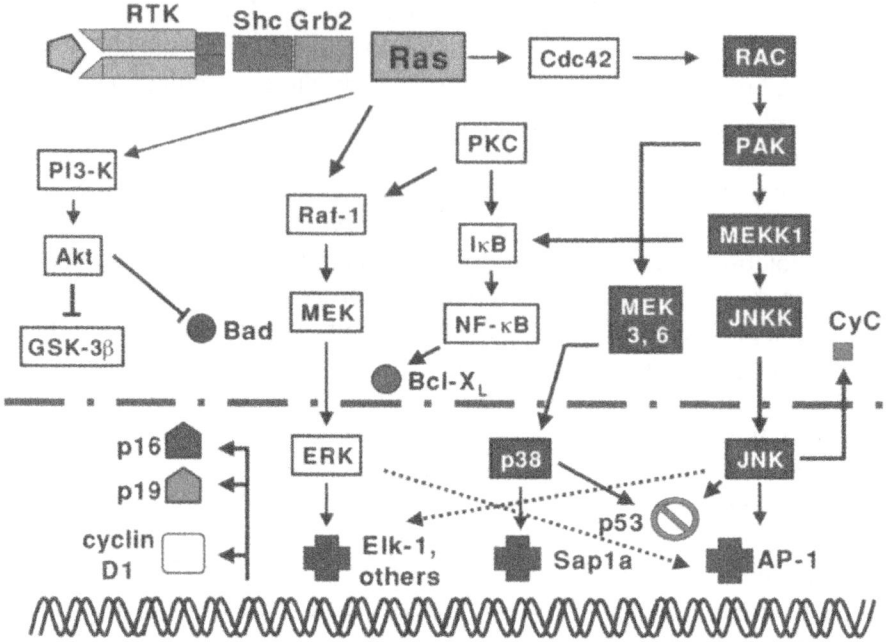

Fig. 6. The Ras signaling network transduces proliferation, senescence, and apoptosis signals. The figure presents a schematic and simplified diagram of key Ras signaling pathways and some of their effectors. RTK, receptor tyrosine kinase (e.g., a growth factor receptor). Shc is an example of adaptor molecule that recruits Ras through Grb2. Pathways represented in white boxes tend to generate survival and/or proliferation signals. For example, the PI-3 kinase pathway inactivates Bad and has an overall anti-apoptotic effect, while the ERK pathway transactivates cyclin D_1, thus stimulating cell cycle progression and cross-talks with NF-κB, which generally but not always mediates survival signals. Growth arrest and senescence can be induced by Ras activation through transactivation of p16[ink4a] and p19[arf], which in turn stabilizes p53. Pathways that have been linked to apoptosis induction are represented in dark gray. Both JNK and p38 can directly activate p53. In addition, JNK is reported to be necessary for cytochrome c (cyc) release from the mitochondria. Dotted lines indicate effects that are not definitively established.

respond to cell-permeable agents. Examples include steroid hormone receptors, retinoid receptors, fatty acid-modulated PPAR transcription factors, and so on. The importance of these signals to cancer is exemplified by the therapeutic usefulness of estrogen receptor antagonists in breast cancer, androgen ablation in prostate cancer, and retinoid-receptor agonists in hematopoietic and skin malignancies.

Other signals utilize transmembrane receptors that lead to the activation and nuclear translocation of latent cytoplasmic transcription factors or transcriptional co-regulators. Examples include the JAK-STAT signaling utilized by many cytokine receptors *(65,66)* and the SMAD transcription factors that transduce signals from TGF family receptors *(67–69)*. In both cases receptor engagement leads to phosphorylation and activation of latent transcription factors which then migrate to the nucleus and act as homo- or heterodimers that induce or repress specific genes after recruiting chromatin-remodeling complexes. Constitutive activation of cytokine receptors can induce transformation in a variety of models *(64)*. Conversely, inactivation of TGF-β or its downstream SMAD transcription factors is a common event in colon cancers, indicating that this pathway acts as a tumor suppressor. One possible mechanism for this may the fact that TGF-β induces the expression of CKI p15^{ink4b}. Thus, loss or inactivation of TGF-β signaling impairs the G_1 restriction point.

NF-κB transcription factors consist of homo- and heterodimers of several related subunits (p50, p52, p65, c-Rel, and Rel-B) that are constitutively bound to inhibitory molecules (IκB). Receptor engagement triggers phosphorylation, ubiquitination and degradation of the inhibitor, releasing NF-κB to the nucleus. At least one member of the family, c-Rel, is a proven proto-oncogene. NF-κB factors modulate cell cycle and apoptosis through multiple mechanisms that are currently under active investigation (*see* above) and NF-κB inhibitory drugs are considered promising candidates for clinical development.

A common theme in all the cases described so far (and in other families of transcriptional regulators such as the helix-loop-helix group) is that transcription factors of the same family can form different homo- and heterodimers that have differential and sometimes opposite effects on gene expression. Additionally, heterodimers between transcription factors of related but different families can also be formed, as in the case of retinoid receptors with PPAR or orphan nuclear receptors *(70)*, further increasing the possible combinations. The overall effect is that many different gene regulatory complexes can be obtained from combinations of relatively few related subunits.

Other signaling pathways communicate with the nucleus indirectly, through complex cascades of protein association and post-translational modifications that ultimately converge on nuclear transcription factors. Here the potential for signal amplification through enzymatic cascades is great, as is the variety of possible cross-talks. From the perspective of a cancer biologist, perhaps the most important of such signaling cascades is the Ras signaling network (Fig. 6), members of which are directly or indirectly involved in a great number of human malignancies *(64)*. Ras itself is thought to be constitutively active due to mutations in a quarter of all human tumors *(4,18)*. We have already seen how Ras activation can induce senescence via upregulation of CKIs and p53. Depending on cellular context, the Ras signaling network generates cell cycle progression signals, survival signals, apoptosis signals, and senescence signals, the balance of which determines the ultimate outcome *(64,71–74)*. Ras (of which several isoforms are known, such as H-Ras, K-Ras, and N-Ras) and its homologues Rho,

Rac, and Cdc42 are small proteins with GTPase activity, which are active when GTP-bound and inactive when bound to GDP. The exchange of GTP for GDP and the rate of GTP hydrolysis are controlled by regulatory molecules (nucleotide exchange factors and GTPase activating factors). Ras proteins are covalently modified with isoprenoid chains that may aid in membrane association, and this fact has been exploited for the development of drugs that block Ras prenylation, thereby inhibiting Ras *(75–77)*. Well-studied examples of Ras activation occur upon engagement of certain growth factor tyrosine kinases such as the EGF receptor. Ligand-bound receptors dimerize, phosphorylate each other, and recruit a cascade of adaptor proteins that recognize phosphotyrosine residues via SH2 (Sarc-homology-2) domains and often bind each other through SH3 domains that recognize proline-rich sequences. In other cases, such as T-cell receptor engagement, nonreceptor tyrosine kinase are recruited by the activated receptor and in turn phosphorylate and recruit adaptor molecules. The ultimate consequence is the formation of multimolecular complexes at the plasma membrane, which in turn recruit the GTP-bound form of Ras proteins. The duration of the signal is controlled by the rate of GTP hydrolysis, which inactivates Ras proteins until a new GTP molecule is bound. Active Ras proteins recruit and activate upstream protein kinases, which in turn phosphorylate and activate downstream protein kinases. These enter the nucleus where they phosphorylate a variety of transcription factors, thereby modulating gene expression. Protein phosphatases such as PP-2A control the half-life of the active kinases. Both upstream and downstream kinases participate in cross-talk with other signaling networks by phosphorylating intermediates of these networks. Ras signaling can affect cell cycle and apoptosis through distinct but cross-talking MAP (mitogen-activated protein) kinase cascades (Fig. 6). The Raf-MEK-ERK cascade converges on transcription factors including Ets family molecules such as Elk, AP-1, and others and generally stimulates cell cycle progression, at least in part through the upregulation of cyclin D_1 expression. Conversely, the JNKK-JNK (c-Jun-N-terminal kinase) cascade converges on a group of transcription factors which includes among others the Jun/Fos AP-1 family and often induce apoptosis in response to cell stress through multiple mechanisms. We have already seen how JNK can activate p53 *(11)*. Recently, JNK has been shown to be required for cytochrome c release from mitochondria one of the main apoptosis inducing factors (*see* above) *(78)*. Similarly, the p38 MAP kinase cascade can activate p53 *(11)* and has been implicated in apoptosis induction, while the PI3-K-Akt cascade transduces a universal survival signal via the inactivation of Bad *(79)*. The Ras signaling network tranduces signals from a large variety of sources, including growth factor, hormone and cytokine receptors, adhesion molecules, and others. Cross-talk has been documented with essentially all other major signaling pathways, including for example NF-κB (which can be activated by Ras through Raf), protein kinase C (which can activate Raf downstream of Ras), and more

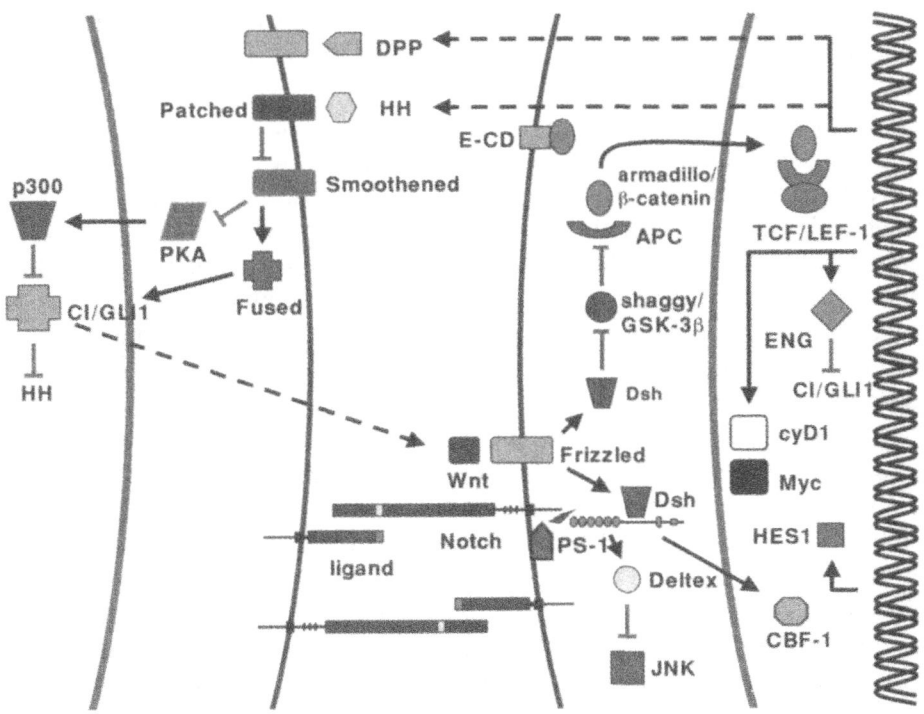

Fig. 7. The Notch, Wnt, and Hedgehog signaling networks. Schematic representation of the interaction between these 3 signaling networks. *See* text for explanation. PS-1, presenilin 1. Dsh, Dishevelled. E-CD, E-cadherin. PKA, protein kinase A. TCF-LEF activation induces cell cycle progression at least in part through cyclin D1 (cyD1) and Myc upregulation. The mechanisms of transformation induced by Gli1 and Notch are still unknown, but inhibitory effects on apoptosis have been documented for Notch-1. Only one Wnt, one Notch, and one Notch ligand are shown for simplicity. Mammals have at least 4 Notch genes, two families of Notch ligands, and a large number of Wnt and Wnt-like secretory molecules.

recently, with the SMAD network *(80)*. Physiologically, it is not surprising that a "master" signaling network is utilized to transduce both growth and growth arrest/apoptosis signals. Cell growth in a healthy organism is never unlimited, and the Ras signaling network provides for elegant feedback mechanisms that can induce and terminate growth. The overall effect of activating the Ras signaling network depend on the overall cellular context, and this is especially important in cancer. Constitutive activation of Ras in a cell with functional senescence, G_1 restriction point and p53 responses ultimately leads to apoptosis or senescence. Conversely, when the G_1 restriction point and p53 are disabled, Ras activation results in a constitutive proliferation signal and neoplastic transformation since the growth arrest/senescence pathways are interrupted.

Another group of signals whose importance in human malignancies is being increasingly recognized include molecules that mediate cell–cell communications and control the timing of complex differentiation programs during development and postnatal life in all metazoa. Signals that control the timing and direction of differentiation were originally identified because of their major developmental effects in invertebrates. Often, these signals are involved in establishing precise "boundaries" between populations of initially equivalent cells that proliferate and differentiate toward different phenotypes. Thus, these signals affect differentiation, growth, and apotosis simultaneously through cascades of transcription factors that are still poorly understood. Three interconnected signaling networks that have proven relevance to human cancer are described below (Fig. 7).

The Wnt family of molecules, vertebrate homologues of Drosophila Wingless, signal through multi-pass transmembrane receptors denominated Frizzled to intracellular mediator Dishevelled *(64)*. Dishevelled blocks the protein kinase shaggy/zeste white 3 or GSK-3β (glycogen synthase kinase 3β), preventing it from phosphorylating APC (the gene mutated in adenomatous poliposis coli). As a consequence, APC becomes unable to sequester β-catenin/armadillo, leading to an increase in free β-catenin, which enters the nucleus and modulates the activity of transcription factors of the TCF/LEF group. This in turn induces the expression of several target genes, including oncogenes such as c-Myc and c-Jun and growth promoting genes such as cyclin D_1. Other targets include transcriptional repressors such as Engrailed, and cytokines such as Decapentaplegic (of the TGF family) and Hedgehog. Hedgehog is secreted and acts on neighboring cells, binding to the membrane receptor Patched. This interaction prevents Patched from inhibiting the other transmembrane receptor Smoothened, which in turn, through the protein kinase Fused inhibits protein kinase A, ultimately leading to activation of transcription factor Cubitus Interruptus/Gli1. Among the genes upregulated by Gli1 is Wingless/Wnt, thus closing the loop of intercellular cross talk. During development, this loop would work to create an active boundary between a group of cells that secrete Wingless and repress Hedgehog and a neighboring group of cells that proliferate, secrete Hedgehog and repress Wingless. Many of these molecules are now known to be involved in cancer *(64,81,82)*. Wnt-1 is a well-known protooncogene for MMTV induced mammary carcinomas in mice. Mutations that inactivate APC are involved in the progression of colon cancer. Mutations in β-catenin that lead to its accumulation and nuclear migration are thought to be involved in tumor progression. β-catenins are also effectors of cell adhesion molecules E-cadherins, which induce β-catenin phosphorylation by Src-family tyrosine kinases. Reduced expression or mutation of E-cadherins are often observed in tumors. Mutations in Patched signaling pathway cause hereditary nevoid basal cell carcinomas and are common in sporadic basal cell carcinomas. Patched mutations favor transformation most likely by leading to unrestrained Gli1 activity. Gli1 is often amplified in various human tumors *(83–87)*.

The Notch signaling network consists of heterodimeric transmembrane Notch receptors that are activated by ligands expressed on the surface of neighboring cells *(88)*. Drosophila has one Notch gene and two ligands, Delta and Serrate, while mammals have four Notch genes and two families of ligands, the Delta-like and Jagged (Serrate-like) families. A constitutively active, truncated form of human Notch-1 generated by a 9:7 chromosomal translocation is associated with T-cell acute lymphoblastic leukemia (T-ALL) and causes a similar syndrome in mice. Constitutive activation of Notch receptors leads to neoplastic transformation in vitro and in a variety of animal models, and increased expression of Notch receptors, ligands, and downstream effectors has been observed in various solid human tumors *(89,90)*. The mechanism of Notch-induced transformation is still unclear. However, inhibition of apoptosis by Notch-1 has been documented in several experimental systems *(91–93)*. Notch signaling is extremely complex and incompletely understood *(88–90,94,95)*. At least two different transduction mechanisms have been discovered. First, upon ligand binding Notch receptors are cleaved and release an intracellular subunit that migrates to the nucleus where it acts as a transcriptional coactivator by converting a constitutive repressor, CBF-1/Suppressor of Hairless into a transcriptional activator. Genes upregulated by CBF-1 include a variety of helix-loop-helix transcriptional inhibitors such as HES-1, which in turn regulate other transcription factors, as well as at least one of the NF-kB components, p52. In addition, through its interaction with the cytoplasmic protein Deltex, Notch downregulates JNK, thus establishing a cross-talk with the Ras network. Moreover, by binding and sequestering Dishevelled Notch cross-talks with the Wingless network. Notch and Wingless responses thus tend to dampen each other. Conversely, a Wingless-responding, Hedgehog secreting cell upregulates Notch ligands, thus activating Notch in the neighboring Wingless secreting, Hedgehog-responsive cells (Fig. 7). Depending on the cellular context, the overall effect of Notch activation can be cell cycle progression and induction of proliferation or cell cycle arrest, inhibition, or induction of apoptosis and a delay or induction of specific differentiation programs *(88,94–96)*. The links between Notch signaling and the cell-cycle and apoptotic machinery are being actively investigated.

7. CONCLUSIONS: THERAPEUTIC IMPLICATIONS AND FUTURE DIRECTIONS

Antineoplastic agents directly or indirectly utilize the cellular signaling network to affect the balance between cell cycle and cell death. Both stress signals and differentiation signals are relevant to cancer therapy and chemoprevention. Creating a cell stress that triggers apoptosis is the primary mode of action of radiotherapy and most chemotherapy agents. Radiation and DNA damaging drugs such as alkylating agents, platinum compounds, and anthracyclines trigger a DNA damage emergency apoptosis (*see* above), as do topoisomerase inhibitors by preventing religation of cleaved DNA. Anti-metabolites such as metothrexate and asparaginase create a metabolic stress that triggers apoptosis preferentially in cancer cells. Cytoskelatal poisons such as taxanes interfere with the correct assembly of the mitotic apparatus and trigger apoptosis through mitotic spindle checkpoints. Even more modern drugs such as histone deacetylase inhibitors most likely trigger a cell stress response by randomly and inappropriately derepressing gene expression. The ultimate aim of anti-angiogenic agents is to induce hypoxic metabolic stress in cancers by preventing the formation of new blood vessels. This is expected to result in growth arrest and/or apoptosis in cancer cells.

Differentiation-inducing therapeutic and preventive agents such as retinoids, vitamin D3 analogs, short chain fatty acids, hybrid polar drugs, cyclooxigenase-2 inhibitors, and so on aim to deliver a signal that modulates gene expression, ultimately tipping the balance against growth and survival and in favor of a differentiation program that results in either growth arrest or apoptosis. A somewhat intermediate position is occupied by agents that interrupt a constitutive growth and survival signal without causing nonspecific metabolic stress. These include estrogen receptor antagonists, androgen inhibitors, growth factor receptor antagonists and blocking monoclonal antibodies such as Trastuzumab (Herceptin), and so forth. Corticosteroids trigger both cell cycle arrest and an apoptotic program in responsive cells. Tyrosine kinase inhibitors and farnesyl- and geranylgeranyltransferase inhibitors that block Ras family proteins have pleiotropic effects on signaling networks that transduce growth and survival signals, ultimately resulting in either growth arrest or apoptosis.

Over the past few decades, through a largely empirical approach, medical oncology has identified groups of agents that affect the key pathways of cell cycle and apoptosis control. A key goal of contemporary cancer research is to build on existing and newly accumulated molecular knowledge to develop a next generation of mechanism-based, rationally designed anti-neoplastic agents. These will specifically target key intermediates of cell fate decision pathways. Therapeutic regimens will be dictated from the gene expression pattern or "molecular signature" of specifc cancers, which will identify the most appropriate targets.

Twenty years of molecular oncology have revealed that cancer results from accumulated genetic damage to crucial component of the cell fate machinery. Unfortunately, the number of different combinations of mutations that can result in neoplastic transformation is quite large. The reasons for such a diversity of oncogenic mechanisms lie in the very nature of cell fate decision mechanisms. Evolution has produced a remarkably complex information processing machinery that regulates cell fate decisions. This machinery functions as a highly interconnected, adaptable network. Interconnectedness is achieved through cross-talk, redundancy, multifunctionality, and context-dependence. Cross-talk implies that intermediates of a given signaling pathway activate or inhibit intermediates of another, parallel pathway. Redundancy implies that similar proteins can often perform the same or partially overlapping functions so that the loss of one gene can be compensated by another. For example, p73 can partially replace p53 in inducing apoptosis in response to unrestrained E2F activity. Bcl-X_L and Bcl-2 both protect from apoptosis by similar mechanisms. As a result, mutations in many related genes (for examples, members of the Ras family or the receptor tyrosine kinase family) can potentially have the same deleterious effect on cell fate. Multifunctionality implies that an individual protein often performs many different functions by interacting with multiple intracellular targets. For example Rb and E2F participate in both cell cycle control and apoptosis control. Mutations that affect a multifunctional protein can disable or constitutively activate multiple functions of this protein or selectively affect specific functions. Thus, a single mutation can simultaneously damage several control processes. Context-dependence refers to the fact that the consequence of activating or disabling a specific gene depend on the activity of other cellular components. Thus, for example, a mutation that constitutively activates Ras can result in cell senescence, apoptosis, or continuous proliferation, depending on the functional status of Rb, p53, and other signaling molecules.

Another cause of genetic complexity in human cancers is the intrinsic genomic instability of neoplastic cells, due in part to loss of DNA damage responses. This causes further accumulation of mutations and genetic heterogeneity as the disease progresses and allows selection of treatment-resistant cells. The end result is a malignant lesions in which the initial oncogene and/or tumor-suppressor gene mutations, added to the additional mutations accumulated during tumor progression have a multitude of direct and indirect effects on gene-expression patterns. High-throughput genomics technologies such as DNA arrays are beginning to yield gene expression profiles of common cancers (97–100). These studies are revealing that large numbers of genes are differentially expressed in cancers compared to nonmalignant tissues, and that morphologically similar cancers can have diverse gene-expression fingerprints. Similar techniques applied to proteins are technically more challenging but are under development (101).

This daunting intricacy suggests that specifically correcting the genetic lesions in each human cancer would hardly be a viable treatment strategy, at least until the development of highly efficient means of delivering and targeting gene therapy vectors in vivo. However, this does not mean that the rational design of new cancer treatments is an unattainable goal. In fact, correcting each genetic lesion in each cancer is not likely to be necessary to achieve therapeutic success. On the contrary, the very interconnectedness of the cell signaling networks implies that while the number of genes whose mutations can cause cancer is very large, the number of key *pathways* into which these genes fall is much smaller. Ultimately, the vast number of oncogenes and tumor-suppressor genes identified to date all converge on a few crucial mechanisms that regulate cell cycle progression, apoptosis, and senescence. Mutations in many different molecules that are part of the same signaling network can result in the same phenotype. For example, activation of the ERK arm of the MAP kinase cascade can conceivably result from mutations in growth factor receptors that activate Ras family GTPases, in adaptor molecules involved in Ras recruiting, in Ras proteins, in nucleotide exchange factors and GTPase activators that modulate the activity of Ras or in any of the downstream protein kinases that are activated by Ras. Similarly, overexpression of cyclin D_1, loss of $p16^{ink4a}$ or $p21^{cip1/waf1}$, loss or Rb, overexpression of Id2 triggered by c-Myc, and other mutations all ultimately result in a disabled G_1 restriction point and unrestrained E2F activity.

Clinical and basic research have produced clear indications on the nature of the pathways crucial to cancer progression. It has become clear that essentially all human malignancies have a disabled G_1 restriction point. Approximately one-half of all human cancers have functional loss of p53, and p53-negative recurrences are common after treatment with DNA-damaging agents of cancers that were originally p53 positive. Approximately one-quarter of all human cancers carry mutations in Ras genes, and many more carry mutations that indirectly result in activation of Ras signaling, such as autocrine overproduction of growth factors or constitutive activation of growth factor receptors. Overexpression of anti-apoptotic genes such as Bcl-2 and Bcl-X_L or constitutive survival signals are commonly encountered. Recently, the experimental neoplastic transformation of primary human cells has been achieved *(102)* by expression of just four key oncoproteins disrupting key signaling pathways. Complete transformation required the disabling of the senescence checkpoint by expression of telomerase, inactivation of the G_1 restriction point and of p53 by SV40 large and small T oncoproteins and a constitutively active Ras mutant to provide a chronic growth stimulus and anchorage-independence.

Thus, a promising strategy for the rational design of cancer treatments lies in the identification of the key *pathways* (as opposed to individual genes) that are affected in each malignancy, and of the optimal attack points within each pathway to develop specific antagonist or agonist drugs. Appropriate combinations of agents could be developed to specifically target two or more key pathways. For example, a cell permeable E2F inhibitor would act downstream of mutations affecting cyclin D_1, Rb, $p16^{ink4a}$, $p21^{cip1/waf1}$ or in principle any other step in the G_1 restriction point. Such an agent would likely be useful in combination with other growth-arresting strategies such as angiogenesis inhibitors, telomerase inhibitors or receptor tyrosine kinase inhibitors. On the other hand, inhibition of E2F, especially in a p53-positive tumor, could actually decrease the effects of a treatment intended to cause apoptosis, such as a DNA-damaging agents. Another potentially useful strategy may lie in manipulating natural signals that affect multiple pathways simultaneously, such as the Wnt or Notch signaling networks.

A significant amount of information is already available on the workings of the key functional pathways that control cell fate, and rapid progress is being made in areas that remain incompletely understood. Over the next few years, large-scale genomics and proteomics studies will rapidly amass information on gene and protein expression patterns in human tumors and in experimental tumor models (103,104). A molecular taxonomy of human tumors based on gene-expression patterns is within reach of today's technology. Perhaps more importantly, data mining to identify functional hyerarchies of gene and protein interactions (105–107), coupled with experimental validation of putative inter-actions, will fill the gaps in our knowledge of cell fate determination networks and give us a clear and complete picture of the intricate machinery that regulates the choice between cell cycle and apoptosis in normal and malignant cells. Based on this knowledge, pathway-specific treatments that target key functional targets utilizing rationally designed drugs, biologics, or combination thereof will become a standard therapeutic approach. One such target-specific agent, the Her2-Neu specific monoclonal antibody Trastuzumab (Herceptin) is already FDA-approved for the treatment of advanced breast cancer (108,109). Ratio-nally designed receptor-tyrosine kinase inhibitors (110) and the Bcr-Abl kinase inhibitor STI571 (111,112) are in clinical development for the treatment of solid tumors and chronic myeloid leukemia, respectively. The promising results obtained so far with these agents suggest that the future of cancer treatment may have already begun.

ACKNOWLEDGMENTS

The author is grateful to Dr. Brian Nickoloff for critical reading of this manu-script, to the NIH (grants RO1CA84065-01 and R43 CA83157), and to the Illi-nois Department of Public Health for supporting his work. The author apologizes to all the investigators whose primary references could not be quoted for reasons of space.

REFERENCES

1. Herwig S, Strauss M. The retinoblastoma protein: a master regulator of cell cycle, differen-tiation and apoptosis. *Eur J Biochem* 1997;246:581–601.
2. Harbour JW, Dean DC. Rb function in cell-cycle regulation and apoptosis. *Nat Cell Biol* 2000;2:E65–E67.
3. Yamasaki L. Balancing proliferation and apoptosis in vivo: the Goldilocks theory of E2F/DP action. *Biochim Biophys Acta* 1999;1423:M9–M15.
4. Lundberg AS, Weinberg RA. Control of the cell cycle and apoptosis. *Eur J Cancer* 1999;35:1886–1894.
5. Harbour JW, Dean DC. The Rb/E2F pathway: expanding roles and emerging paradigms. *Genes Dev* 2000;14:2393–2409.

6. Zhang HS, Gavin M, Dahiya A, Postigo AA, Ma D, Luo RX, et al. Exit from G1 and S phase of the cell cycle is regulated by repressor complexes containing HDAC-Rb-hSWI/SNF and Rb-hSWI/SNF. *Cell* 2000;101:79–89.

7. Lasorella A, Noseda M, Beyna M, Iavarone A. Id2 is a retinoblastoma protein target and mediates signalling by Myc oncoproteins. *Nature* 2000;407:592–598.

8. Dang CV. c-Myc target genes involved in cell growth, apoptosis, and metabolism. *Mol Cell Biol* 1999;19:1–11.

9. O'Connell MJ, Walworth NC, Carr AM. The G2-phase DNA-damage checkpoint. *Trends Cell Biol* 2000;10:296–303.

10. Shackelford RE, Kaufmann WK, Paules RS. Cell cycle control, checkpoint mechanisms, and genotoxic stress. *Environ Health Perspect* 1999;107 Suppl 1:5–24.

11. Sionov RV, Haupt Y. The cellular response to p53: the decision between life and death. *Oncogene* 1999;18:6145–6157.

12. Gardner RD, Burke DJ. The spindle checkpoint: two transitions, two pathways. *Trends Cell Biol* 2000;10:154–158.

13. Fang G, Yu H, Kirschner MW. Control of mitotic transitions by the anaphase-promoting complex. *Philos Trans R Soc Lond B Biol Sci* 1999;354:1583–1590.

14. Taylor SS. Chromosome segregation: dual control ensures fidelity. *Curr Biol* 1999;9: R562–R564.

15. Chan GK, Jablonski SA, Sudakin V, Hittle JC, Yen TJ. Human BUBR1 is a mitotic checkpoint kinase that monitors CENP-E functions at kinetochores and binds the cyclosome/APC. *J Cell Biol* 1999;146:941–954.

16. Peters JM. Subunits and substrates of the anaphase-promoting complex. *Exp Cell Res* 1999;248:339–349.

17. Hayflick L. The illusion of cell immortality. *Br J Cancer* 2000;83:841–846.

18. Lundberg AS, Hahn WC, Gupta P, Weinberg RA. Genes involved in senescence and immortalization. *Curr Opin Cell Biol* 2000;12:705–709.

19. Campisi J. Cancer, aging and cellular senescence. *In Vivo* 2000;14:183–188.

20. Collins K. Mammalian telomeres and telomerase. *Curr Opin Cell Biol* 2000;12:378–383.

21. Griffith JD, Comeau L, Rosenfield S, Stansel RM, Bianchi A, Moss H, et al. Mammalian telomeres end in a large duplex loop. *Cell* 1999;97:503–514.

22. Bailey SM, Meyne J, Chen DJ, Kurimasa A, Li GC, Lehnert BE, et al. DNA double-strand break repair proteins are required to cap the ends of mammalian chromosomes. *Proc Natl Acad Sci USA* 1999;96:14899–14904.

23. Bringold F, Serrano M. Tumor suppressors and oncogenes in cellular senescence. *Exp Gerontol* 2000;35:317–329.

24. Dai CY, Enders GH. p16 INK4a can initiate an autonomous senescence program. *Oncogene 2000* 2000;19:1613–1622.

25. Lee G, Park BS, Han SE, Oh J, You Y, Baek J, et al. Concurrence of replicative senescence and elevated expression of p16(INK4A) with subculture-induced but not calcium-induced differentiation in normal human oral keratinocytes. *Arch Oral Biol 2000* 2000;45:809–818.

26. Fuxe J, Akusjarvi G, Goike HM, Roos G, Collins VP, Pettersson RF. Adenovirus-mediated overexpression of p15INK4B inhibits human glioma cell growth, induces replicative senescence, and inhibits telomerase activity similarly to p16INK4A [In Process Citation]. *Cell Growth Differ* 2000;11:373–384.

27. Groth A, Weber JD, Willumsen BM, Sherr CJ, Roussel MF. Oncogenic Ras induces p19ARF and growth arrest in mouse embryo fibroblasts lacking p21Cip1 and p27Kip1 without activating cyclin D-dependent kinases. *J Biol Chem* 2000;275:27473–27480.

28. Ferbeyre G, de SE, Querido E, Baptiste N, Prives C, Lowe SW. PML is induced by oncogenic ras and promotes premature senescence. *Genes Dev* 2000;14:2015–2027.

29. Chaturvedi V, Qin JZ, Denning MF, Choubey D, Diaz MO, Nickoloff BJ. Apoptosis in proliferating, senescent, and immortalized keratinocytes. *J Biol Chem* 1999;274: 23358–23367.
30. Karlseder J, Broccoli D, Dai Y, Hardy S, de LT. p53- and ATM-dependent apoptosis induced by telomeres lacking TRF2. *Science* 1999;283:1321–1325.
31. Saretzki G, Sitte N, Merkel U, Wurm RE, von ZT. Telomere shortening triggers a p53-dependent cell cycle arrest via accumulation of G-rich single stranded DNA fragments. *Oncogene* 1999;18:5148–5158.
32. VonZglinicki T. Role of oxidative stress in telomere length regulation and replicative senescence. *Ann NY Acad Sci* 2000;908:99–110.
33. Cerni C. Telomeres, telomerase, and myc. An update. *Mutat Res* 2000;462:31–47.
34. Urquidi V, Tarin D, Goodison S. Role of telomerase in cell senescence and oncogenesis. *Annu Rev Med* 2000;51:65–79.
35. Herbert B, Pitts AE, Baker SI, Hamilton SE, Wright WE, Shay JW, et al. Inhibition of human telomerase in immortal human cells leads to progressive telomere shortening and cell death. *Proc Natl Acad Sci USA* 1999;96:14276–14281.
36. Zhang X, Mar V, Zhou W, Harrington L, Robinson MO. Telomere shortening and apoptosis in telomerase-inhibited human tumor cells. *Genes Dev* 1999;13:2388–2399.
37. Kass-Eisler A, Greider CW. Recombination in telomere-length maintenance. *Trends Biochem Sci* 2000;25:200–204.
38. Kerr JF, Wyllie AH, Currie AR. Apoptosis: a basic biological phenomenon with wide-ranging implications in tissue kinetics. *Br J Cancer* 1972;26:239–257.
39. Hengartner MO. The biochemistry of apoptosis. *Nature* 2000;407:770–776.
40. Rich T, Allen RL, Wyllie AH. Defying death after DNA damage. *Nature* 2000;407:777–783.
41. Savill J, Fadok V. Corpse clearance defines the meaning of cell death. *Nature* 2000;407: 784–788.
42. Krammer PH. CD95's deadly mission in the immune system. *Nature* 2000;407:789–795.
43. Meier P, Finch A, Evan G. Apoptosis in development. *Nature* 2000;407:796–801.
44. Yuan J, Yankner BA. Apoptosis in the nervous system. *Nature* 2000;407:802–809.
45. Nicholson DW. From bench to clinic with apoptosis-based therapeutic agents. *Nature* 2000;407:810–816.
46. Jacotot E, Ferri KF, Kroemer G. Apoptosis and cell cycle: distinct checkpoints with overlapping upstream control. *Pathol Biol (Paris)* 2000;48:271–279.
47. Raleigh JM, O'Connell MJ. The G(2) DNA damage checkpoint targets both Wee1 and Cdc25. *J Cell Sci* 2000;113:1727–1736.
48. Hansen R, Oren M. p53; from inductive signal to cellular effect. *Curr Opin Genet Dev* 1997;7:46–51.
49. King KL, Cidlowski JA. Cell cycle regulation and apoptosis. *Annu Rev Physiol* 1998;60: 601–617.
50. Brady HJ, Gil-Gomez G. The cell cycle and apoptosis. *Results Prob Cell Differ* 1999;23: 127–144.
51. Kauffmann-Zeh A, Rodriguez-Viciana P, Ulrich E, Gilbert C, Coffer P, Downward J, et al. Suppression of c-Myc-induced apoptosis by Ras signalling through PI(3)K and PKB. *Nature* 1997;385:544–548.
52. Zha J, Harada H, Yang E, Jockel J, Korsmeyer SJ. Serine phosphorylation of death agonist BAD in response to survival factor results in binding to 14-3-3 not BCL-X(L). *Cell* 1996;87:619–628.
53. Mayo MW, Baldwin AS. The transcription factor NF-kappaB: control of oncogenesis and cancer therapy resistance. *Biochim Biophys Acta* 2000;1470:M55–M62.
54. Barkett M, Gilmore TD. Control of apoptosis by Rel/NF-kappaB transcription factors. *Oncogene* 1999;18:6910–6924.
55. Pahl HL. Activators and target genes of Rel/NF-kappaB transcription factors. *Oncogene* 1999;18:6853–6866.

56. Webster GA, Perkins ND. Transcriptional cross talk between NF-kappaB and p53. *Mol Cell Biol* 1999;19:3485–3495.
57. Shao J, Fujiwara T, Kadowaki Y, Fukazawa T, Waku T, Itoshima T, et al. Overexpression of the wild-type p53 gene inhibits NF-kappaB activity and synergizes with aspirin to induce apoptosis in human colon cancer cells. *Oncogene* 2000;19:726–736.
58. Ryan KM, Ernst MK, Rice NR, Vousden KH. Role of NF-kappaB in p53-mediated programmed cell death. *Nature* 2000;404:892–897.
59. Marin MC, Kaelin WGJ. p63 and p73: old members of a new family. *Biochim Biophys Acta* 2000;1470:M93–M100.
60. Levrero M, De LV, Costanzo A, Gong J, Wang JY, Melino G. The p53/p63/p73 family of transcription factors: overlapping and distinct functions. *J Cell Sci* 2000;113:1661–1670.
61. Irwin M, Marin MC, Phillips AC, Seelan RS, Smith DI, Liu W, et al. Role for the p53 homologue p73 in E2F-1-induced apoptosis. *Nature* 2000;407:645–648.
62. Lissy NA, Davis PK, Irwin M, Kaelin WG, Dowdy SF. A common E2F-1 and p73 pathway mediates cell death induced by TCR activation. *Nature* 2000;407:642–645.
63. Stiewe T, Putzer BM. Role of the p53-homologue p73 in E2F1-induced apoptosis. *Nat Genet* 2000;26:464–469.
64. Hunter T. Oncoprotein networks. *Cell* 1997;88:333–346.
65. Imada K, Leonard WJ. The Jak-STAT pathway. *Mol Immunol* 2000;37:1–11.
66. Williams JG. STAT signalling in cell proliferation and in development. *Curr Opin Genet Dev* 2000;10:503–507.
67. Zimmerman CM, Padgett RW. Transforming growth factor beta signaling mediators and modulators. *Gene 2000* 2000;249:17–30.
68. Massague J, Wotton D. Transcriptional control by the TGF-beta/Smad signaling system. *EMBO J* 2000;19:1745–1754.
69. Attisano L, Wrana JL. Smads as transcriptional co-modulators. *Curr Opin Cell Biol* 2000;12:235–243.
70. Rogers MB. Life-and-death decisions influenced by retinoids. *Curr Top Dev Biol* 1997; 35:1–46.
71. Downward J. Ras signalling and apoptosis. *Curr Opin Genet Dev* 1998;8:49–54.
72. Frame S, Balmain A. Integration of positive and negative growth signals during ras pathway activation in vivo. *Curr Opin Genet Dev* 2000;10:106–113.
73. Olson MF, Marais R. Ras protein signalling. *Semin Immunol* 2000;12:63–73.
74. rez-Sala P, Rebollo A. Novel aspects of Ras proteins biology: regulation and implications. *Cell Death Differ* 1999;6:722–728.
75. Scharovsky OG, Rozados VR, Gervasoni SI, Matar P. Inhibition of ras oncogene: a novel approach to antineoplastic therapy. *J Biomed Sci* 2000;7:292–298.
76. Adjei AA. Signal transduction pathway targets for anticancer drug discovery. *Curr Pharm Des* 2000;6:361–378.
77. Pincus MR, Brandt-Rauf PW, Michl J, Carty RP, Friedman FK. ras-p21-induced cell transformation: unique signal transduction pathways and implications for the design of new chemotherapeutic agents. *Cancer Invest* 2000;18:39–50.
78. Tournier C, Hess P, Yang DD, Xu J, Turner TK, Nimnual A, et al. Requirement of JNK for stress-induced activation of the cytochrome c-mediated death pathway. *Science 2000* 2000;288:870–874.
79. Krasilnikov MA. Phosphatidylinositol-3 kinase dependent pathways: the role in control of cell growth, survival, and malignant transformation. *Biochemistry (Mosc)* 2000;65:59–67.
80. Mulder KM. Role of Ras and Mapks in TGFbeta signaling. *Cytokine Growth Factor Rev* 2000;11:23–35.
81. Polakis P. Wnt signaling and cancer. *Genes Dev* 2000;14:1837–1851.
82. Behrens J. Control of beta-catenin signaling in tumor development. *Ann NY Acad Sci* 2000;910:21–33.

83. Booth DR. The hedgehog signalling pathway and its role in basal cell carcinoma. *Cancer Metastasis Rev* 1999;18:261–284.
84. Matise MP, Joyner AL. Gli genes in development and cancer. *Oncogene* 1999;18:7852–7859.
85. Wicking C, Smyth I, Bale A. The hedgehog signalling pathway in tumorigenesis and development. *Oncogene* 1999;18:7844–7851.
86. Ruiz. Gli proteins and Hedgehog signaling: development and cancer. *Trends Genet* 1999;15:418–425.
87. Hahn H, Wojnowski L, Miller G, Zimmer A. The patched signaling pathway in tumorigenesis and development: lessons from animal models. *J Mol Med* 1999;77:459–468.
88. Artavanis-Tsakonas S, Rand MD, Lake RJ. Notch signaling: cell fate control and signal integration in development. *Science* 1999;284:770–776.
89. Jang M-S, Zlobin A, Miele L. Notch signaling as a target in multimodality cancer therapy. *Curr Opin Mol Ther* 2000;2:55–65.
90. Zlobin A, Jang M-S, Miele L. Toward the rational design of cell fate modifiers: Notch signaling as a target for novel biopharmaceuticals. *Curr Pharm Biotechnol* 2000;1:83–106.
91. Deftos ML, He Y-W, Ojata EW, Bevan MJ. Correlating Notch signaling with thymocyte maturation. *Immunity* 1998;9:777–786.
92. Jehn BM, Bielke W, Pear WS, Osborne BA. Protective effects of notch-1 on TCR-induced apoptosis. *J Immunol* 1999;162:635–638.
93. Shelly LL, Fuchs C, Miele L. Notch-1 prevents apoptosis in murine erythroleukemia cells and is necessary for differentiation induced by hybrid polar drugs. *J Cell Biochem* 1999; 73:164–175.
94. Miele L, Osborne B. Arbiter of differentiation and death: Notch signaling meets apoptosis. *J Cell Physiol* 1999;181:393–409.
95. Osborne B, Miele L. Notch and the immune system. *Immunity.* 1999; 11:653-663.
96. Milner LA, Bigas A. Notch as a mediator of cell fate determination in hematopoiesis: evidence and speculation. *Blood* 1999; 93:2431-2448.
97. Perou CM, Sorlie T, Eisen MB, van de Rijn M, Jeffrey SS, Rees CA, et al. Molecular portraits of human breast tumours. *Nature* 2000; 406:747-752.
98. Alizadeh AA, Eisen MB, Davis RE, Ma C, Lossos IS, Rosenwald A, et al. Distinct types of diffuse large B-cell lymphoma identified by gene expression profiling. *Nature* 2000; 403:503–511.
99. Leethanakul C, Patel V, Gillespie J, Pallente M, Ensley JF, Koontongkaew S, et al. Distinct pattern of expression of differentiation and growth-related genes in squamous cell carcinomas of the head and neck revealed by the use of laser capture microdissection and cDNA arrays. *Oncogene* 2000;19:3220–3224.
100. Carlisle AJ, Prabhu VV, Elkahloun A, Hudson J, Trent JM, Linehan WM, et al. Development of a prostate cDNA microarray and statistical gene expression analysis package. *Mol Carcinog* 2000;28:12–22.
101. VonEggeling F, Davies H, Lomas L, Fiedler W, Junker K, Claussen U, et al. Tissue-specific microdissection coupled with ProteinChip array technologies: applications in cancer research. *Biotechniques* 2000;29:1066–1070.
102. Hahn WC, Counter CM, Lundberg AS, Beijersbergen RL, Brooks MW, Weinberg RA. Creation of human tumour cells with defined genetic elements. *Nature* 1999;400:464–468.
103. Celis JE, Kruhoffer M, Gromova I, Frederiksen C, Ostergaard M, Thykjaer T, et al. Gene expression profiling: monitoring transcription and translation products using DNA microarrays and proteomics. *FEBS Lett* 2000;480:2–16.
104. Marx J. Medicine. DNA arrays reveal cancer in its many forms. *Science* 2000;289:1670–1672.
105. Harkin DP. Uncovering functionally relevant signaling pathways using microarray-based expression profiling. *Oncologist* 2000;5:501–507.
106. Butte AJ, Tamayo P, Slonim D, Golub TR, Kohane IS. Discovering functional relationships between RNA expression and chemotherapeutic susceptibility using relevance networks. *Proc Natl Acad Sci USA* 2000;97:12182–12186.

107. Butte AJ, Kohane IS. Mutual information relevance networks: functional genomic clustering using pairwise entropy measurements. *Pac Symp Biocomput* 2000;418–429.
108. Stebbing J, Copson E, O'Reilly S. Herceptin (trastuzamab) in advanced breast cancer. *Cancer Treat Rev* 2000;26:287–290.
109. Green MC, Murray JL, Hortobagyi GN. Monoclonal antibody therapy for solid tumors. *Cancer Treat Rev* 2000;26:269–286.
110. Bridges AJ. The rationale and strategy used to develop a series of highly potent, irreversible, inhibitors of the epidermal growth factor receptor family of tyrosine kinases. *Curr Med Chem* 1999;6:825–843.
111. O'Dwyer ME, Druker BJ. Status of bcr-abl tyrosine kinase inhibitors in chronic myelogenous leukemia. *Curr Opin Oncol* 2000;12:594–597.
112. Thiesing JT, Ohno-Jones S, Kolibaba KS, Druker BJ. Efficacy of STI571, an abl tyrosine kinase inhibitor, in conjunction with other antileukemic agents against bcr-abl-positive cells. *Blood* 2000;96:3195–3199.

6 CDK Inhibitors as Targets of Chemoprevention Agents

Joanna K. Sax, BS and
Wafik S. El-Deiry, MD, PhD

CONTENTS

1. INTRODUCTION

Chemoprevention is a promising approach in the use of natural or synthetic compounds to inhibit neoplastic development prior to or during the preneoplastic period. The goal of chemopreventive drug development is to identify safe and effective chemopreventive agents for clinical use *(1)*. Agents with chemopreventive potential are tested in preclinical toxicity and pharmacokinetic studies and then moved forward to Phase I, II, and III clinical trials *(1)*. Although many drugs may not prevent cancer completely, delaying the onset of cancer for 15–20 years may significantly increase the standard of living for an individual. For example, delaying the onset of cancer from age 55–70 or 75 provides a large window of prevention in a person's life and therefore warrants the investigation

From: *Cancer Drug Discovery and Development:*
Cell Cycle Inhibitors in Cancer Therapy: Current Strategies
Edited by: A. Giordano and K. J. Soprano © Humana Press Inc., Totowa, NJ

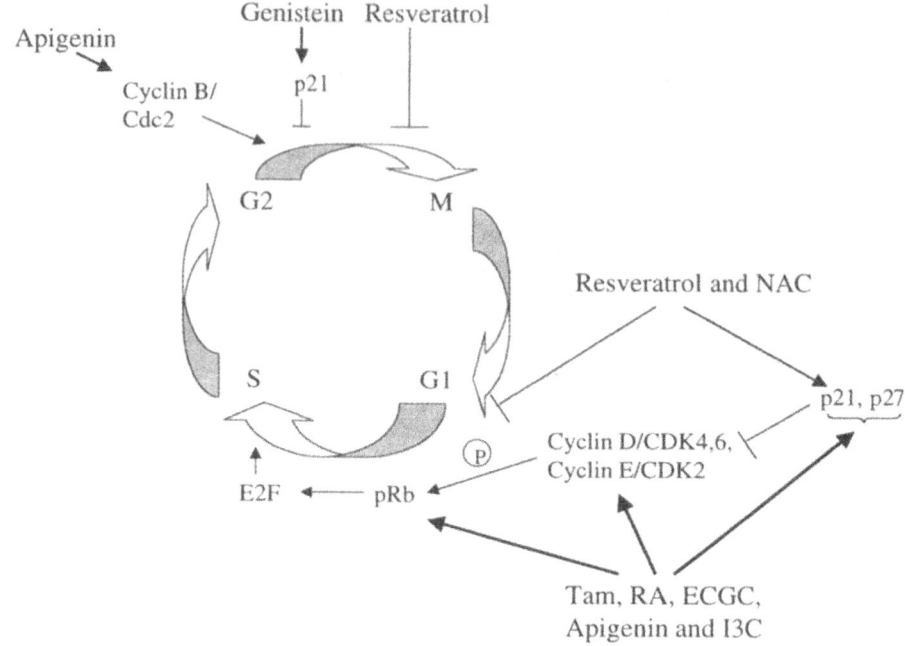

Fig. 1. Potential cell cycle targets of various chemopreventive agents. Shown schemati-
cally is the mammalian cell cycle with phases as indicated (G_1, S, G_2, and M). The
components regulating cell cycle transition include: E2F, pRb protein, cyclin D/CDK4,6
complexes, cyclin E/CDK2 complexes, cyclin B/Cdc2 complexes, and negative regulators of the CIP/KIP and Ink4 families. Chemopreventive agents appear to target various
regulators at critical junctions. Tamoxifen (Tam), Retinoic Acid (RA), Indole-3-Carbinol
(I3C), and Apigenin appear to target pRb protein phosphorylation, CDK kinase activity,
expression of various G_1 cyclins and CDKs (*see* Table 1) and expression of p21 and p27.
The effect of Apigenin on p27 has not yet been examined; however, apigenin also appears
to affect cyclin B/cdc2 at the G_2/M transition. Resveratrol and N-acetyl-cysteine (NAC)
appear to induce a G_1 arrest and to target p21. NAC also targets p16. Resveratrol also
induces a G_2 arrest. Genistein appears to induce a G_2 arrest and affect p21 expression.

of novel approaches into the efficacy of chemopreventive agents. Although
current investigations into the targets of many chemopreventive agents spans a
diverse range of cellular functions such as, inhibition of ras oncogene, epidermal
growth factor receptor (EGFR), angiogenesis, and many more *(2)*; for the purposes of this chapter, we are going to focus on agents that target components
involved in cell proliferation and differentiation.

2. CDK INHIBITORS, CELL CYCLE, AND CANCER

In mammalian cells, the cell cycle is regulated by a number of related enzymes
that possess kinase activity, known as cyclin-dependent kinases (CDKs). The

activity of each CDK is modulated by its interaction with both cell-cycle specific cyclins and CDK inhibitors (CDKI). When CDKs are active in G1, they can phosphorylate the product of the tumor-suppressor retinoblastoma gene (pRb), which subsequently releases the pRb protein from its binding partner, E2F, which can then activate transcription of genes important in cell cycle progression (Fig. 1).

The progression of cells from G_1 to S is a tightly coordinated system that is regulated by the interaction of CDKs with a G_1 specific cyclin or CDKI. There are two families of CDKIs, Ink4, and CIP/KIP. The Ink4 family consists of p16, p15, p18, and p19. p21, p27, and p57 are members of the CIP/KIP family. In response to DNA damage, CDKI expression is upregulated and cell cycle progression is delayed until the DNA is repaired and the cell can then resume progression through the cell cycle. The regulated delay of the cell cycle at a checkpoint or the induction of apoptosis if the damage cannot be repaired is required to inhibit the selection and uncontrolled proliferation of aberrant cells. Cells that are able to escape these regulatory mechanisms may survive and potentially cause cancer (reviewed in McDonald and El-Deiry (2000) and Ozoren and El-Deiry (2000)) *(3,4)*. Therefore, the discovery and development of novel chemopreventive drugs that specifically target CDKIs may provide a novel approach to containing the proliferation of pre-neoplastic cells before they are able to cause tumorigenesis.

3. TAMOXIFEN

Perhaps the most well-known chemopreventive agent, Tamoxifen (Tam) is used for the prevention of breast cancer, as well as other types of cancer. Tam, a nonsteroidal antiestrogen, is a competitive inhibitor of estradiol *(5)*. Originally synthesized by Imperial Chemical Industries PLC as an antifertility drug, its antiestrogenic properties facilitated the development of Tam in the treatment of breast cancer *(5,6)*. Breast cancer is a major burden worldwide and the most common cancer affecting women in developed countries *(7)*. The need to prevent and treat breast cancer led to the development of a randomized clinical trial to evaluate the effectiveness of Tam as a chemopreventive agent for women who are at increased risk for the disease *(8)*. The National Surgical Adjuvant Breast and Bowel Project chemopreventive trial found that administration of Tam for at least five years decreased the incidence of invasive and noninvasive breast cancer *(8)*.

The known efficacy of Tamoxifen as an anti-cancer agent has prompted many researchers to address Tam in the treatment of several types of cancer and develop laboratory models to begin to look at the putative cellular mechanisms. Long-term Tam administration was found to suppress stimulation of mouse mammary tumorigenesis by progesterone and be more effective than ovariectomy in mice

(9). In radiation-induced mammary carcinomas, administration of tamoxifen suppressed the emergence of mammary tumors in rats *(10)*. The ability to show suppressive effects of Tamoxifen in a mouse model *(9)* and rat models where mammary tumorigenesis is induced by radiation or carcinogens *(10–12)* provides possible ways to try to understand the cellular and molecular mechanisms behind breast tumorigenesis and the role of tamoxifen in prevention and treatment.

In vitro studies using cell lines derived from patients with hormone-dependent breast cancer have shown variable effects depending on the concentration of Tam used in each study *(5,13–15)*. A cytostatic effect has been observed using low concentrations of Tam on estrogen receptor positive cells where the cells arrested in early G_1 of the cell cycle, whereas at higher concentrations a cytotoxic effect, characterized by cell death, was observed in both estrogen receptor positive and negative cells *(5)*. Changes in the cell cycle components that act in G_1 have been associated with changes in proliferation rates in both normal and transformed mammary epithelial cells *(16)*. The activation of CDKs in G_1 by binding to their respective cyclins activates the kinase activity of the CDK and leads to subsequent phosphorylation of specific substrates and cell cycle progression. The abundance of G_1 cyclins and CDKIs govern the cell cycle progression. Because Tam was seen to arrest cells at G_1, the natural sequence of events is to attempt to determine the molecular mechanism behind the cell cycle arrest.

Interestingly, Tam has been shown to cause a G_1 arrest in both estrogen receptor positive (ER) positive and ER negative cells. Tamoxifen has been shown to cause a G_1 arrest in ER positive MCF-7 cells and Western blots did not reveal a change in protein expression level of CDK 2, 4, 6, Cyclin D_1 and E, and p21. However, treatment with Tam caused a decrease in Retinoblastoma (Rb) protein level and an increase in the relative levels of hypophosphorylated Rb *(17)*. Cover et al. (1999) found a decrease on CDK2 specific activity with increasing concentrations of Tam, which may account for the hypophosphorylated state of Rb *(17)*. Although still unclear, a cell cycle component may be causing the decrease in CDK2 activity, which could be a CDKI besides p21, that is, an as of yet unidentified target of Tam.

The mechanism for Tam's activity on ER negative cells remains unclear. Tam appears to inhibit protein kinase C in a dose-dependent manner *(18)*, modulate the activity of phospholipases and lipid signaling pathways *(19)*, inhibit calmodulin-dependent cAMP phosphodiesterase *(20)*, retard glycosphingolipid metabolism *(21)*, and increase expression of transforming growth factor-β (TGF-β) *(22)*, all of which may impact on cell growth or cell proliferation. Lee et al. (1999) *(23)* used ER negative lung cancer cells to study the ER independent effect of Tamoxifen on the cell cycle. They found that Tam induced a G_1 growth arrest in these cells and that G_1 cyclin expression and G_1 CDK expression was unaltered (except CDK2 expression in H322 cells was attenuated). However, the expression of CDKIs, p21 and p27, were strongly activated in the ER-negative cells. Tam treatment induced G_1 arrest with a corresponding increase in CDKI expression associated with increase cyclin/CDK/CDKI complex formation, reduction of CDK activity, and accumulation of hypophosphorylated Rb protein *(23)*. To further elucidate the molecular mechanism of Tamoxifen's role in G1 arrest in ER negative tumor cells, Lee et al. *(24)* used deletion analysis and found an Sp1 binding site in the p21 promoter region that is important for Tam's trans- activation. The authors hypothesize that perhaps Tam enhances the transcrip- tional activity of Sp1 or Sp3 to p21 expression, possibly by phosphorylation of these ubiquitous transcription factors *(24)*. The Sp1 transcription factor has been previously shown to be phosphorylated and activated in response to epidermal growth factor (EGF) receptor activation *(25)*. This may suggest that perhaps Tam activates the mitogen-activated protein kinase (MAPK) cascade, which can lead to phosphorylation of Sp1; however, Lee et al. showed that inhibition of MAPK- related kinases with chemical inhibitors does not attenuate Tam induced p21 expression *(24)*. Future studies in this area are needed to delineate the putative signaling pathway induced by treatment with Tam, leading to activation of Sp1 or other targets and upregulation of p21.

One important question that remains is why p21 is upregulated upon treatment with tamoxifen in certain cell types and whether expression of the ER may be inhibiting upregulation of p21. Additionally, what is the response of cell lines or tissues that are p21 null to treatment with Tamoxifen. Moreover, the regulated expression of other CIP/KIP and Ink4 family members in response to tamoxifen treatment should be addressed in studies using cell lines that are ER-positive and -negative.

4. RETINOIDS

Retinoic Acid (RA) is a metabolite of vitamin A and it has been known for 75 years that vitamin A deficiency in the rat model causes distinct effects on both cell proliferation and differentiation *(26)*. Because cancer is a problem of both cell differentiation and cell proliferation, it is no wonder that RA has made its way to being tested for chemopreventive measures. Clinical trials over the past 20 years have shown that RAs have been effective in controlling progression of early carcinogenesis *(27)*. RAs have been shown to be effective in treating promyelocytic leukemia, oral premalignant lesions, squamous cell carcinoma of the head and neck, and certain skin cancers *(27–32)*. Controlling cell prolifera- tion and differentiation through the use of natural agents may be an important way to manage cancer rather than using drugs that primarily kill cells and are very toxic to the individual *(26)*.

The two issues for use of RA in chemoprevention are the practical develop- ment of retinoids in prevention and treatment of cancer and determining the molecular mechanism underlying RAs inhibition of carcinogenesis *(26)*. The efficacy of using retinoids in cancer chemoprevention can be tested in a variety of ways in the laboratory through cellular and molecular techniques.

Trans Retinoic Acid and its stereoisomer, 9-*cis* RA, have been shown to have profound effects on cell growth and proliferation of human hematopoetic cells, as well as other cell types *(33–35)*. All-*trans* RA inhibits cell growth and induces cell differentiation in human myeloma cell lines as well as cells from patients with acute promyelocytic leukemia (APL) *(33,36–40)*. However, the mechanism promoting cell differentiation and inhibiting cell growth has remained unclear. Treatment of human myeloma cell lines with trans RA down regulated expression of interleukin-6 (IL-6) receptor expression, which is a major growth factor receptor in myeloma cells *(41,42)*. Chen et al. *(39)* tried to rescue the growth arrest phenotype caused by treatment with trans RA by overexpressing IL-6Rα in OPM-2 human myeloma cells. Treatment with RA actually enhanced expression of IL-6Rα in the transfectants. However, the clonogenic growth of the IL-6Rα transfectants remained inhibited by treatment with trans RA. Surprisingly, addition of exogenous IL-6 failed to overcome the growth arrest effects caused by trans RA. These data suggest that RA mediated growth arrest is not mediated solely through the IL-6R, but through additional pathways *(39)*. To investigate the post retinoic acid receptor pathway and the role of cell cycle components, Chen et al. *(39)* found that incubation with trans RA caused dephosphorylation of the retinoblastoma protein in OPM-2 cells. Additionally, expression of p21 increased after a 24-h exposure to trans RA, while the protein levels of CDK2, CDK4, and p27 remained unchanged *(39)*. The dephosphorylation of Rb and the increased expression of p21 are consistent with the finding that treatment with trans RA causes a G_1 arrest in OPM-2 cells. These results do not rule out the possibility that the IL-6 pathway may in some way be related to p21 expression, however, that hypothesis remains to be tested.

Incubation of cells of hematopoetic origin with trans RA induces G_1 arrest, upregulation of p21 expression, and dephosphorylation of pRb. However, it is important to elucidate the pathway leading to these events. In an elegant study, Naderi and Blomhoff (1999) *(43)* addressed the mechanisms underlying the growth inhibitory effects of retinoids on human B-lymphocytes. Human B cells were stimulated into mid to late G_1 by anti-IgM antibodies and then treated with retinoic acid. Treatment with retinoic acid was shown to inhibit Rb phosphorylation, decrease CDK activity, and increase the association of p21 with CDK2, transiently increase the expression of p21, and increase mRNA levels of cyclin E, cyclin A, and p21 *(43)*. Treatment of the B cells with Ro13-7410 (TTNPB), a RAR-selective agonist, mimicked the key events affected by treatment with trans RA, i.e., inhibited both pRb phosphorylation and cyclin E expression and induced a transient increase in p21 levels. However, treatment of B cells with the RARa antagonist, Ro 41-5253, prevented the RA-mediated inhibition of pRb phosphorylation and induction of p21. These studies imply that RA mediates

Table 1
Structure and Possible Cell Cycle Targets of Various Chemopreventive Agents*

Name	Structure	Possible Targets[#]
Tamoxifen		G1 arrest, pRb, CDK2 kinase activity, p21, and p27
All trans Retinoic Acid		G1 arrest, pRb, CDK activity, association of p21 and CDK2, p21, p27, cyclin E and A
Genistein		G2 arrest p21
Resveratrol		G1 and G2 arrest, p21, bax
Apigenin		G1 and G2 arrest, cyclin B/Cdc2, CDK2 kinase activity, cyclin D1, pRb, and p21
(–)–Epigallocatechin gallate		G1 arrest, pRb, CDK 2 & 4 kinase activity, p21, and p27
Indole-3-Carbinol		G1 arrest, Cdk6, pRb, p21, and p27
N-acetyl-L-cysteine		G1 arrest, p16, and p21

*There are targets, in addition to cell cycle components, that these compounds may affect.
#See text for references.

growth inhibition on B cells through the nuclear receptors *(43)*. Significantly, patients with APL carry a 15:17 chromosomal translocation that fuses RARa (on chromosome 17) to PML, a transcription factor (on chromosome 15) *(44–46)*. The fusion protein, PML-RAR, may interfere with promyelocytic differentiation possibly by behaving as a dominant negative oncogene in the nonliganded state *(45,46)*. Therefore, treatment with RA may relieve this inhibition by possibly promoting myelocyte differentiation *(45)*. In fact, treatment of APL patients with trans RA can achieve remission for some time *(47,48)*. Clearly, elucidating the upstream components of RAs inhibition of the cell cycle is important to piece together the puzzle of how and why RA may inhibit cell proliferation and cell differentiation and may be very beneficial in the treatment of APL patients.

Interestingly, treatment with RA induces expression of cyclin E, cyclin A, and p21 in B cells and it is important to address the molecular mechanisms responsible for RAs role in transcriptional regulation of the cell cycle machinery (Fig. 1 and Table 1). Treatment of the myelomonocytic cell line, U937, with trans RA induces p21 mRNA and protein expression *(44)*. Using p21 promoter/reporter fusions transiently transfected into human keratinocyte HaCaT cells, which are readily transfected and are p53 null, Liu et al. *(44)* found transcriptional activation of p21 fusions in response to treatment with trans RA. Using deletion constructs, visual scans and in vitro gel mobility shift assays, Liu et al. were able to determine a retinoic acid response element (RARE), in the p21 promoter *(44)*. RARE are composed of direct repeats of the core AGGTCA half-site spaced by 5 nucleotides, whereas other hormone response elements for the vitamin D receptor and thyroid hormone receptor are composed of the direct repeats spaced by 3 or 4 nucleotides, respectively (reviewed in Mangelsdorf and Evans [1995]) *(49)*. Liu et al. showed that purified RAR and RXR can bind to RARE and complexes containing RARs are also able to bind selectively to the RARE in the p21 promoter *(44)*. Therefore, RAs-mediated growth arrest followed by lymphocyte differentiation may be mediated by the induction of p21, through both signaling pathways and transcriptional activation.

Retinoic acid also affects cells of nonlymphoid origin. For example, treatment of the human lung squamous carcinoma cell line, CH27, with RA mediates a time- and dose-dependent growth arrest in G_1 *(50)*. The RA-mediated G_1 arrest is associated with increase in protein levels of RARb and the cell cycle inhibitor, p27. Hsu et al. hypothesized that reduction of CDK2 kinase activity and induction of p27 causes the G_1 arrest *(50)*. Additionally, the growth of cultured gastric cell lines was inhibited by treatment with 9-*cis*-RA and the growth arrest was accompanied by a transient induction of p21 expression *(51)*. Interestingly, the growth of the MKN-7 gastric cell line, which does not transcribe RARs or RXR-a, was not inhibited by treatment with 9-*cis*-RA *(51)*. Retinoic acid has also been shown to inhibit cell cycle progression in MCF-7 human breast cancer cells by reducing expression of specific cell cycle regulatory proteins such as cyclin D3,

CDK4, pRb protein, E2F1, and p21 and there was not an induction of p16 or p27 expression (Fig. 1 and Table 1) *(52)*. Clearly, understanding the molecular mechanisms of RA-mediated growth arrest may further aid efforts to prevent or treat many forms of malignancies.

5. GENISTEIN

Epidemiological studies have shown that cultures with diets rich in soy products have a lower incidence/mortality rate in certain types of cancer *(53–55)*. Genistein is an isoflavone that occurs naturally in soy products *(56)*. Recent studies looking at the action of purified isoflavones on several types of established cancer cell lines found genistein to exert chemopreventive as well as chemotherapeutic benefits *(57–59)*.

Genistein is believed to possess potential chemopreventive effects in a variety of ways. When administered to prepubertal rats, genistein decreased the formation of 7, 12-dimethylbenzanthracene (DMBA) induced mammary tumors, possibly by facilitating the differentiation of terminal buds to lobules *(55,60,61)*. Genistein also appears to possess chemopreventive activity in prostate cancer; although the mechanism is unclear, it is believed that genistein may generally decrease androgen levels in men *(62,63)*. Genistein also appears to have hormone-independent effects, such as inhibition of protein tyrosine kinase activity *(64,65)*, eukaryotic DNA topoisomerase II activity *(66)*, reactive oxygen species (ROS) formation *(67,68)*, and induction of apoptosis and cell cycle arrest *(58,69–71)*. Although much work has examined possible mechanisms of action genistein exerts on cell proliferation and differentiation, for the purposes of this chapter we will focus on the cell cycle and cell death controls. However, it should be mentioned that the many pathways genistein effects undoubtedly may be connected to expression and inhibition of certain cell cycle-regulatory components.

The efficacy of genistein in chemoprevention has been tested in rodent models. The induction of mammary cancer in rats using the DMBA carcinogen is a powerful model to study both chemopreventive and chemotherapeutic effects of various agents. It has been shown in the DMBA rat model that virgin rats are more susceptible to the effects of DMBA than multiparous rats *(72–74)*. It is thought that the maturation of the terminal end buds to lobules in the mammary gland as a result of each complete pregnancy offers protection against chemical carcinogenesis, explaining why virgin rats have a higher incidence of carcinomas *(73,75,76)*. Lamatiniere et al. *(56)* treated rats with genistein the first week postpartum, before exposure to DMBA, to determine whether genistein exerts chemopreventive benefits at this stage in development. This study found that not only did treatment with genistein suppress mammary carcinogenesis, but that genistein-treated animals showed enhanced maturation of terminal ductal structure and reduced cell proliferation in the mammary gland through an altered endocrine system *(56)*. Interestingly, urine is a significant route for the excretion of many isoflavones *(77)*. Therefore, a recent study by Zhou et al. (1998) looked at the effects of soy isoflavones, particularly genistein, on bladder cancer. Using a syngeneic murine model, the MB49 bladder carcinoma was used in C57BL/6J mice. Mice with genistein supplementation showed reduced tumor proliferation and increased tumor cell apoptosis compared to control animals *(58)*. Both the DMBA rat and bladder mouse models beg the question of what is happening at the cellular and molecular level. These data suggest genistein may be involved in both cell differentiation and proliferation and warrants further studies into the molecular mechanisms associated with cellular control.

Tumor cell lines are an effective way to study the effect of genistein on cell proliferation and apoptosis at the cellular and molecular level. In 1993, Matsukawa and colleagues looked at the effect of genistein on cell cycle progression. This study analyzed the cell cycle progression and kinetics of a human gastric cancer cell line and found a G_2/M arrest upon treatment with genistein that was reversible upon removal of the isoflavone *(71)*. The Matsukawa study was published the same year that the discovery of p21 and its role in cell cycle inhibition was published; however, this group did not look at the effect on CDKIs associated with the G_2/M arrest. Although genistein was shown to inhibit proliferation and effect tyrosine signaling pathways in cell lines *(71,78)*, an examination of the effect of treatment with genistein directly on cell cycle components was not addressed until several years later. Shao and colleagues showed that genistein causes a G_2/M arrest in both ER positive and ER negative breast cancer cell lines and this inhibition in cell cycle associated with the induction of p21 expression in a p53-independent manner. Additionally, increasing time and dose treatment with genistein induced apoptosis in all breast cancer cell lines treated *(69)*. These data suggest that genistein has cytostatic properties at lower concentrations and cytotoxic properties at higher concentrations.

After showing that genistein has anti-proliferative actions on breast cancer cells, Shao et al. (1998) went on to show that treatment of MCF-7 and MDA-MB-231 cells with genistein inhibited in vitro invasion of these cells. Additionally, in xenograft studies with these breast cancer cell lines, genistein inhibited tumor growth, induced p21 expression, and stimulated apoptosis (Fig. 1) *(70)*. The anti-invasive effects of genistein may be attributed to regulation of extracellular matrix (ECM) proteases and their inhibitors, which are implicated in tumor invasion and metastasis *(69)*. Genistein also induced the expression of p21 in the xenograft models; however, it is not clear whether this induction is related causally to apoptosis *(70)*.

Genistein is yet another example of a compound found in the diet of cultures that have a lower incidence of specific cancers. However, it should be noted that treatment with genistein in a colon cancer rat model caused an increase in colon tumor incidence *(79)*. Additionally, there is much work left to be done to determine the mechanism of action genistein exerts on many areas of cell growth.

6. RESVERATROL

Resveratrol (3,5,4'-trihydroxystilbene) occurs naturally in a variety of plants including grapes, peanuts, and pine nuts. Classified as an antibiotic of plant origin, its role in plant physiology seems to be as an anti-fungal agent and is produced by plants as a defense mechanism *(80)*. Human consumption of resveratrol is believed to predominantly come from red wine. Recent studies have addressed the association of moderate wine consumption with protection from heart disease. It is thought resveratrol may be protective against oxidation of lipoproteins *(81)*, inhibit platelet aggregation, and alter eicosanoid synthesis *(80)*. Additionally, resveratrol is thought to possess chemopreventive activity by inhibiting events associated with cancer progression *(82)*.

Resveratrol, along with other anti-inflammatory agents such as aspirin, indomethacin, piroxicam, and sulindac, possess the ability to inhibit cyclo-oxygenase (COX) *(82–84)*. COX inhibition is important in chemoprevention because the products of COX catalysis can stimulate cell growth and suppress the immune system *(82,85)*. Resveratrol was identified as a potent inhibitor of COX, and its activity is specific to COX-1 *(82)*.

Based on the findings that resveratrol may be involved in the inhibition of events required for tumor initiation, Jang et al. (1997) studied the effects of resveratrol in the carrageenan-induced model of inflammation in rats. Treatment with resveratrol significantly reduced pedal edema in both the acute and chronic phases *(82)*. Based on the potential of resveratrol to inhibit tumor promotion, Jang et al. (1997) also showed that treatment with resveratrol effects events associated with tumor initiation, such as inhibition of free-radical formation, an antimutagenic effect, and induction of quinone reductase activity (which can detoxify carcinogens) *(82)*.

The potential of resveratrol's chemopreventive activity has been addressed in cultured mouse mammary gland and animal models. Administration of resveratrol, to a mouse mammary gland culture model of carcinogenesis, inhibited the development of DMBA-induced preneoplastic lesions, suggesting that resveratrol may prevent the initiation of tumor formation *(82)*. In a two-stage mouse skin cancer model, application of resveratrol in a dose-dependent manner during promotion, reduced skin carcinogenesis *(82)*. Moreover, no signs of toxicity were observed in these studies. To test the effect of resveratrol in an already established rat tumor model, Carbo et al. *(86)* administered resveratrol to rats bearing the Yoshida AH-130 ascites hepatoma, a fast-growing tumor. Treatment of these rats with resveratrol lowered tumor growth and analysis of the tumors showed a slight accumulation in G_2/M phase of the cell cycle *(86)*. The effect of resveratrol in rodent models of both chemoprevention and chemotherapeutic warrants further study into the mode of action at the cellular level.

The structure of resveratrol is similar to the synthetic estrogen diethylstilbestrol. Therefore, recent studies have investigated whether resveratrol may function through the estrogen receptor. Gehm et al. (1997) reported that not only can resveratrol bind to the estrogen receptor, but also it functions as an agonist for ER-mediated transcription. Using a luciferase reporter assay with an estrogen-response element upstream of the thymidine kinase promoter, resveratrol produced dose-dependent transcriptional activation in MCF-7 ER positive cells (87). This transcriptional activation could be inhibited by estrogen agonists. Moreover, the transcriptional activation of estrogen responsive constructs was likely dependent on the presence of the estrogen receptor because the effect was not observed in the ER-negative cell line MDA-MB-231 (87). However, this study did not address additional potential cellular effects besides ER responsiveness in the ER-negative cell line.

Lu and Serrero (88) reported that resveratrol behaves as an ER antagonist in the presence of estrogen and thereby inhibits the growth of human breast cancer cells. Resveratrol inhibited the growth of MCF-7 cells in a dose-dependent manner (88). However, when MCF-7 cells were grown in estrogen-depleted PFMEM media, resveratrol acted as a weak growth stimulator, but in the presence of estrogen, resveratrol antagonized the growth-stimulatory effect of estrogen (88). These studies show that resveratrol does indeed bind to the ER and that in the absence of estrogen, resveratrol behaves as a partial agonist; however, in the presence of estrogen, resveratrol behaves as an antagonist. The molecular mechanisms and functions of these behaviors will require future studies.

Resveratrol is able to exert its anti-cancer effects on cell lines other than human breast. Treatment of human prostate cancer cell lines with resveratrol inhibits cell growth (89). Specifically, a disruption in the transition between G_1 and S phase of the cell cycle was seen in three androgen-nonresponsive prostate cancer cell lines and apoptosis was observed in the androgen-responsive LNCap cell line, upon resveratrol treatment (89). Interestingly, treatment with resveratrol resulted in a progressive reduction in both intracellular and secreted PSA in all cell lines tested (89) and future studies will address the effect of resveratrol on PSA.

Previous studies have established that treatment with resveratrol either inhibits the establishment of tumors or also causes growth arrest in both animal models and tumor cell lines. Therefore, Tessitore et al. (2000) investigated the expression of two genes involved in cell proliferation and apoptosis, p21 and bax, in an azoxymethane-induced colon carcinogenesis model. Resveratrol was administered to the rats through drinking water before carcinogen treatment. Aberrant crypt foci (ACF) were isolated and analyzed for the cell cycle genes, p21 and bax. Treatment with resveratrol caused an enhancement of bax expression in the ACF, but not in the surrounding mucosa, suggesting enhanced apoptosis contributes to reduced growth of the foci *(90)*. p21 expression was found in all ACF in both control and resveratrol-treated rats. Surprisingly, p21 expression was not detected in the non-ACF mucosa in resveratrol treated animal while p21 expression was found in all the non-ACF mucosa in control rats. The authors hypothesized that the loss of p21 expression in resveratrol treated rats may give pre-neoplastic lesions a growth disadvantage because cells lacking p21 have been reported to undergo apoptosis in response to DNA damaging agents *(90,91)*.

Resveratrol has a promising future as a chemopreventive agent given its ease of consumption, low toxicity, and recent findings as an anti-cancer agent in laboratory models. However, many questions remain as to the cellular and molecular mechanisms by which it works. The evidence that resveratrol is able to inhibit cell proliferation warrants the characterization of the cell cycle machinery and in particular, CDKIs as potential targets.

7. FLAVANOIDS

Flavanoids naturally occur in plants and vegetables and have been shown to have chemopreventive benefits in laboratory models. Three examples of flavanoids studied in the prevention of cancer are grape polyphenols, apigenin, and Epigallocatechin-3-gallate (EGCG).

Grapes are rich in polyphenols, with approx 60–70% of the polyphenols in the seeds *(92)*. The polyphenols in the grape seeds are flavan–3-ol derivatives *(92,93)*. These are a different class of derivatives than the previously discussed resveratrol, which is a trihydroxy-stilbene *(93)*.

A study by Damianaki et al. (2000) tested four compounds found in red wine thought to possess antiproliferative activity. Three of the four compounds were the flavanoids: catechin, epicatechin, and quercetin, with the fourth compound, resveratrol. Treatment of both ER-positive and ER-negative breast cancer cell lines with each compound showed varying results. All three flavanoids decreased cell proliferation in a dose-dependent manner, with epicatechin the most potent in the three cell lines tested, MCF7, T47D, and MDA-MB-231. Resveratrol had previously been shown to bind to the estrogen receptor, and perhaps the mode of action of the polyphenols on proliferation may act in a similar fashion. However, all three of these polyphenols showed different profiles in binding to the ER in MCF7 and T47D cells, suggesting that the mode of action of these compounds may not only be due to estrogen receptor binding; moreover, they exert antiproliferative activity in ER-negative cells, suggesting multiple modes of action *(93)*.

Polyphenols found in grape seeds can modulate anti-tumor behavior in some cancer models. In the DMBA initiated, TPA promoted SENCAR mouse skin two-stage carcinogenesis model, topical application of a grape seed polyphenolic compound significantly inhibited TPA tumor promotion *(92)*. Using high-performance liquid chromatography (HPLC), physiochemical properties, and spectral analysis, polyphenolic fractions from the grape seeds were identified. Five individual polyphenols, catechin, procyanidin B2, procyanidin B5, procyanidin C1, and procyanidin B5-3'-gallate were assessed for antioxidant activity. The inhibition potential towards lipid peroxidation increased with the increased degree in polymerization within the polyphenol structure and the position of linkage between inter-flavin units also influenced lipid peroxidation activity *(92)*. These results show that grape seed polyphenols possess anti-tumor promoting activity in the mouse skin tumorigenesis model and that the activity may be due to anti-oxidant activity. However, the molecular mechanism by which grape seed polyphenols inhibit skin tumorigenesis remains to be elucidated.

Recent evidence suggests that treatment of prostate cancer cells, DU145, with grape seed polyphenolic fraction (GSP) modulates mitogenic signaling, induces G_1 arrest and apoptosis in both a time- and dose-dependent manner *(94)*. Treatment of DU145 with GSP inhibited the activation of ERK1/2, which are MAPK extracellular signal-regulated protein kinases that are thought to be constitutively active in human prostate carcinomas. Moreover treatment with GSP resulted in a significant induction of p21, a decrease in CDK4 protein expression, a G_1 cell cycle arrest, and induction of apoptotic death *(94)*. It appears that GSP has cytostatic effects at lower concentrations by inducing growth arrest, while it has cytotoxic effects at higher concentrations by inducing apoptosis. Future studies need to be directed at the mechanism by which cell cycle arrest is induced and define how the apoptotic pathway is modulated.

Green and black tea are another source for flavanoids. Like the polyphenolic fractions isolated from grape seeds, tea contains the polyphenol epigallocatechin-3-gallate (ECGC) present in the leaves and stems of tea plants. Studies with ECGC derived from tea show it exerts many of the same pharmacological and biochemical properties as those derived from grape seeds. For example, ECGC contains antioxidant activity *(95)*, inhibits mitotic signal transduction through modulation of growth factor receptor binding *(96)*, and induces cell cycle arrest and apoptosis *(97)*.

To investigate the effects of ECGC on cell cycle progression, Liang et al. *(98)* treated MCF-7 breast cancer cells with ECGC and analyzed proteins involved in cell cycle progression and arrest. Treatment with ECGC induced a G_1 arrest that could be characterized by the hypophosphorylation of pRb, inhibition of CDK2 and CDK 4 kinase activity, and induction of p21 and p27 (Fig. 1 and Table 1) *(98)*. Further studies showed that p21 induction occurred through both p53-dependent and -independent pathways *(98)*. These results suggest that ECGC in tea may play an important role in inhibiting growth of tumors and inducing cell cycle arrest in cancer cells. It would be an important study to compare the effects of ECGC on primary cells and tumor cells in tissue culture and determine its pharmacological and biochemical properties in order to have a broader understanding of the potential of ECGC to be used as a chemopreventive agent.

Apigenin is another naturally occurring flavanoid found in fruits and vegetables. Previously, apigenin was shown to significantly inhibit chemical and UV-B light induced skin tumorigenesis in mice when applied topically *(99)*. To investigate the molecular mechanism responsible for inhibition of skin tumorigenesis, mouse skin derived cell lines, C50 and 308, and human HL-60 leukemia cells were cultured in media containing apigenin. A G_2/M arrest was induced upon treatment with apigenin and the mechanism appeared to be due in part to inhibition of the mitotic kinase activity of p34cdc2 and perturbation of cyclin B1 levels (Fig. 1) *(100)*. Additionally, treatment of rat neuronal cells, B104, with apigenin induced a G_2/M arrest. This effect was dose-dependent and reversible when apigenin was removed from the media *(101)*.

More recently, Lepley and Pelling *(102)* have shown that treatment with apigenin can induce a G_1 arrest, in addition to the G_2 arrest previously shown. Treatment of human diploid fibroblasts (HDF) with apigenin caused both a G_1 and G_2 arrest, with the G_1 arrest more clearly defined by using HDF cells first synchronized in G_0 and then released from quiescence. When cells arrested in G_1, they were characterized by a decrease in CDK2 kinase activity, increase in cyclin D_1 levels (which signified that cells were arrested in G_1 and not G_0), hypophosphorylation of pRb in a dose-dependent manner, and a dose-dependent induction of p21 in a p53-dependent manner (Table 1) *(102)*. However, the mechanism by which apigenin increases and decreases expression cell cycle regulatory components remains to be elucidated. A report by Kuo and Yang stated that apigenin may interfere with the MAPK pathway *(103)*. Thus apigenin may exert its effect on the cell cycle through alterations in signal transduction pathways that ultimately impact on cell cycle transitions *(102)*.

Transformation of normal cells to cancer cells involves the loss of checkpoint controls. Perhaps treatment with flavanoids can effect the cell cycle machinery in such a way that normal cells are less likely to lose control of checkpoints and thus serve as beneficial chemopreventive agents.

8. INDOLE-3-CARBINOL

Indole-3-Carbinol (I3C) is a naturally occurring component of cruciferous vegetables such as Brussel sprouts, broccoli, cabbage, and cauliflower. Humans who consume increased quantities of these vegetables have a decreased risk to develop cancer *(104)*. In animal models, I3C has been shown to provide chemopreventive effects by inducing various cytochrome P450 (CYP) isoenzymes that are responsible for the oxidative metabolism of certain carcinogens *(105,106)* and the metabolism of estradiol *(106)*.

In several different rodent mammary tumor models, I3C has been shown to possess chemopreventive effects. In both the DMBA- and methylnitrosourea (MNU)-induced animal models, long-term administration of I3C retarded tumor growth both by fewer tumors and longer latency periods for tumor development as compared to controls without I3C treatment *(105)*. Treatment with I3C induced various drug metabolizing enzymes in the livers of these animals, which could account for the inhibition of DMBA-induced mammary carcinogenesis. However, the results obtained using the direct acting carcinogen, MNU, suggest additional mechanisms for tumor suppression, such as a decrease in serum estrogen levels because mammary tumors induced by MNU are estrogen-responsive *(105)*. Bradlow et al. (1991) addressed whether dietary consumption of I3C altered the incidence of spontaneous mammary tumors in C3H/OuJ mice. I3C consumption significantly decreased mammary tumor incidence in all dose groups and prolonged tumor latency in the high-dose group *(106)*. Moreover, this study determined that dietary intake of I3C in mice increased the cytochrome P450 content in hepatic microsomes and increased estradiol 2-hydroxylation. It is thought the effect of increased 2-hydroxylation may protect the mice from mammary tumors by inactivating endogenous estrogens *(106)*. Estradiol is metabolized via two distinct pathways; one yields 16α-hydroxyesterone, whereas the other pathway yields 2-hydroxyestrone *(107)*. 16α-hydroxyesterone covalently binds to the estrogen receptor and exerts effects similar to estradiol *(107)*. Women who have elevated levels of 16α-hydroxyesterone have been associated with increased risk for breast cancer *(108)*. Attempts to decrease 16α-hydroxylation have been unsuccessful, which have led to efforts to increase the other pathway of estradiol metabolism, 2-hydroxylation *(107)*.

In order to address whether I3C may effect estradiol metabolism, Tiwari et al. *(109)* treated ER positive MCF-7 cells and ER negative MDA-MB-231 with I3C and compared the biochemical events associated with I3C treatment and a relationship, if any, with estrogen responsiveness. Treatment with I3C caused a more pronounced antiproliferative effect on the MCF-7 cells which was associated with a selective increase in the C-2 hydroxylation pathway leading to 2-hydroxylation and the induction of P-4501A1; changes in C-2 hydroxylation and induction of P-4501A1 were not observed in the MDA-MB-231 cells *(109)*. Because these cells were not treated with a carcinogen, the mechanism by which I3C induces C-2 hydroxylation must be an independent characteristic of I3C.

Carcinogenesis is a multistep process that requires early events of initiation, followed by promotion, and then detectable tumorigenesis. Telang et al. *(110)* developed a system to study mammary carcinogenesis by using human mammary epithelial cells, 184-B5, (184-B5 that can be initiated for carcinogenesis by expression of the oncogene HER-2/neu (184-B5/HER) or by treatment with the chemical carcinogen benzo[a]pyrene (BP) (184-B5/BP)). Treatment of 184-B5/BP and 184-B5/HER with I3C decreased cell proliferation, increased the amount of 2-hydroxyesterone, decreased the amount of 16α-hydroxyesterone, and induced apoptosis *(110)*. Based on these results, the decrease in E_2 metabolite ratio appeared to correspond with tumorigenesis *(110)*, however, the molecular mechanism behind the antiproliferative effects of I3C remains to be elucidated.

To study the mechanism by which I3C decreases cell proliferation, Cover et al. *(111)* used MCF-7 and MDA-MB-231 cells to examine the cell cycle machinery in response to I3C treatment. Treatment of MCF-7 cells with I3C induced a G_1 arrest, decreased protein and mRNA levels of CDK6, inhibited the phosphorylation of pRb, and induced expression of p21 and p27 (Fig. 1) *(111)*. Interestingly, treatment of MCF-7 cells with I3C did not effect cell viability or ER responsiveness. Moreover, the same effects on cell cycle arrest and the cell cycle machinery were observed in MDA-MB-231 cells upon treatment with I3C, suggesting that I3C can effect the proliferation of the cell in a previously undefined antiproliferative pathway *(111)*. It is worthy to note that the inhibition of CDK6 expression and kinase activity correlated with the G_1 arrest, while induction of p21 and p27 occurred after the cells began to display their maximal G_1 arrest, which implicates CDK6 as a direct target of I3C and possibly p21 and p27 as secondary targets *(111)*.

Although the molecular mechanisms responsible for the effects of I3C on carcinogenesis remain to be further elucidated, chemoprevention clinical trials with I3C are underway. One clinical trial initially addressed whether the dietary intake of I3C can alter the estrogen metabolite ratio in favor of 2-hydroxyesterone vs. 16α-hydroxyesterone and act in a protective manner to decrease breast cancer incidence *(112)*. Clinical findings revealed that the vast majority of women treated with I3C for 1 mo increased the 2-hydroxyesterone:16α-hydroxyesterone metabolite ratio and the increase was maintained over the 3-mo time period *(112)*. A later study by Wong et al. (1997) aimed to determine a safe dose schedule of I3C that would result in a significant increase in urinary 2-hydroxyesterone to 16α-hydroxyesterone. Results of this study showed that 300 mg of I3C daily oral intake achieved the estrogen metabolite goal with no significant toxicity *(113)*. These clinical trials did not look at the changes in molecular mechanisms induced by treatment with I3C, such as alterations in the cell cycle machinery. A more detailed study will be required to determine whether treatment with I3C actually exerts chemopreventive behavior.

9. *N*-ACETYLCYSTEINE

N-acetylcysteine (NAC) is a small molecule that is known to possess antitumor activity in organs such as skin, lung, liver, and colon *(114–117)*. NAC is clinically used for the treatment of chronic bronchitis and paracetamol poisoning *(118,119)*. NAC can act as an anti-oxidant, block both DNA strand breakage and mutagenesis, and induce p53-dependent apoptosis *(120–122)*.

Because agents that induce apoptosis often cause cell cycle arrest as well, Liu et al. *(120)* investigated the effect of NAC on cell cycle progression in the 308 papilloma cell line. Treatment of 308 cells with NAC prolonged cell cycle progression through G_1 and induced both p16 and p21 (Fig. 1 and Table 1) *(120)*. Knock-out cells in p53, p21, or p16 were used to determine which protein is important for G_1 arrest upon treatment with NAC. Both p53 and p21 knock-out cells retained the full G_1 arrest, whereas only 40% of the arrest was lost in p16 knock-out cells *(120)*. The pathway or protein responsible for the remaining 60% remains to be elucidated. Treatment with higher doses of NAC induced apoptosis *(120)*, which raises the issue of determining the concentration of NAC to use to act as a cytostatic or cytotoxic agent.

Humans are exposed to many carcinogens throughout their lives. Discovering chemopreventive agents that induce expression of tumor-suppressor genes, such as p21 and p16, may be a beneficial way to prevent the transition from normal cells to cancer cells.

10. SULINDAC AND FLAVOPIRIDOL

Both Sulindac and Flavopiridol appear to have chemopreventive promise. Although these two compounds have not been shown to target CDKIs specifically, they have been shown to influence the cell through a number of mechanisms, including cell cycle arrest and apoptosis.

Sulindac is a non-steroidal anti-inflammatory (NSAID) that has been shown to inhibit both cyclooxygenase isoforms (COX-1 and COX-2) *(123,124)*. COX mediated synthesis of prostaglandins have been shown to possess growth-promoting properties. Treatment of APC[Min/+] mice, which have germline mutations of the mouse homologue APC *(125)* with sulindac decreased the number of polyps as compared to the control mice *(126)*. Although the exact mechanism of chemoprevention of intestinal neoplasia is unclear, it has been shown that sulindac and derivatives thereof can inhibit growth and induce apoptosis in other cancer models such as human prostate cancer cell lines *(127)* and human hepatocellular carcinoma cell lines *(128)*.

Flavopiridol is a flavone derivative that can induce cell cycle arrest and apoptosis in numerous transformed cell lines *(129–132)*. Although studies using flavopiridol do not show that it can target CDKIs directly, it has been shown to reduce CDK2 and CDK4 kinase activity in human breast carcinoma cell lines *(131)*, downregulate cyclin D_1 in esophageal and breast carcinoma cell lines *(129,132)*, and induce apoptosis in non-small cell lung cancer (NSCLC) and esophageal cancer cell lines *(129,130)*. Continued efforts with flavopiridol will determine the mechanism of cell cycle arrest and apoptosis, and these findings can be applied to murine models of carcinogenesis.

As an increasing number of chemopreventive agents are discovered and studied, we learn that they can not be catalogued into distinct categories such as cell cycle inhibitors or tyrosine kinase inhibitors because each agent appears to have multiple putative targets that may or may not relate to one another and continued efforts will elucidate these important mechanisms.

11. CONCLUSIONS

Although additional chemopreventive agents exist that are beyond the scope of this chapter, the compounds discussed within are examples of those compounds that affect cell cycle, cell death, and differentiation pathways. All the chemopreventive agents discussed earlier cause either a G_1 arrest, G_2 arrest, or both. Many of them target the CDK inhibitors directly, the kinase activity of cell cycle CDKs, or phosphorylation of the pRb protein (Fig. 1 and Table 1). Tamoxifen and RA have been shown to enhance transcription of p21 through a Sp1 binding site and a RARE element in the p21 promoter, respectively. Treatments with Genistein, Resveratrol, Apigenin, ECGC, I3C, and NAC have been shown to induce expression of p21, although the molecular mechanism behind these effects remain unclear. Tamoxifen, RA, ECGC, and I3C have been shown to alter expression of p27, and NAC alters expression of p16. However, again, the molecular mechanisms behind these changes in expression remain to be elucidated.

Many of these chemopreventive agents have pleiotropic effects within the cell. They may influence a variety of cellular actions ranging from signaling pathways to reactive oxygen species formation. It is important to take these many pathways into account when delineating the mechanisms of action chemopreventive agents have on cells. Some pathways may cross-communicate, while others may cause opposing effects. Continued studies of the cellular effects and molecular mechanisms of each chemopreventive agent will lead to a greater understanding and increase the promise of chemopreventive therapy.

REFERENCES

1. Kelloff GJ, Boone CW, Crowell JA, et al. New agents for cancer chemoprevention. *J Cell Biochem Suppl* 1996;26:1–28.
2. National Cancer Institute, Division of Cancer Prevention, 1999 Annual Report. www.nci.nih.gov.
3. McDonald ER, 3rd, El-Deiry WS. Cell cycle control as a basis for cancer drug development. *Int J Oncol* 2000;16:871–886.
4. Ozoren NaE-D, Wafik S. Introduction to cancer genes and growth control, in *DNA Alterations in Cancer*, Ehrlich M., ed. Eaton Publishing, Natick, MA, 2000, pp. 3-43.
5. Legha SS. Tamoxifen in the treatment of breast cancer. *Ann Intern Med* 1988;109:219–228.
6. Harper MJ, Walpole AL. Contrasting endocrine activities of cis and trans isomers in a series of substituted triphenylethylenes. *Nature* 1966;212:87.

7. Forbes JF. The control of breast cancer: the role of tamoxifen. *Semin Oncol* 1997;24: S1-5–S1-19.

8. Fisher B, Costantino JP, Wickerham DL, et al. Tamoxifen for prevention of breast cancer: report of the National Surgical Adjuvant Breast and Bowel Project P-1 Study. *J Natl Cancer Inst* 1998;90:1371–1388.

9. Jordan VC, Lababidi MK, Langan-Fahey S. Suppression of mouse mammary tumorigenesis by long-term tamoxifen therapy. *J Natl Cancer Inst* 1991;83:492–496.

10. Welsch CW, Goodrich-Smith M, Brown CK, et al. Effect of an estrogen antagonist (tamoxifen) on the initiation and progression of gamma-irradiation-induced mammary tumors in female Sprague-Dawley rats. *Eur J Cancer Clin Oncol* 1981;17:1255–1258.

11. Jordan VC. Effect of tamoxifen (ICI 46,474) on initiation and growth of DMBA-induced rat mammary carcinomata. *Eur J Cancer* 1976;12:419–424.

12. Gottardis MM, Jordan VC. Antitumor actions of keoxifene and tamoxifen in the N-nitrosomethylurea-induced rat mammary carcinoma model. *Cancer Res* 1987;47:4020–4024.

13. Reddel RR, Murphy LC, Sutherland RL. Effects of biologically active metabolites of tamoxifen on the proliferation kinetics of MCF-7 human breast cancer cells in vitro. *Cancer Res* 1983;43:4618–4624.

14. Taylor CM, Blanchard B, Zava DT. Estrogen receptor-mediated and cytotoxic effects of the antiestrogens tamoxifen and 4-hydroxytamoxifen. *Cancer Res* 1984;44:1409–1414.

15. Darbre PD, Curtis S, King RJ. Effects of estradiol and tamoxifen on human breast cancer cells in serum-free culture. *Cancer Res* 1984;44:2790–2793.

16. Hamel PA, Hanley-Hyde J. G1 cyclins and control of the cell division cycle in normal and transformed cells. *Cancer Invest* 1997;15:143–152.

17. Cover CM, Hsieh SJ, Gram EJ, et al. Indole-3-carbinol and tamoxifen cooperate to arrest the cell cycle of MCF-7 human breast cancer cells. *Cancer Res* 1999;59:1244–1251.

18. O'Brian CA, Liskamp RM, Solomon DH, et al. Triphenylethylenes: a new class of protein kinase C inhibitors. *J Natl Cancer Inst* 1986;76:1243–1246.

19. Kiss Z. Tamoxifen stimulates phospholipase D activity by an estrogen receptor-independent mechanism. *FEBS Lett* 1994;355:173–177.

20. Rowlands MG, Parr IB, McCague R, et al. Variation of the inhibition of calmodulin dependent cyclic AMP phosphodiesterase amongst analogues of tamoxifen; correlations with cytotoxicity. *Biochem Pharmacol* 1990;40:283–289.

21. Cabot MC, Giuliano AE, Volner A, et al. Tamoxifen retards glycosphingolipid metabolism in human cancer cells. *FEBS Lett* 1996;394:129–131.

22. Knabbe C, Lippman ME, Wakefield LM, et al. Evidence that transforming growth factor-beta is a hormonally regulated negative growth factor in human breast cancer cells. *Cell* 1987;48:417–428.

23. Lee TH, Chuang LY, Hung WC. Tamoxifen induces p21WAF1 and p27KIP1 expression in estrogen receptor-negative lung cancer cells. *Oncogene* 1999;18:4269–4274.

24. Lee TH, Chuang LY, Hung WC. Induction of p21WAF1 expression via Sp1-binding sites by tamoxifen in estrogen receptor-negative lung cancer cells. *Oncogene* 2000;19:3766–3773.

25. Merchant JL, Du M, Todisco A. Sp1 phosphorylation by Erk 2 stimulates DNA binding. *Biochem Biophys Res Commun* 1999;254:454–461.

26. Sporn MB, Roberts AB. Role of retinoids in differentiation and carcinogenesis. *J Natl Cancer Inst* 1984;73:1381–1387.

27. Hsu SL, Chen MC, Chou YH, et al. Induction of p21(CIP1/Waf1) and activation of p34(cdc2) involved in retinoic acid-induced apoptosis in human hepatoma Hep3B cells. *Exp Cell Res* 1999;248:87–96.

28. Lotan R. Retinoids in cancer chemoprevention. *FASEB J* 1996;10:1031–1039.

29. Chomienne C, Fenaux P, Degos L. Retinoid differentiation therapy in promyelocytic leukemia. *FASEB J* 1996;10:1025–1030.

30. Smith MA, Parkinson DR, Cheson BD, et al. Retinoids in cancer therapy. *J Clin Oncol* 1992;10:839–864.
31. Hong WK, Lippman SM, Itri LM, et al. Prevention of second primary tumors with isotretinoin in squamous-cell carcinoma of the head and neck. *N Engl J Med* 1990;323:795–801.
32. Kraemer KH, DiGiovanna JJ, Mashell AN, et al. Prevention of skin cancer in xeroderma pigmentosum with the use of oral isotretinoin. *N Engl J Med* 1988;318:1633–1637.
33. Muto A, Kizaki M, Yamato K, et al. 1,25-Dihydroxyvitamin D3 induces differentiation of a retinoic acid-resistant acute promyelocytic leukemia cell line (UF-1) associated with expression of p21(WAF1/CIP1) and p27(KIP1). *Blood* 1999;93:2225–2233.
34. Lotan R. Effects of vitamin A and its analogs (retinoids) on normal and neoplastic cells. *Biochim Biophys Acta* 1980;605:33–91.
35. Douer D, Koeffler HP. Retinoic acid enhances growth of human early erythroid progenitor cells in vitro. *J Clin Invest* 1982;69:1039–1041.
36. Breitman TR, Selonick SE, Collins SJ. Induction of differentiation of the human promyelocytic leukemia cell line (HL-60) by retinoic acid. *Proc Natl Acad Sci USA* 1980;77:2936–2940.
37. Sakashita A, Kizaki M, Pakkara S, et al. 9-cis-retinoic acid: effects on normal and leukemic hematopoiesis in vitro. *Blood* 1993;81:1009–1016.
38. Kizaki M, Ikeda Y, Tanasaki R, et al. Effects of novel retinoic acid compound, 9-cis-retinoic acid, on proliferation, differentiation, and expression of retinoic acid receptor-alpha and retinoid X receptor-alpha RNA by HL-60 cells. *Blood* 1993;82:3592–3599.
39. Chen YH, Lavelle D, DeSimone J, et al. Growth inhibition of a human myeloma cell line by all-trans retinoic acid is not mediated through downregulation of interleukin-6 receptors but through upregulation of p21(WAF1). *Blood* 1999;94:251–259.
40. Chen YH, Desai P, Shiao RT, et al. Inhibition of myeloma cell growth by dexamethasone and all-trans retinoic acid: synergy through modulation of interleukin-6 autocrine loop at multiple sites. *Blood* 1996;87:314–323.
41. Sidell N, Taga T, Hirano T, et al. Retinoic acid-induced growth inhibition of a human myeloma cell line via down-regulation of IL-6 receptors. *J Immunol* 1991;146:3809–3814.
42. Ogata A, Nishomoto N, Shima Y, et al. Inhibitory effect of all-trans retinoic acid on the growth of freshly isolated myeloma cells via interference with interleukin-6 signal transduction. *Blood* 1994;84:3040–3046.
43. Naderi S, Blomhoff, HK. Retinoic acid prevents phosphorylation of pRB in normal human B lymphocytes: regulation of cyclin E, cyclin A, and p21(Cip1). *Blood* 1999;94:1348–1358.
44. Liu M, Iavarone A, Freedman LP. Transcriptional activation of the human p21(WAF1/CIP1) gene by retinoic acid receptor. Correlation with retinoid induction of U937 cell differentiation. *J Biol Chem* 1996;271:31723–31728.
45. Kakizuka A, Miller WH, Jr., Umesono JK, et al. Chromosomal translocation t(15;17) in human acute promyelocytic leuke-mia fuses RAR alpha with a novel putative transcription factor, PML. *Cell* 1991;66:663–674.
46. de The H, Lavau C, Marchio A, et al. The PML-RAR alpha fusion mRNA generated by the t(15;17) translocation in acute promyelocytic leukemia encodes a functionally altered RAR. *Cell* 1991;66:675–684.
47. Huang ME, Ye YC, Chen SR, et al. Use of all-trans retinoic acid in the treatment of acute promyelocytic leukemia. *Blood* 1988;72:567–572.
48. Warrell RP Jr., Frankel SR, Miller WH Jr., et al. Differentiation therapy of acute promyelocytic leukemia with tretinoin (all-trans-retinoic acid). *N Engl J Med* 1991;324:1385–1393.
49. Mangelsdorf DJ, Evans RM. The RXR heterodimers and orphan receptors. *Cell* 1995; 83:841–850.
50. Hsu SL, Hsu WJ, Liu MC, et al. Retinoic acid-mediated G1 arrest is associated with induction of p27(Kip1) and inhibition of cyclin-dependent kinase 3 in human lung squamous carcinoma CH27 cells. *Exp Cell Res* 2000;258:322–331.

51. Naka K, Yokozaki H, Domen T, et al. Growth inhibition of cultured human gastric cancer cells by 9-cis-retinoic acid with induction of cdk inhibitor Waf1/Cip1/Sdi1/p21 protein. *Differentiation* 1997;61:313–320.

52. Zhu WY, Jones CS, Kiss A, et al. Retinoic acid inhibition of cell cycle progression in MCF-7 human breast cancer cells. *Exp Cell Res* 1997;234:293–299.

53. Severson RK, Nomura AM, Grove JS, et al. A prospective study of demographics, diet, and prostate cancer among men of Japanese ancestry in Hawaii. *Cancer Res* 1989;49:1857–1860.

54. Lee HP, Gourley L, Duffy SW, et al. Dietary effects on breast-cancer risk in Singapore. *Lancet* 1991;337:1197–1200.

55. NCI D. Chemoprevention Branch and Agent Development Committee. Clinical Development Plan: Genistein. *J Cell Biochem* 1996;26S:114–126.

56. Lamartiniere CA, et al. Genistein suppresses mammary cancer in rats. *Carcinogenesis* 1995;16:2833–2840.

57. Su SJ, Yeh TM, Lei HY, et al. The potential of soybean foods as a chemoprevention approach for human urinary tract cancer. *Clin Cancer Res* 2000;6:230–236.

58. Zhou JR, Mukherjee P, Gugger ET, et al. Inhibition of murine bladder tumorigenesis by soy isoflavones via alterations in the cell cycle, apoptosis, and angiogenesis. *Cancer Res* 1998;58:5231–5238.

59. Yanagihara K, Ho A, Toge T, et al. Antiproliferative effects of isoflavones on human cancer cell lines established from the gastrointestinal tract. *Cancer Res* 1993;53:5815–5821.

60. Murrill WB, Brown NM, Zhang JX, et al. Prepubertal genistein exposure suppresses mammary cancer and enhances gland differentiation in rats. *Carcinogenesis* 1996;17:1451–1457.

61. Brown NM, Lamartiniere CA. Xenoestrogens alter mammary gland differentiation and cell proliferation in the rat. *Environ Health Perspect* 1995;103:708–713.

62. Evans BA, Griffiths K, Morton MS. Inhibition of 5 alpha-reductase in genital skin fibroblasts and prostate tissue by dietary lignans and isoflavonoids. *J Endocrinol* 1995;147:295–302.

63. Ross RK, Bernstein L, Lobo RA, et al. 5-alpha-reductase activity and risk of prostate cancer among Japanese and US white and black males. *Lancet* 1992;339:887–889.

64. Akiyama T, Ishida J, Nakagawa S, et al. Genistein, a specific inhibitor of tyrosine-specific protein kinases. *J Biol Chem* 1987;262:5592–5595.

65. Akiyama T, Ogawara H. Use and specificity of genistein as inhibitor of protein-tyrosine kinases. *Methods Enzymol* 1991;201:362–370.

66. Okura A, Arakawa H, Oka H, et al. Effect of genistein on topoisomerase activity and on the growth of [Val 12]Ha-ras-transformed NIH 3T3 cells. *Biochem Biophys Res Commun* 1988;157:183–189.

67. Wei H, et al. Inhibition of tumor promoter-induced hydrogen peroxide formation in vitro and in vivo by genistein. *Nutr Cancer* 1993;20:1–12.

68. Wei H, Cai Q, Rahn RO. Inhibition of UV light- and Fenton reaction-induced oxidative DNA damage by the soybean isoflavone genistein. *Carcinogenesis* 1996;17:73–77.

69. Shao ZM, Alpaugh ML, Fontana JM, et al. Genistein inhibits proliferation similarly in estrogen receptor-positive and negative human breast carcinoma cell lines characterized by P21WAF1/CIP1 induction, G2/M arrest, and apoptosis. *J Cell Biochem* 1998;69:44–54.

70. Shao ZM, Wu J, Shen ZZ, et al. Genistein exerts multiple suppressive effects on human breast carcinoma cells. *Cancer Res* 1998;58:4851–4857.

71. Matsukawa Y, Marui N, Sakai T, et al. Genistein arrests cell cycle progression at G2-M. *Cancer Res* 1993;53:1328–1331.

72. Welsch CW. Host factors affecting the growth of carcinogen-induced rat mammary carcinomas: a review and tribute to Charles Brenton Huggins. *Cancer Res* 1985;45:3415–3443.

73. Russo IH, Russo J. Developmental stage of the rat mammary gland as determinant of its susceptibility to 7,12-dimethylbenz[a]anthracene. *J Natl Cancer Inst* 1978;61:1439–1449.

74. Grubbs CJ, Peckham JC, Cato KD. Mammary carcinogenesis in rats in relation to age at time of N-nitroso-N-methylurea administration. *J Natl Cancer Inst* 1983;70:209–212.

75. Russo J, Russo IH. DNA labeling index and structure of the rat mammary gland as determinants of its susceptibility to carcinogenesis. *J Natl Cancer Inst* 1978;61:1451–1459.

76. Russo J, Russo IH. Biological and molecular bases of mammary carcinogenesis. *Lab Invest* 1987;57:112–137.

77. Adlercreutz H, Fotsis T, Bannwart C, et al. Isotope dilution gas chromatographic-mass spectrometric method for the determination of lignans and isoflavonoids in human urine, including identification of genistein. *Clin Chim Acta* 1991;199:263–278.

78. Clark JW, Santas-Moore A, Stevenson LE, et al. Effects of tyrosine kinase inhibitors on the proliferation of human breast cancer cell lines and proteins important in the ras signaling pathway. *Int J Cancer* 1996;65:186–191.

79. Rao CV, Wang CX, Simi B, et al. Enhancement of experimental colon cancer by genistein. *Cancer Res* 1997;57:3717–3722.

80. Soleas GJ, Diamandis EP, Goldberg DM. Resveratrol: a molecule whose time has come? And gone? *Clin Biochem* 1997;30:91–113.

81. Frankel EN, Waterhouse AL, Kinsella JE. Inhibition of human LDL oxidation by resveratrol. *Lancet* 1993;341:1103–1104.

82. Jang, M., Cai L, Udeani GO, et al. Cancer chemopreventive activity of resveratrol, a natural product derived from grapes. *Science* 1997;275:218–220.

83. Waddell WR, Ganser GF, Cerise EJ, et al. Sulindac for polyposis of the colon. *Am J Surg* 1989;157:175–179.

84. Thun MJ, Namboodiri MM, Heath Jr CW. Aspirin use and reduced risk of fatal colon cancer. *N Engl J Med* 1991;325:1593–1596.

85. Plescia OJ, Smith AH, Grinwich K. Subversion of immune system by tumor cells and role of prostaglandins. *Proc Natl Acad Sci USA* 1975;72:1848–1851.

86. Carbo N, Costelli P, Baccino FM, et al. Resveratrol, a natural product present in wine, decreases tumour growth in a rat tumour model. *Biochem Biophys Res Commun* 1999; 254:739–743.

87. Gehm BD, McAndrews JM, Chien PY, et al. Resveratrol, a polyphenolic compound found in grapes and wine, is an agonist for the estrogen receptor. *Proc Natl Acad Sci USA* 1997;94:14138–11443.

88. Lu R, Serrero G. Resveratrol, a natural product derived from grape, exhibits antiestrogenic activity and inhibits the growth of human breast cancer cells. *J Cell Physiol* 1999;179: 297–304.

89. Hsieh TC, Wu JM. Differential effects on growth, cell cycle arrest, and induction of apoptosis by resveratrol in human prostate cancer cell lines. *Exp Cell Res* 1999;249:109–115.

90. Tessitore L, Davit A, Sarotto I, et al. Resveratrol depresses the growth of colorectal aberrant crypt foci by affecting bax and p21(CIP) expression. *Carcinogenesis* 2000;21:1619–1622.

91. Waldman T, Lengauer C, Kinzler KW, et al. Uncoupling of S phase and mitosis induced by anticancer agents in cells lacking p21 [see comments]. *Nature* 1996;381:713–716.

92. Zhao J, Wang J, Chen Y, et al. Anti-tumor-promoting activity of a polyphenolic fraction isolated from grape seeds in the mouse skin two-stage initiation-promotion protocol and identification of procyanidin B5-3'-gallate as the most effective antioxidant constituent. *Carcinogenesis* 1999;20:1737–1745.

93. Damianaki A, Bakogeorgan E, Kampa M, et al. Potent inhibitory action of red wine polyphenols on human breast cancer cells. *J Cell Biochem* 2000;78:429–441.

94. Agarwal C, Sharma Y, Agarwal R. Anticarcinogenic effect of a polyphenolic fraction isolated from grape seeds in human prostate carcinoma DU145 cells: modulation of mitogenic signaling and cell-cycle regulators and induction of G1 arrest and apoptosis. *Mol Carcinog* 2000;28:129–138.

95. Xu Y, Ho CT, Amin SG, et al. Inhibition of tobacco-specific nitrosamine-induced lung tumorigenesis in A/J mice by green tea and its major polyphenol as antioxidants. *Cancer Res* 1992;52:3875–3879.

96. Ahmad N, Feyes DK, Nieminen AL, et al. Green tea constituent epigallocatechin-3-gallate and induction of apoptosis and cell cycle arrest in human carcinoma cells. *J Natl Cancer Inst* 1997;89:1881–1886.

97. Liang YC, et al. Suppression of extracellular signals and cell proliferation through EGF receptor binding by (-)-epigallocatechin gallate in human A431 epidermoid carcinoma cells. *J Cell Biochem* 1997;67:55–65.

98. Liang YC, Lin-Sh, et al. Inhibition of cyclin-dependent kinases 2 and 4 activities as well as induction of Cdk inhibitors p21 and p27 during growth arrest of human breast carcinoma cells by (-)-epigallocatechin-3-gallate. *J Cell Biochem* 1999;75:1–12.

99. Birt DF, Mitchell D, Gold B, et al. Inhibition of ultraviolet light induced skin carcinogenesis in SKH-1 mice by apigenin, a plant flavonoid. *Anticancer Res* 1997;17:85–91.

100. Lepley DM, et al. The chemopreventive flavonoid apigenin induces G2/M arrest in keratinocytes. *Carcinogenesis* 1996;17:2367–2375.

101. Sato F, Matsukawa Y, Matsumoto K, et al. Apigenin induces morphological differentiation and G2-M arrest in rat neuronal cells. *Biochem Biophys Res Commun* 1994;204:578–584.

102. Lepley DM, Pelling JC. Induction of p21/WAF1 and G1 cell-cycle arrest by the chemopreventive agent apigenin. *Mol Carcinog* 1997;19:74–82.

103. Kuo ML, Yang, NC. Reversion of v-H-ras-transformed NIH 3T3 cells by apigenin through inhibiting mitogen activated protein kinase and its downstream oncogenes. *Biochem Biophys Res Commun* 1995;212:767–775.

104. Young TB, Wolf DA. Case-control study of proximal and distal colon cancer and diet in Wisconsin. *Int J Cancer* 1988;42:167–175.

105. Grubbs CJ, Steele VE, Casebolt T, et al. Chemoprevention of chemically-induced mammary carcinogenesis by indole-3-carbinol. *Anticancer Res* 1995;15:709–716.

106. Bradlow HL, Michnovicz J, Telang NT, et al. Effects of dietary indole-3-carbinol on estradiol metabolism and spontaneous mammary tumors in mice. *Carcinogenesis* 1991;12:1571–1574.

107. NCI D, Chemoprevention Branch and Agent Development Committee. Clinical Development Plan: Indole-3-Carbinol. *J Cell Biochem* 1996;26S:127–136.

108. Schneider J, Kinne D, Fracchia A, et al. Abnormal oxidative metabolism of estradiol in women with breast cancer. *Proc Natl Acad Sci USA* 1982;79:3047–3051.

109. Tiwari RK, Guo L, Bradlow HL, et al. Selective responsiveness of human breast cancer cells to indole-3-carbinol, a chemopreventive agent. *J Natl Cancer Inst* 1994;86:126–131.

110. Telang NT, Katdare M, Bradlow HL, et al. Inhibition of proliferation and modulation of estradiol metabolism: novel mechanisms for breast cancer prevention by the phytochemical indole-3-carbinol. *Proc Soc Exp Biol Med* 1997;216:246–252.

111. Cover CM, Hsieh SJ, Tran SH, et al. Indole-3-carbinol inhibits the expression of cyclin-dependent kinase-6 and induces a G1 cell cycle arrest of human breast cancer cells independent of estrogen receptor signaling. *J Biol Chem* 1998;273:3838–3847.

112. Bradlow HL, Michnovicz JJ, Halper M, et al. Long-term responses of women to indole-3-carbinol or a high fiber diet. *Cancer Epidemiol Biomarkers Prev* 1994;3:591–595.

113. Wong GY, Bradlow L, Sepkovic D, et al. Dose-ranging study of indole-3-carbinol for breast cancer prevention. *J Cell Biochem Suppl* 1997;29:111–116.

114. Steele VE, Kelloff GT, Wilkinson BP, et al. Inhibition of transformation in cultured rat tracheal epithelial cells by potential chemopreventive agents. *Cancer Res* 1990;50:2068–2074.

115. Pereira MA, Khoury MD. Prevention by chemopreventive agents of azoxymethane-induced foci of aberrant crypts in rat colon. *Cancer Lett* 1991;61:27–33.

116. Izzotti A, D'gostini F, Bagnasco M, et al. Chemoprevention of carcinogen-DNA adducts and chronic degenerative diseases. *Cancer Res* 1994;54:1994s–1998s.

117. De Flora S, Astengo M, Serra D, et al. Inhibition of urethan-induced lung tumors in mice by dietary N-acetylcysteine. *Cancer Lett* 1986;32:235–241.

118. Holdiness MR. Clinical pharmacokinetics of N-acetylcysteine. *Clin Pharmacokinet* 1991;20:123–134.

119. Smilkstein MJ, Knapp GL, Kulig KW, et al. Efficacy of oral N-acetylcysteine in the treatment of acetaminophen overdose. Analysis of the national multicenter study (1976 to 1985). *N Engl J Med* 1988;319:1557–1562.

120. Liu M, Wikonkal NM, Brash DE. Induction of cyclin-dependent kinase inhibitors and G(1) prolongation by the chemopreventive agent N-acetylcysteine. *Carcinogenesis* 1999;20:1869–1872.

121. Chan JY, Stout DL, Becker FF. Protective role of thiols in carcinogen-induced DNA damage in rat liver. *Carcinogenesis* 1986;7:1621–1624.

122. Solen G. Radioprotective effect of N-acetylcysteine in vitro using the induction of DNA breaks as end-point. *Int J Radiat Biol* 1993;64:359–366.

123. Gupta RA, DuBois RN. Aspirin, NSAIDS, and colon cancer prevention: mechanisms? *Gastroenterology* 1998;114:1095–1098.

124. Williams CS, Mann M, DuBois RN. The role of cyclooxygenases in inflammation, cancer, and development. *Oncogene* 1999;18:7908–7916.

125. Su LK, Kinzler KW, Vogelstein B, et al. Multiple intestinal neoplasia caused by a mutation in the murine homolog of the APC gene [published erratum appears in *Science* 1992 May 22;256(5060):1114]. *Science* 1992;256:668–670.

126. Torrance CJ, Jackson PE, Montgomery E, et al. Combinatorial chemoprevention of intestinal neoplasia [see comments]. *Nat Med* 2000;6:1024–1028.

127. Lim JT, Piazza GA, Han EK, et al. Sulindac derivatives inhibit growth and induce apoptosis in human prostate cancer cell lines. *Biochem Pharmacol* 1999;58:1097–1107.

128. Rahman MA, Dhar DK, Masunaga R, et al. Sulindac and exisulind exhibit a significant antiproliferative effect and induce apoptosis in human hepatocellular carcinoma cell lines. *Cancer Res* 2000; 60:2085–2089.

129. Schrump DS, Matthews W, Chen GA, et al. Flavopiridol mediates cell cycle arrest and apoptosis in esophageal cancer cells. *Clin Cancer Res* 1998;4:2885–2890.

130. Shapiro GI, Koesner DA, Malvanga CB, et al. Flavopiridol induces cell cycle arrest and p53-independent apoptosis in non-small cell lung cancer cell lines. *Clin Cancer Res* 1999;5:2925–2938.

131. Carlson BA, Dubay MM, Sausville EA, et al. Flavopiridol induces G1 arrest with inhibition of cyclin-dependent kinase (CDK) 2 and CDK4 in human breast carcinoma cells. *Cancer Res* 1996;56:2973–2978.

132. Carlson B, Lahusen T, Singh S, et al. Down-regulation of cyclin D1 by transcriptional repression in MCF-7 human breast carcinoma cells induced by flavopiridol. *Cancer Res* 1999;59:4634–4641.

7

Cell Cycle Regulatory Genes as Targets of Retinoids

Kenneth J. Soprano, PhD,
Sijie Zhang, MD, PhD,
Dongmei Zhang, PhD,
William F. Holmes, MS,
Valeria Masciullo, MD, PhD,
Antonio Giordano, MD, PhD,
and Dianne R. Soprano, PhD

CONTENTS

From: *Cancer Drug Discovery and Development:*
Cell Cycle Inhibitors in Cancer Therapy: Current Strategies
Edited by: A. Giordano and K. J. Soprano © Humana Press Inc., Totowa, NJ

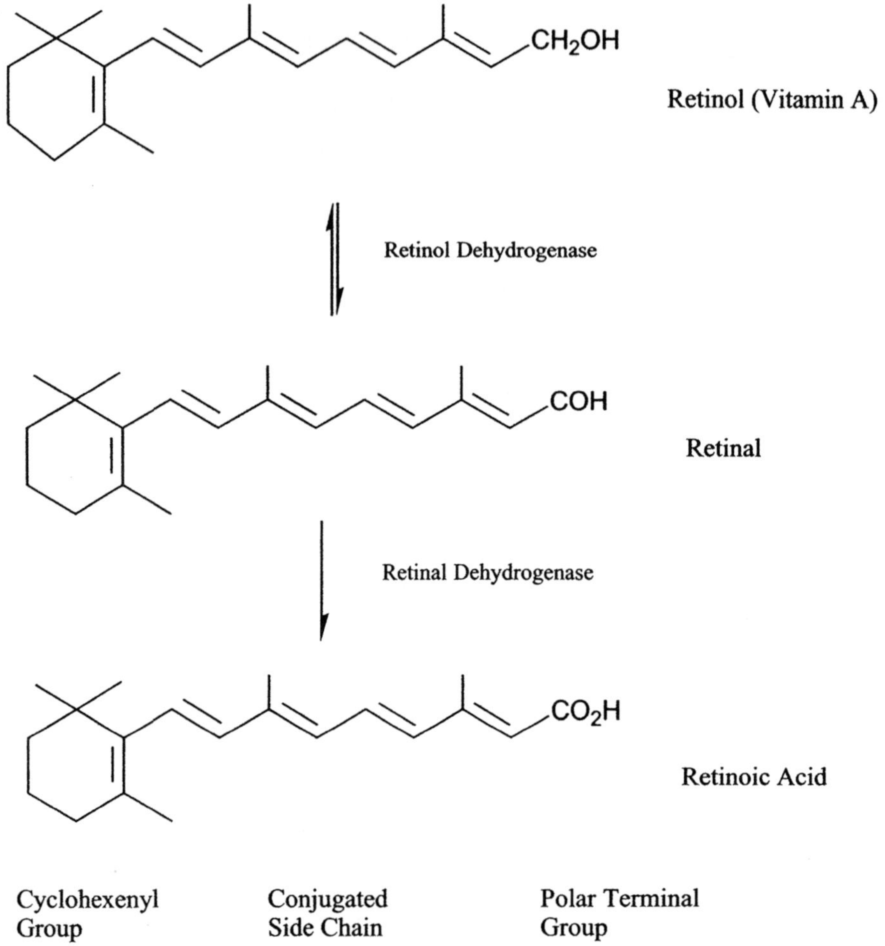

Cyclohexenyl   Conjugated   Polar Terminal
Group   Side Chain   Group

Fig. 1. Chemical structures of retinol, retinal, and retinoic acid, the major metabolic forms of Vitamin A. There are three functional moieties of retinoids: a polar end, a conjugated side chain, and a cyclohexenyl ring. The different polar end determines the nature of the specific retinoid. Retinol is the major transport form of vitamin A. Retinal is the light-sensitive pigment in the retina, and retinoic acid performs all of the other functions of vitamin A. Although the conversion of retinol to retinal is reversible, the conversion of retinal to retinoic acid is irreversible.

1. RETINOIDS

Retinoids are a large group of natural and synthetic derivatives of vitamin A. There are more than 4000 different compounds in this group. Vitamin A and its derivatives play an essential role in vision, immuno-modulation, reproduction, maintaining epithelial tissue, cell growth, and differentiation. Retinol, retinal, and retinoic acid (RA) are among the most important natural retinoids. Retinol is the alcohol form, and is the major transport form of vitamin A. Retinal is the aldehyde form. It is produced by an enzymatic oxidation of retinol in a variety of tissues or by a direct cleavage of dietary β-carotene in small intestine and liver. Retinal can be converted back to retinol through a reduction reaction. In contrast, further oxidation of retinal into retinoic acid (RA) is an irreversible step (Fig. 1). RA is effective therapeutically in the treatment of a variety of diseases involving cell proliferation, abnormal differentiation, and inflammation. 11-cis-retinal is the chromophore in the visual protein, rhodopsin. With the exception of vision and reproduction, all of the action of vitamin A can be accomplished by retinoic acid. 9-cis and 13-cis RA are natural isomers of all-*trans* RA (ATRA).

1.1. Absorption and Transportation of Vitamin A

Vitamin A is an essential fat-soluble nutrient. The major pathways for vitamin A adsorption and transport are summarized in Fig. 2. β-carotene is a major dietary source of vitamin A. It is present in green-leaf vegetables, carrots, sweet potatoes, and egg yolks. Each molecule of β-carotene is broken down into two molecules of retinal by intestinal 15-15' β-carotene oxygenase. The retinal is further reduced to retinol by a NADPH dependent enzyme. The second dietary source of vitamin A is retinyl esters, found in milk, meat, and liver. Retinyl ester is hydrolyzed into retinol in the small intestine. Retinol is then absorbed by the intestinal mucosa through passive diffusion and complexes with cellular retinol-binding protein II (CRBP II). Retinol is then converted back to retinyl-ester by lecithin-retinol acyl-transferase. Chylomicrons deliver retinyl-ester to various tissues, mainly liver, but also to other tissues such as bone marrow, peripheral blood cells, spleen, adipose tissue, and kidney. Retinyl ester is the major storage form of vitamin A. Liver is the major storage organ. However, in many other organs, low concentrations of retinyl ester are also stored. When the body is in need of retinol, retinyl ester is hydrolyzed to retinol and transported to different organs. Retinol enters the circulation by complexing with retinol-binding proteins (RBP). Once inside a cell, retinol is converted to retinal. Retinal is then oxidized to retinoic acid. The conversion of retinal to retinoic acid is catalyzed by a NAD dependent aldehyde dehydrogenase: retinaldehyde-2 (Raldh2). Retinoic acid enters the cell nucleus and interacts with retinoic acid receptors (RAR) and retinoid X receptors (RXR). Most cellular functions of retinoic acid are mediated through RAR/RXR receptors.

1.2. Intracellular and Extracellular Retinoid Binding Proteins

Retinoids are transported in the blood and within different cellular compartments by various proteins. Retinoids interact with these proteins via noncovalent bonds. In the plasma, small quantities of retinoic acid are transported by binding with albumin. The majority of retinol travels to different tissues by conjugating with retinol binding proteins (RBP). RBP is a protein of approx 21 KD. It binds

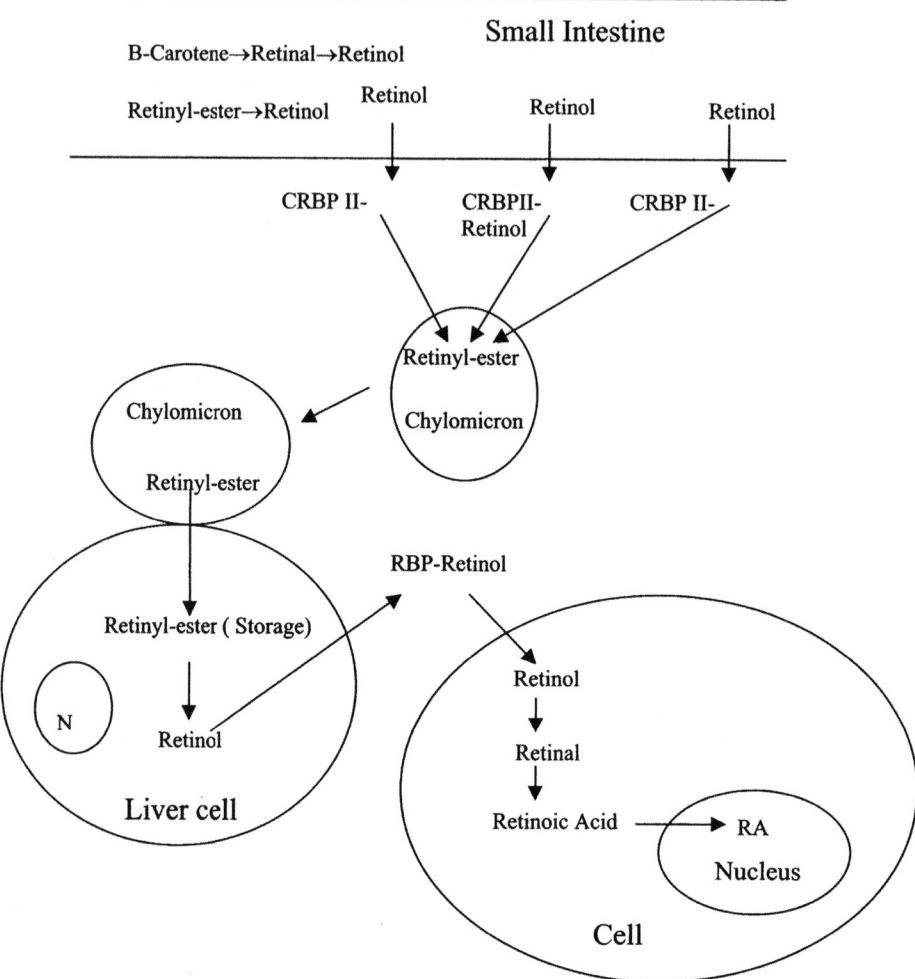

Fig. 2. Absorption and transportation of Vitamin A. β-Carotene and retinyl-ester are the major dietary sources of vitamin A. Retinol is the digestive product of β-Carotene and retinyl-ester. After retinol passes through the small intestinal mucosa by passive diffusion, it binds with CRBP-II, then forms retinyl-ester again. Chylomicrons deliver the retinyl-esters to liver cells for storage. The major storage form of vitamin A is retinyl-ester. Retinyl-ester is broken down into retinol, and then retinol binds with RBP. In the plasma, RBP delivers retinol to target cell cytoplasm. Retinol is converted into retinal and then into retinoic acid in the cytoplasm. Retinoic acid then enters the cell nucleus.

and transports a single retinol molecule within its hydrophobic pocket. RBP further complexes with transthyretin (TTR, also called pre-albumin), a thyroxin-binding protein, to form a 55KD tetramer of identical subunits. Transthyretin transports both retinol and thyroid hormone. The TTR complex is thought to prevent the loss of RBP through glomerular filtration. Furthermore, the binding affinity of retinol to RBP doubles after RBP complexes with TTR *(1)*. The exact mechanism of retinol entrance into target cells is still a mystery. Hypothesized mechanisms include passive diffusion or a RBP receptor mediated process *(2)*. However, the presence of a RBP receptor has yet to be definitively demonstrated on responsive cells.

Within the cytoplasm, retinol interacts with cellular retinol-binding protein (CRBP), and retinoic acid binds with cellular retinoic acid binding protein (CRABP). Both proteins have two isoforms: CRBP I, CRBP II, and CRABP I, CRABP II, respectively.

CRBP protects cell membranes from retinoids *(3)*. Cell membrane function depends on its composition. It is vulnerable to the influence of daily fluctuation of vitamin A concentration. Although cell membranes have an enormous capacity to sequester retinol, membranes have little retinal *(4)*. The concentration of CRBP far exceeds retinol and retinal *(4)*. CRBP also has high affinity for retinol and retinal *(5)*. These two factors ensured sequestration of retinal and retinol by CRBP within cytoplasm instead of cell membrane. CRBP also protects retinoids from nonenzymatic chemical transformations. Retinol usually undergo spontaneous isomerization and oxidation, binding with CRBP totally stopped the process *(6)*. By using *in situ* hybridization, Kuppumbatti and colleagues observed a loss of CRBP expression in 24% of breast cancer specimens compared with normal breast tissue and normal tissue adjacent to the carcinomas. They found that the loss of CRBP expression is similar between ductal carcinoma *in situ* (27%) and invasive lesions (22%). These investigators suggested it might be an early event in breast carcinogenesis *(7)*.

In humans, CRABP I is mainly distributed in the reproductive system, including testis, epididymis, vas deferens, seminal vesicles, ovary, oviduct, and uterus. It is also found in the brain and the spinal cord. CRABP II is mainly found in skin. It has been proposed that CRABP I and CRABP II might: 1) regulate intracellular concentration of retinoic acid, and 2) function as transport proteins that carry retinoic acid from cytoplasm into nucleus *(8,9)*. However, knock-out mice with deletion of both CRABP I and CRABP II were essentially normal *(10)*. Therefore, the exact functions of CRABP I and CRABP II are still not very clear.

1.3. Retinoid Nuclear Receptors: RAR and RXR

Retinoids mediate their effect mainly by binding to their nuclear receptors: retinoic acid receptor (RAR) and retinoid-X-receptor (RXR). RAR/RXR are ligand dependent transcription factors. They belong to the superfamily of nuclear hormone receptors (NHR). There are three RAR subtypes (RAR-α, RAR-β, and RAR-γ) and three RXR subtypes (RXR-α, RXR-β, and RXR-γ).

RAR/RXR proteins contain six functional domains based on homology among themselves and with other nuclear hormone receptors *(11)* (Fig. 3). The A/B

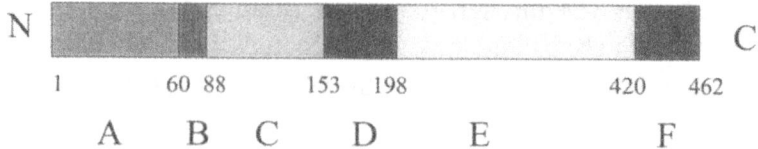

N ... C

1   60 88   153   198   420   462

A   B   C   D   E   F

Fig. 3. Different domains of RAR/RXR. Domain A/B is the ligand independent transactivation (AF-1) domain. Domain C is the DNA binding domain, which contains a pair of zinc fingers. Domain C targets the receptor to specific DNA sequences known as retinoic acid response elements (RARE). Domain D is the hinge region that is the binding site of nuclear receptor co-activators and co-repressors. Domain E is the ligand binding, dimerization, and ligand-dependent transactivation (AF-2) region. Domain F has unknown functions.

Domain is the ligand independent transactivation (AF-1) domain. Domain C is the DNA binding domain, which contains a pair of zinc fingers. It targets the receptor to specific DNA sequences known as retinoic acid response elements (RARE). Domain D is the hinge region that is the binding site of nuclear receptor co-activators and co-repressors. Domain E is the ligand binding, dimerization, and ligand-dependent transactivation (AF-2) region. The functions of the F Domain have yet to be determined. RXR proteins do not have the F domain. The C and E domain is highly conserved among the three subtypes of RAR. These domains share 94–97% homology. These domains are also highly conserved among subtypes of RXR (91–97% homology). Furthermore, the homology of the C and E domain between species is higher than between RAR and RXR subtypes within a given species. The D domain is also well-conserved within RAR or RXR subtypes of a given species, but the similarity between species is even greater. The B domain of the RAR subtypes is also well-conserved. The A domain is not related at all *(11)*.

RAR binds both all-trans retinoic acid (ATRA) and 9-cis retinoic acid (9-cis RA), whereas RXR only binds 9-cis RA. Upon ligand binding, RAR and RXR can form either heterodimers (RAR/RXR) or homodimers (RXR/RXR). They interact with retinoic acid-response elements (RAREs) in the promoter region of response genes to enhance or repress DNA transcription. RXR also forms heterodimers with many other nuclear hormone receptors including: thyroid hormone receptor (TR), vitamin D_3 receptor (VDR), peroxisome proliferator-activated receptor (PPAR), and others. The binding of RXR with these nuclear hormone receptors enhances receptors' binding to their corresponding hormone response elements (HRE). Heterodimers bind more efficiently and selectively than homodimers to their cognate elements.

The RARs and RXRs are encoded by different genes located on different chromosomes. In human, RAR-α is located at chromosome 17q21.1. RAR-β is located at chromosome 3p24. RAR-γ is located at chromosome 12q13. RXR-α is located at chromosome 9q34.3. RXR-β is located at chromosome 6p21.3. Finally, RXR-γ is located at chromosome 1q22-q23. Each subtype also has different isoforms due to alternative splicing and differential usage of two promoters. RAR-α has seven isoforms, RAR-β has four isoforms, and RAR-γ has seven. The distinct function of each isoform is currently under active research in our laboratory.

Temporal and spatial distribution of the different RAR/RXR isoforms has raised a question whether each receptor isoform has its own unique function. In knock-out mice studies in which a single isoform has been deleted, there is no observable defect. This suggests functional redundancy between different isoforms (12–14). However, mice with a complete RAR-α gene deletion have degenerative testicular germinal epithelium. RAR-γ knock-out mice show keratinizing squamous metaplasia of seminal vesicle and prostate. Harderian gland, which provides lubrication for the eyelids, also fails to develop in RAR-γ knock-out mice. RXR-α null mutation mice have major cardiac malformation (15). Therefore, each RAR/RXR subtype must have its unique functions.

1.4. Co-Repressor and Co-Activator of RAR/RXR

Co-repressors and co-activators, which interact with nuclear hormone receptors, were identified by the yeast two-hybrid system. Two co-repressors that bind to unliganded RAR have been isolated: N-CoR (nuclear receptor co-repressor) and SMRT (silencing mediator for RAR and TR). Both of these co-repressors only bind with receptor in the absence of ligand. Co-repressors complex with histone deacetylase induce changes in chromatin, causing DNA to be inaccessible to the transcriptional machinery. Upon ligand binding, the co-repressors are released and co-activators are recruited. Several co-activators have been identified that interact directly with RARs/RXRs in an agonist ligand-dependent manner. They have been shown to enhance the activity of AF-2 regions. Some of these co-activators, such as SRC-1, CBP/p300, and ACTR, possess an intrinsic histone acetyltransferase activity (16–19). They also interact with the histone acetyltransferase p/CAF (20). Acetylation of histone will open up the condensed chromatin so the DNA becomes accessible to the basal transcriptional machinery. Furthermore, CBP and p300 also interact with RNA helicase A that in turn binds RNA polymerase II (21). Therefore, co-activators act as mediators to make compacted DNA more accessible and to recruit the basal transcriptional machinery for transcription.

1.5. Retinoic Acid Response Elements

Retinoic acid response elements (RARE) are nucleotide sequences that are located in the promoter region of many RA response genes. They usually consist of two direct repeats of the six-nucleotide sequence, AGGTCA. These two direct repeats are separated by various numbers of nucleotides. The RAR/RXR heterodimer preferentially interacts with two direct repeats that are separated by either five or two nucleotides (called DR5 or DR2 elements). RXR/RXR homodimers and RXR/PPAR heterodimers bind to DR1 elements. RXR/VD$_3$ binds to DR3, and RXR/T$_3$ binds to DR4 elements. RXR occupies the 5' hexameric motif on DR2, DR3, DR4, and DR5, and its partner PPAR, VDR, TR, and RAR occupy the 3' motif *(22)*. Upon binding of the RARE with heterodimer or homodimer, gene transcription is either activated or repressed depending on the binding dimer and the spacing between the two direct repeats.

2. RETINOIDS AND CANCER

Epidemiological studies have long suggested an inverse correlation between cancer development and dietary consumption of vitamin A or beta-carotene *(23)*. In 1925, Wolbach and Howe observed a histological similarity between the epithelium of vitamin A-deficient organs and neoplastic tissue *(24)*. In 1955, Lasnitzki treated atypical prostate epithelial cells with retinoic acid resulting in induction of normal morphology in these cells *(25,26)*. Vitamin A-deficient animals were susceptible to chemical carcinogens. The incidence of cancer is very high among them *(27)*.

Retinoids play an important role in maintaining epithelial tissue. Epithelial tissue covers internal and external body surfaces. Cancers that arise from epithelial tissues are termed carcinomas. Carcinoma is the most common form of neoplastic disease. Vitamin A deficiency induces transformation of simple columnar epithelium into a pseudo-stratified form, then into stratified squamous epithelium, and finally into stratified keratinizing squamous epithelium. This transformation is the pre-neoplastic lesion of many mucous secreting epithelial carcinomas. The transformation process is reversible by administration of vitamin A.

Retinoids suppress the transforming effects of chemical, physical, and viral carcinogens. Retinoids inhibit mouse embryo cell transformation induced by 3-methylcholanthrene (MCA) or by γ-rays. The inhibitory effect is observed even when adding retinoids after 7 d of MCA treatment or after 96 h of radiation *(28,29)*. Retinoids also inhibit anchorage-independent growth of malignant cells *(30)*. ATRA inhibits the growth of HPV16 transformed human epidermal keratinocytes by inhibiting the expression of HPV16 oncogenes E6 and E7 *(31)*.

2.1. Head and Neck Cancer

In 1986, one study reported that 13-cis-retinoic acid (2 mg/Kg/d) reversed oral pre-malignant lesions in 67% patients compared with 10% treated by placebo *(32)*. In another study, patients with oral pre-malignant lesions were initially treated with a 3-mo induction course of 13-cis-retinoic acid (1.5 mg/kg/d), then a 9-mo maintenance dosage of 13-cis-RA (0.5 mg/kg/d) or β-carotene (30 mg/ kg/d). This study demonstrated that even in the low-dosage maintenance phase, fewer patients (8%) developed malignant oral lesions than the placebo group (55%) *(33)*. In a study of 103 head and neck cancer patients treated for 12 mo with 13-cis-retinoic acid (50–100 mg/m^2/d) or placebo following surgery and/or radiotherapy, there was a significantly lower rate of developing second primary tumors in retinoid-treated patients (4 vs 24%). However, the primary disease recurrence or survival was the same in both groups *(34)*. Therefore, 13-cis-retinoic acid can prevent the development of second primary cancers. It has no effect against cancer initiation, primary disease recurrence, or survival *(35)*.

2.2. Lung Cancer

In 1975, an epidemiological study of 8,278 Norwegian men showed a lower incidence of lung cancer in patients with higher vitamin A index. The vitamin A index is calculated based on the reported consumption of vegetables and dairy products *(36)*. In one uncontrolled trial, chronic smokers with squamous metaplasia of the bronchial epithelium were treated with etretinate (25 mg/d) for 6 mo. A reduction in the extent of squamous metaplasia was observed in most treated patients *(37)*. In one prospective study of 1,954 middle-aged men followed for 19 yr, the incidence of lung cancer was inversely related to the intake of dietary β-carotene *(38)*. Retinyl palmitate, a natural retinoid derivative, was tested in 307 patients with stage I non-small cell lung carcinoma after surgery. Half of the patients were treated with retinyl palmitate and the other half received no treatment. After 1 yr, 18 patients in the retinyl palmitate group developed a second primary tumor compared with 29 in the control group *(39)*. Intragastric injection of 5 mg retinyl palmitate twice weekly reduced both incidence and multiplicity of respiratory tumors in hamsters *(40)*.

2.3. Breast Cancer

Hislop and colleagues have found that the incidence of proliferative benign breast disease was inversely related with vitamin A supplementation and frequent green vegetable consumption *(41)*. Moon and colleagues have shown that fenretinide was one of the most active chemopreventive agents in early mammary carcinogenesis model studies *(42)*. 4-Hydroxyphenylretinamide (4-HPR) is a synthetic retinoid that binds neither RAR nor RXR, yet it prevents prostate, bladder, and breast cancer. It accumulates in the rodent mammary gland *(43)*. In vitro, it induces apoptosis in several cancer cell lines. It also inhibits carcinogenesis of chemical compounds in the mammary gland of rats and enhances the anticancer effect of tamoxifen *(43–46)*.

2.4. Skin Cancer

In several Phase II and Phase III clinical trials, both topical and systemic retinoids have effectively reversed premalignant skin lesions *(47)*. 13-cis-retinoic acid or etretinate has significantly reduced the number of skin cancers in xeroderma pigmentosum patients and transplant patients *(47,48)*. Patients with skin premalignancy treated with retinol (25,000 IU/d) resulted in a remarkable reduction of squamous cell carcinomas compare with the control group *(49)*.

2.5. Acute Promyelocytic Leukemia

Acute promyelocytic leukemia (APL) is a subtype of acute myeloid leukemia (AML). Patients with APL have an accumulation of undifferentiated hematopoietic blast cells and a severe hemorrhagic syndrome caused by a coagulation disorder. In 1977, Rowley et al. observed that APL patients were consistently associated with a translocation of chromosome 15 and 17 *(50)*. Subsequently, RAR-α was mapped to chromosome 17q21. The breakpoint on chromosome 15 contained a gene with unknown function at that time. It was named PML (promyelocytic leukemia). PML later was found to act as a growth suppressor and a proto-oncogene factor that inhibits transformation *(51)*. The translocated chromosomes encode PML/RAR-α and RAR-α/PML fusion genes and their transcripts. Early studies suggested that treatment of APL patients with 13-cis-RA could induce APL cell differentiation *(52)*. In the late 1980s, Chinese scientists began trials of all-trans-RA in the treatment of APL patients. They reported complete remission of APL patients treated with all-trans retinoic acid (45–100 mg/m^2/d) *(53,54)*. The success of treating APL patients with ATRA highlighted the fact that cell differentiation therapy is a potent and practical method for the treatment of human cancer.

2.6. Ovarian Cancer

The National Cancer Institute sponsored a randomized clinical trial at the Istituto Nazionale Tumori of Milan, Italy begun on March 1, 1987. The purpose of the study was to determine the chemopreventive effect of 4-HPR on the prevention of a second incidence of primary breast cancer of women who already had breast cancer. 1422 patients were treated with oral 4-HPR at 200 mg per day for 5 yr. Another 1427 patients received no treatment at all. All patients (2849) had surgery for T1-T2 breast cancer without axillary-node involvement. None of them had evidence of local recurrence or distant metastases before the study. After five years, a total of 43 patients had new primary tumors in sites other than the breast, 21 in the 4-HPR group and 22 in the control group. The types of new primary tumors appear to be equal in both groups, except for ovarian epithelial cancer. During the five years of clinical trial, 6 patients in the control group developed ovarian cancer, and none in the 4-HPR group. Two patients in the 4-HPR group developed ovarian carcinoma after the completion of the trial. One had a stage IIIC ovarian serous adenocarcinoma 10 mo after the trial. The other had an unclassified stage IIIC ovarian carcinoma 30 mo after the trial *(55)*. This study suggested a protective action of 4-HPR against the development of ovarian cancer. However, this protection only occurs as long as a patient continues to be treated with 4-HPR.

Table 1
Effect of RA on Cell Cycle Stage Distribution of Ovarian Carcinoma Cells[a]

Cell line	Treatment	$\%G_0 + G_1$	$\%S$	$\%G_2 + M$
CA-OV3	EtOH	72	13	13
	RA	96	1	2
SK-OV3	EtOH	74	9	17
	RA	72	10	18

[a]In order to determine the effect of RA treatment on cell-cycle distribution, ovarian tumor cell lines were plated at a concentration of 1×10^5 cells per 60 mm tissue-culture dish. On d 1, 3, and 5 after plating, the cells were treated with either RA ($10^{-6} M$) or ethanol. The cells were harvested on d 7 after plating, fixed in 25% ethanol prepared in PBS, and stained with Hoechst 342. Cell cycle distribution was analyzed using an Epics Elite flow cytometer. The proportions of cells with G_0/G_1, S, and G_2/M DNA content were determined by the PARA 1 program supplied by Coulter.

In other studies, 4-HPR increased survival time of nude mice transplanted with a human epithelial ovarian adenocarcinoma cell line. 4-HPR also enhanced the anti-tumor activity of platinum when administered intraperitoneally (56).

Many studies have shown the ability of retinoids to inhibit the growth of ovarian cancer cell lines (57–61). For example, RA treatment of an ovarian surface epithelial cell line, HOC-7, reduced DNA synthesis and downregulated myc gene expression correspond with the growth inhibition (62,63). Our laboratory has also studied the RA growth inhibitory effect on ovarian cancer cells by using two established ovarian tumor cell lines: CA-OV3 and SK-OV3. We isolated single cell clones from a pool of CA-OV3 and SK-OV3 cells and determined their growth sensitivity by four different assays: 1) direct cell counts; 2) autoradiographic determination of DNA synthesis; 3) soft agar assay; 4) dye-based growth assay (MTT Assay). We found that all CA-OV3 subclones were sensitive to RA growth inhibitory effect, although the degree of inhibition varied among these subclones. The growth inhibitory effect of CA-OV3 was dose-dependent. On the other hand, all SK-OV3 subclones were resistant to RA growth-inhibitory effect. Next we examined the cell cycle stage distribution of ATRA-treated ovarian cancer cells by using flow cytometric analysis. We found that RA treatment resulted in a G_1 block in RA sensitive CA-OV3 cells (Table 1). Using cell cycle kinetic analysis, we were able to pinpoint the execution point of RA to a time in mid/late G_1, 2 h prior to the start of S phase (64).

To understand the molecular mechanism by which RA suppresses growth of ovarian tumor cells, expression of RAR-α, RAR-β, RAR-γ, RXR-α, RXR-β, and RXR-γ was examined in CA-OV3 and SK-OV3 cells by using Northern blotting and RNAse protection assay. The results showed that RAR-β and RXR-γ mRNAs were undetectable in either of these two cell lines. While RAR-γ and RXR-β

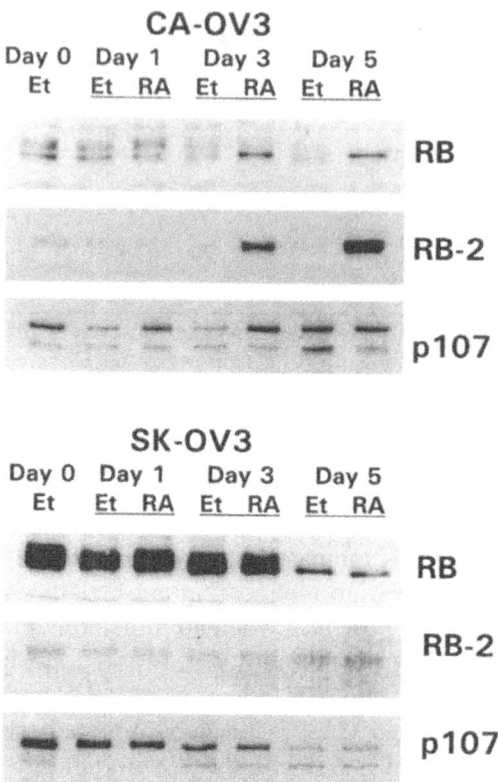

Fig. 4. Western blot analysis of RB protein family expression after RA treatment. Actively proliferating CA-OV3 and SK-OV3 cells were treated with either ethanol or retinoic acid ($10^{-6} M$). On day 0, 1, 3, and 5 of treatment, cells were harvested and protein extracts prepared. Expression of the RB family of proteins was analyzed by polyacrylamide gel electrophoresis followed by Western blotting. Labels to the right indicate the primary antibody used.

mRNA levels were similar in these two cell lines, there were slightly higher levels of RAR-α (~twofold) and RXR-α (three- to fourfold) in RA-sensitive CA-OV3 cells compared to RA-resistant SK-OV3 cells. Furthermore, RAR-α mRNA levels increased in CA-OV3 cells but not in SK-OV3 cells after ATRA treatment *(65)*.

We also found that modulation of RARs and RXRs could alter sensitivity of tumor cells to retinoids. For example, we found that ATRA inhibited cell growth of the RA resistant SK-OV3 cell line by 20%, after they were transfected with either RAR-α or RXR-α cDNA. Furthermore, ATRA could inhibit SK-OV3 cell growth by 50%, if they were transfected with both RAR-α and RXR-α cDNA.

Likewise, the RA sensitive CA-OV3 cells could be made resistant to ATRA growth inhibition after transfection with either anti-sense RAR-α/RXR-α cDNA or dominant negative mutant RAR-β. Similar results were obtained using an oral squamous cell carcinoma model *(66)*. These studies suggested that RAR/RXR play a critical role in modulating RA sensitivity in human tumor cells.

2.7. Metabolites of ATRA

In the cell, all-trans retinoic acid is converted to 4-hydroxy-ATRA by hydroxylation at the fourth position of the β-ionone ring *(67)*. The reaction is catalyzed by a cytochrome P-450-dependent ATRA 4-hydroxylase *(67)*. This metabolite was further catalyzed by another P450-depedent enzyme *(67)*. Epoxidation of ATRA yields 5,6-epoxy-ATRA *(68)*. 4-oxo-ATRA and 5,6-epoxy-retinoic acids inhibit the growth of MCF-7 breast cancer cell to the same extent as ATRA at $10^{-8}M$ and $10^{-7}M$, but lesser extent at $10^{-6}M$. 4-oxo-ATRA has been shown to bind to RAR *(69)*. Both 4-oxo-ATRA and 5,6-epoxy-ATRA can activate RAR-dependent gene transcription in RAR co-transfected CV-1 cells *(70)*.

However, high-performance liquid chromatography (HPLC) studies have shown that the majority of the ATRA is not being converted to its metabolites *(71)*. Therefore, metabolites of ATRA do not seem to be responsible for the growth-suppressing effect of ATRA.

2.8. RAR-β and Cancer

RAR-β is mapped on chromosome 3p21, a region that is often deleted or mutated in many cancers *(72)*. In many cancers, such as: lung (NSCLC), head and neck, breast, ovarian, and others, RAR-β expression is undetectable by using Northern and Western blot *(73,74)*. Its level decreases in the very early stage of carcinogenesis. For example, 50% of oral premalignant leukoplakia lesions have no RAR-β expression. Sixty percent of dysplastic lesions adjacent to head and neck squamous cell carcinomas failed to express RAR-β mRNA *(75)*. Esophageal cancer cells that express RAR-β are sensitive to RA induced growth inhibition and apoptosis. Cells that fail to express RAR-β show no growth inhibition and apoptosis upon RA treatment *(76)*. Re-expression of RAR-β in RAR-β negative cancer cells restored the ability of RA to induce growth inhibition and apoptosis *(77)*. RAR-β expression was upregulated by retinoid treatment, and this upregulation was associated with clinical response *(78)*. Taken together, these data indicate that a reduced expression of RAR-β is associated with carcinogenesis, and upregulation of RAR-β is correlated with tumor growth inhibition and clinical response. Consistent with these observations, our laboratory found that RAR-β mRNA levels were undetectable by Northern blot in both RA-sensitive (CAOV3) and RA-resistant (SKOV3) ovarian tumor cell lines *(65)*.

3. RA MEDIATES GROWTH SUPPRESSION BY TARGETING THE RETINOBLASTOMA PROTEIN FAMILY

Several laboratories including our own have shown that RA blocks cell cycle progression at G_1 (64,79–84). G_1 check point progression is controlled by the retinoblastoma (Rb) protein family and G_1 cyclin/CDK complexes. The Rb family has three members, pRb, p107, and Rb2/p130 (85–87), among which pRb is the most investigated and well-known tumor-suppressor gene. It has been widely reported that RA causes hypophosphorylation of Rb in various cell lines (79,88–95). For example, Wilchen et al. reported hypophosphorylation of Rb in T-47D breast cancer cells upon RA treatment (79). Matsuo and Thiele reported a complete downregulation of G_1 cyclin/CDK activity and hypophosphorylated Rb protein in SMS-KCNR human neuroblastoma cells (88). Spinella et al. found that in the human embryonic carcinoma cell line NT2/D$_1$, RA caused a progressive decline in cyclin D$_1$ and hypophosphorylation of Rb (91). Finally, Naderi and Blomhoff found that RA prevented phosphorylation of Rb in normal human B-lymphocytes when these cells were stimulated with anti-µ and SAC (89). These findings suggest that hypophosphorylation of Rb is a common mechanism mediating inhibition of cell cycle progression upon RA treatment.

While the literature contains many studies on the effects of retinoid treatment on cell cycle gene expression, none of these studies have been performed in ovarian carcinoma cells. As discussed previously, the retinoid sensitivity of the two ovarian adenocarcinoma cell lines we have studied (CA-OV3 and SK-OV3) is well-established (57,64,96–98). We chose to compare one RA-sensitive cell line (CA-OV3) and one RA-resistant cell line (SK-OV3) to identify differences in cell cycle gene expression, which might mediate growth inhibition by RA.

Our Western blot assay results were consistent with reports using other cell models. Figure 3 shows that CA-OV3 cells exhibited significant hypophosphorylation of Rb protein upon RA treatment. In control-treated, actively growing CA-OV3 cells, Rb was present and migrated in a microheterogeneous pattern on sodium dodecyl sulfate polyacrylamide gel electrophoresis (SDS-PAGE), presumably reflecting the presence of multiple phosphorylated forms. However, in response to RA treatment, Rb became hypophosphorylated and migrated as a single, fast-moving band on SDS-PAGE. This pattern became apparent by the third day of RA treatment, which corresponded to the start of growth inhibition.

The most striking finding from our study was that RA treatment resulted in a very significant increase in Rb2/p130 protein in RA-sensitive CA-OV3 cells but not in RA-resistant SK-OV3 cells (Fig. 3). The increase of Rb2/p130 became apparent after 3 d of RA treatment, corresponding to when growth inhibition became apparent. The correspondence between growth inhibition and Rb2/p130 accumulation suggested that Rb2/p130 might be a mediator of RA-induced growth inhibition. Rb2/p130 is the newest member of the retinoblastoma protein family *(86,99,100)*. It is the predominant member of the retinoblastoma protein family seen in quiescent G_0 cells. It complexes with E2F4 and 5, but not with E2F1, 2 and 3 in G_0 and early G_1. As the cells are stimulated to grow, the Rb2/E2F complexes are phosphorylated by G_1 CDKs. Phosphorylated Rb2/p130 is degraded leading to the dissociation of transcriptional repressing Rb2/E2F4 complexes and cell cycle progression (for review *see* refs. *105,136*). In contrast, in cells that are blocked in G_1, the G_1 CDKs do not phosphorylate Rb2/p130. As a result, we would expect to see an increase in Rb2/p130 complexed with E2F4 or 5. This is indeed what was found in our study. Thus, our findings are consistent with the theory that Rb2/p130 is a growth-inhibitory factor that suppresses cell cycle progression. Rb2/p130 also plays an important role in terminal differentiation and embryonic development.

Within the past few years, there are only four reports that describe changes of Rb2/p130 protein level after RA treatment *(95,101–103)*. Two studies described a hypophosphorylation pattern of Rb2/p130 in B-lymphoblastoid cell lines after RA treatment *(95,102)*. One study reported that RA increased the level of nuclear E2F4, p107, and Rb2/p130 in normal human bronchial epithelial (HBE) cells *(103)*. Finally, Hsu et al. found that in human hepatoma Hep3B cells, RA treatment caused Rb2/p130 hyperphosphorylation, p34 (cdc2) activation, and RA-induced cell death *(101)*.

Although our results are very provocative, a number of questions remain to be answered. For example, CA-OV3 cells exhibited both Rb hypophosphorylation and Rb2/p130 accumulation. Is this simply redundancy or do the two members of the retinoblastoma family control different sets of target genes? Because Rb and Rb2/p130 bind to different E2F members, they regulate the expression of different E2F-dependent genes and thus, it is likely that both Rb and Rb2/p130 are needed to fully inhibit cell cycle progression.

Since the regulation of the Rb family is mainly by phosphorylation, control at the transcriptional level does not seem to play an important role. As shown by RNase protection assays, the steady-state RNA level of Rb, p107 and Rb2/p130 did not seem to change significantly after RA treatment in CA-OV3 cells. The highest fold of induction at the mRNA level was for the p16 gene. However, it was no more than twofold. Interestingly, we found that expression of p53, p21, p16, and p15 was extremely low in SK-OV3 cells in comparison to CA-OV3 cells.

In summary, the results from RNase protection assays and Western blot assays suggest that one of the mechanism by which RA causes G_1 arrest is by targeting the retinoblastoma protein family.

4. MECHANISM OF RA MEDIATED RB-RB2/P130 HYPOPHOSPHORYLATION

4.1. Increased p27 Protein Level and Decreased CDK2 Kinase Activity

The functions of all three members of the Rb family are regulated by cell cycle-dependent phosphorylation. Since we observed a significant hypophosphorylation of the Rb protein, we also examined the level of various cyclins, CDKs, and CDK inhibitory proteins. In CA-OV3 cells, cyclin D_1 was the only cyclin that had a significant change in level upon RA treatment. The protein levels of CDK 2, 4, and 6 did not change in response to RA treatment. Interestingly, the protein level of p27 increased significantly after 3 d of RA treatment. None of these changes were observed in the RA resistant SK-OV3 cells. When we examined the kinase activity of CDK 2, 4, and 6 in CA-OV3 cells, we noticed a downregulation of CDK 2 kinase activity after 3 d of RA treatment, corresponding to the increase in p27 level. Although the kinase activity of CDK 4 and 6 also decreased slightly, it did not seem to change as significantly as CDK2. Based on these results, we hypothesized that p27 inhibited CDK2 kinase activity leading to Rb hypophosphorylation in late G_1. This hypothesis was further confirmed by immunoprecipitation assays in which we found that p27 was associated with cyclin E. It has been shown that the cyclin D/CDK 4 and CDK 6 appear to be responsible for early G_1 phosphorylation of Rb, while the cyclin E/CDK2 complex is responsible for mid to late G_1 phosphorylation of pRb (104,105). Since CDK 2 is the partner for cyclin E, increased p27 binding to the cyclin E/CDK 2 complex will lead to decreased cyclinE/CDK2 kinase activity and, as a consequence, hypophosphorylation of Rb in late G_1.

Since Rb hypophosphorylation is very commonly observed in response to RA treatment, as mentioned previously, many groups have tried to explore the mechanism of Rb hypophosphorylation. Research from human breast cancer T-47D cells suggested that retinoids cause hypophosphorylation of pRb, and RA could affect CDK activity without reducing cyclin or CDK levels. It was hypothesized that induction of an inhibitor of CDK4 by RA could account for the observed reduction in CDK activity (79). A number of groups have also found decreased G_1 cyclin/CDK kinase activity in cells growth arrested by RA (88,94,95). This leads to an investigation of the status of CDK inhibitors following RA treatment. Using the myelomonocytic cell line U937, Liu et al. demonstrated that p21[WAF1/CIP1] is a RA-responsive gene. It contains an RARE in its promoter (106). In two other human myeloma cell lines, OPM-2 and C5, the protein level and mRNA level of p21 were also found to be upregulated (107). But other studies also suggested that p27[Kip1] upregulation could be a primary response in RA-treated cells (88,95,108,109). Interestingly this upregulation appears to be at the protein level but not at the mRNA level (88,95,108). Borriello et al. showed that the

accumulation of p27 is due to decreased proteasome-dependent degradation
(108). In another report, the human small cell lung carcinoma cell line H209 that
is RAR-β negative and resistant to RA-induced growth inhibition, was studied.
No change of p27 expression was found upon RA treatment. However, when this
cell line was transfected with RAR-β, the cells showed growth inhibition and p27
upregulation *(109)*. This suggests that RA-induced growth arrest could involve
RAR-β mediated induction of p27.

The increase in p27 protein level and decrease in CDK 2 activity, which we
observed in our ovarian carcinoma model, is consistent with these other reports
(88,95). It appears that p27 upregulation is controlled post-translationally in our
model system. The results from RNAse protection assays did not support direct
induction of transcription of p27. It will be interesting to look at p27 protein
stability in response to RA treatment in our system. Clearly different cell systems
utilize different mechanisms to achieve the same goal: hypophosphorylation of
the retinoblastoma protein family leading to G_1 arrest. In some systems p21 plays
the major role. In others p27 seems to be more important. Sometimes it is the
cyclin or CDK themselves being downregulated by RA. Whether this is due to
cell type specificity or different manipulation of the cells is not known. We did
not detect p21 protein in either CA-OV3 or SK-OV3. Yaginuma and Westphal
found that in the SK-OV3 cell line there were sequence deletions/rearrangements
in at least one allele of the p53 gene and transcripts were not detectable. Sequence
analysis of the entire coding region of the p53 gene revealed point mutations
resulting in codon changes of a highly conserved region of the protein in CA-
OV3 cells *(110)*. Since the transcription of p21 is controlled by p53, abnormal
p53 expression will lead to abnormal p21 expression. This is confirmed by our
RPA results that SK-OV3 cells did not have p53 or p21 mRNA. This might
explain why we could not detect p21 in our system. Since p21 and p27 are more
closely related to each other than to p16 or p15 (the *ink* family), when p21 is not
functional, p27 will likely become a major player. The p53 gene is the most
commonly mutated gene in cancer cells. Therefore p21 will be abnormal in a lot
of tumor cell lines. This might explain why different tumor cell lines utilize
different CDK inhibitory proteins to cause Rb hypophosphorylation.

Many groups have reported a decrease of cyclin D_1 protein level upon RA
treatment, suggesting this might be the cause of Rb hypophosphorylation *(82,
90–93,111)*. Overexpression of cyclin D_1 in human mammary epithelial cells
abolished RA-induced growth inhibition in these cells *(90)*. Langenfeld et al.
(1997) further suggested that RA-induced cyclin D_1 proteolysis might be the
cause of RA induced growth inhibition, because they observed a decline in cyclin
D_1 protein but not mRNA. Moreover, they found that treatment with an ubiquitin-
dependent proteasome inhibitor could prevent this decrease *(111)*. Studies
involving the human embryonic carcinoma cell line NT2/D_1 revealed that RA
accelerates ubiquitination of wild-type cyclin D_1 and causes a reduction in cyclin

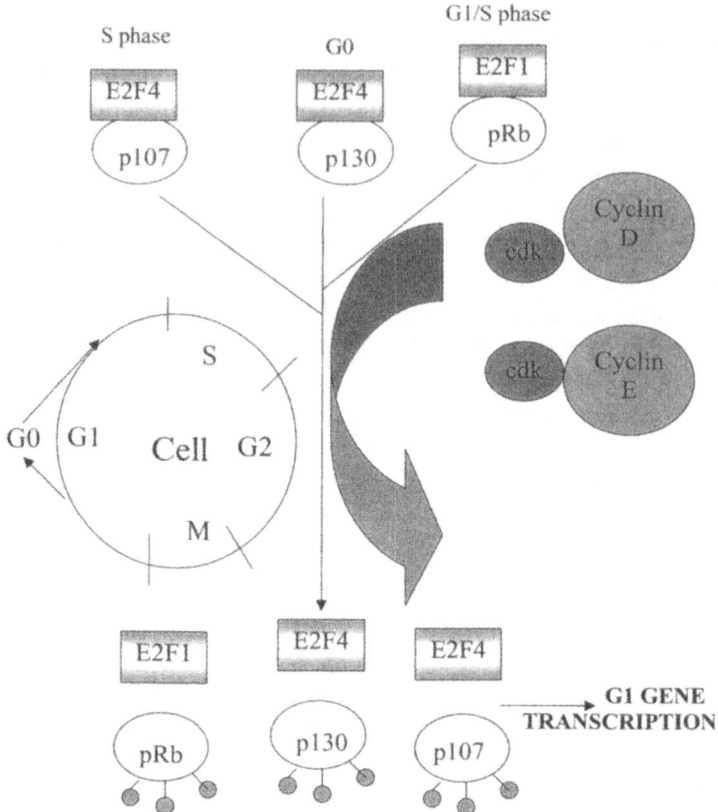

Fig. 5. Model for the regulation of cell cycle progression by the RB protein family.

D_1 protein levels. In contrast, a mutated cyclin D_1 (T286A), which is resistant to phosphorylation and ubiquitination, is not subject to RA-induced protein level decline *(91)*. While the role of retinoic acid in protein degradation is not clear, it has drawn more and more attention. It is interesting to speculate how the same reagent (RA) in one cell model can cause an increase in cell cycle protein stability (as is the case for p27), while in another cell model, it causes a decrease in cell cycle protein stability (as in the case of cyclin D_1). Elucidating how the same treatment (RA) can elicit such opposite effects is likely to be a topic of considerable research interest in the future.

4.2. Low Levels of p27 Protein Expression in Late-Stage RA-Resistant Ovarian Tumors

In a related study, we found that late stage primary ovarian tumors express low levels of p27 protein as determined by Western blot analysis. Giordano and

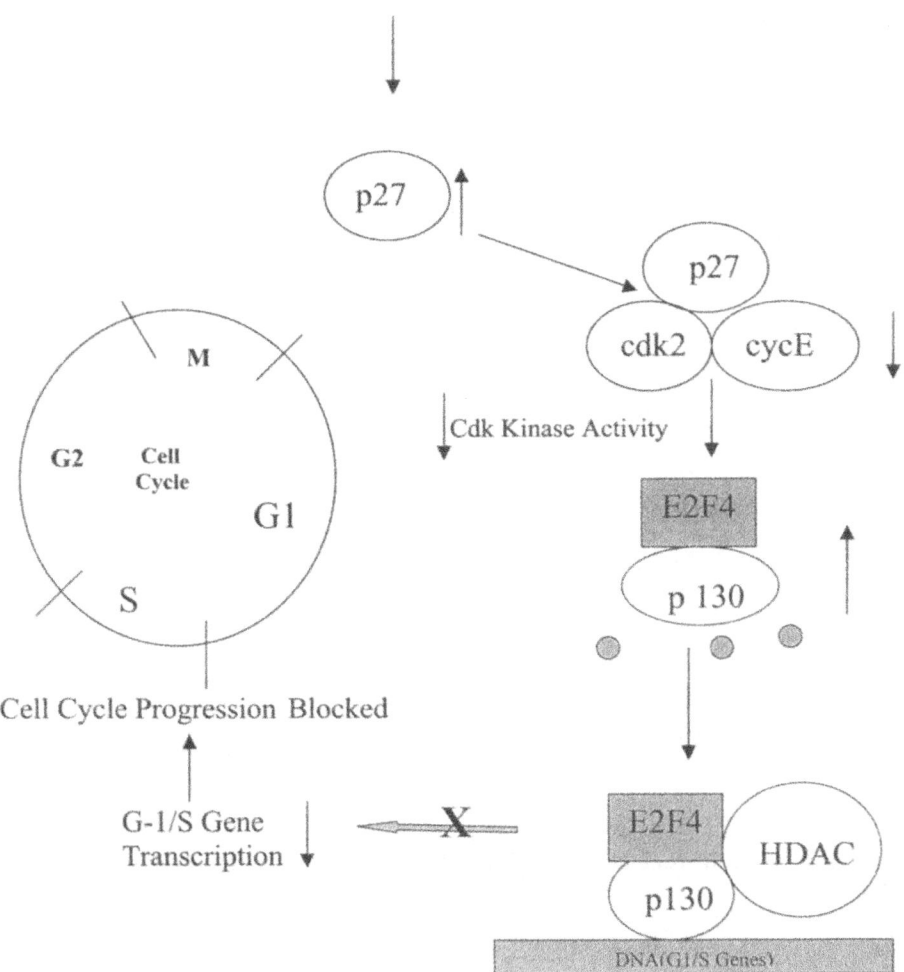

Fig. 6. Model for the regulation of cell cycle progression in retinoid-sensitive cells after RA treatment.

colleagues reported a similar finding using immunohistochemistry analysis. They discovered that the frequent loss of p27 expression in primary ovarian adeno-carcinomas (33%) was much higher than low malignant potential ovarian cancers (6%) *(112)*. Low levels of p27 are associated with poor prognosis in many tumors including breast, prostate, colon, and lung cancers *(113–116)*. Our data along with that of Giordano's laboratory suggests that low p27 expression in late stage ovarian cancer is a frequent event. In human lung squamous carcinoma

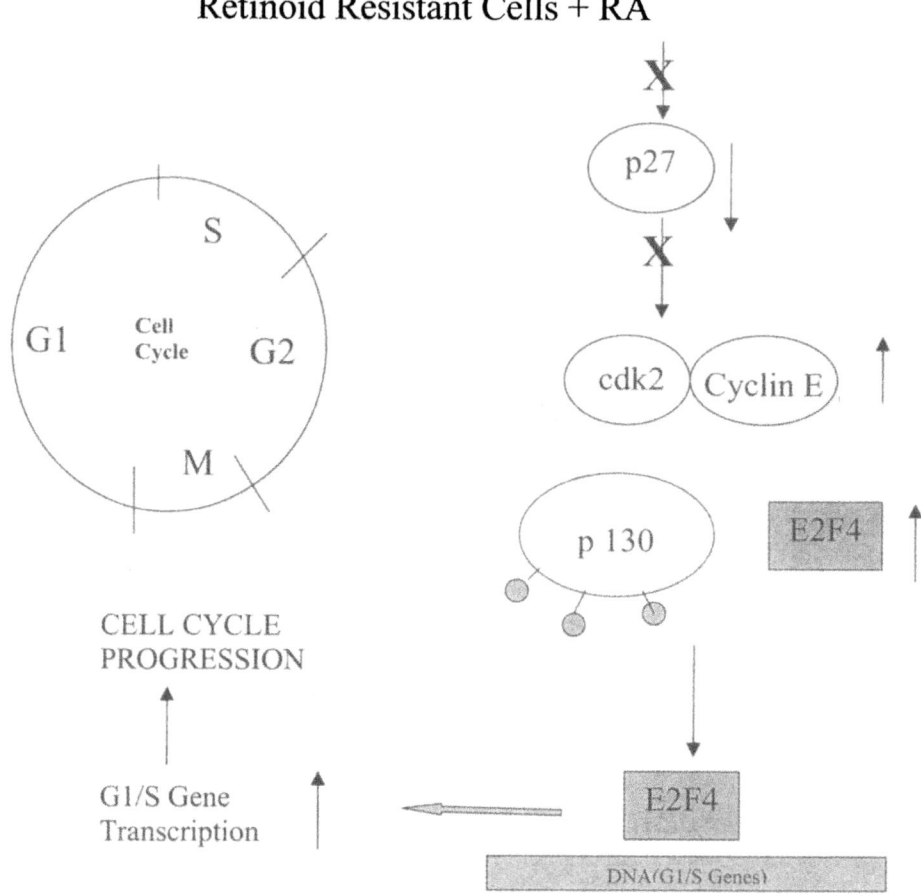

Fig. 7. Model for the regulation of cell cycle progression in retinoid-resistant cells after RA treatment.

CH27 cells, RA-mediated dose- and time-dependent growth arrest in G_1 phase is accompanied by upregulation of p27 *(117)*. Studies have also shown a positive association between survival rate and p27 expression in ovarian cancer patients *(112,118)*.

As mentioned previously, p27 is a cyclin-dependent kinase inhibitor. It is a potent tumor suppressor gene. p27 regulates G_1 progression by inhibiting cyclin E/CDK2 complexes, thus preventing them from phosphorylating members of the RB family including Rb2/p130. Hypophosphorylated Rb2/p130 proteins will bind tightly with E2F4 transcription factors, thus preventing the transcription of genes necessary for cell cycle progression. Hypophosporylated Rb2/p130 also recruits HDAC (Histone Deacetylase) protein, which prevents gene transcription (Figs. 5 and 6). Levels of p27 have been shown to be regulated by ubiquitin-proteasome-dependent degradation mechanisms *(119)*. Low p27 expression in primary ovarian tumors may result from increased degradation by the ubiquitin-proteasome system. In neuroblastoma cells, RA increases p27 levels by downregulating the ubiquitin-proteasome p27-degrading pathway. In the lung cancer cell line, H209, the growth-inhibitory effect of RA is via RAR-β mediated induction of p27 *(109)*. Our laboratory has demonstrated that RA treatment of CAOV3 cells leads to an increase in p27 expression and an increase in hypophosphorylated Rb and Rb2/p130. Interestingly, we found that cell lines prepared from primary ovarian tumors that express low levels of p27 were resistant to the growth-inhibitory effects of RA. We speculate that in late-stage primary ovarian tumors with low p27 levels, the effect of RA is reduced because most of the Rb2/p130 is hyperphosphorylated and Rb2/p130-E2F4 complexes do not form. As a result, cell cycle progression genes continue to be transcribed and cell cycle progression proceeds (Fig. 7). We also speculate that low p27 may be due to low RAR-β level. It will be interesting to see if one can transfect these cells with RAR-β and then determine if p27 level changes after RA treatment.

5. RA CAUSES RB2/P130 ACCUMULATION BY DECREASING DEGRADATION OF THE PROTEIN

As we have mentioned earlier, we found that treatment of CA-OV3 cells with RA caused a 10-fold increase in Rb2/p130 protein level. In order to identify the mechanism of RA-mediated Rb2/p130 induction in CA-OV3 cells, we performed RNAse protection assays (RPA), transcription transactivation assays, and a cycloheximide study. From the RNAse protection assays, we only observed a slight induction of the Rb2/p130 mRNA level after 3 d of RA treatment. The induction was no more than twofold, which could not be considered sufficient to account for the extent of induction observed. The evidence from RPA suggested that RA did not directly induce the transcription of Rb2/p130. In order to confirm this, we utilized transcription transactivation experiments employing CAT reporter plasmid constructs containing various portions of the 5' regulatory region of the Rb2/p130 gene. When we analyzed the sequence of the 5' regulatory region of the Rb2/p130 gene, we found several putative RAREs within the promoter region. If Rb2/p130 was truly a RA-responsive gene, we would have expected to see induction of CAT activity upon RA treatment. However, the results of these experiments showed that RA treatment did not increase the transcription of the Rb2/p130 gene. Therefore we concluded that the RA mediated Rb2/p130 induction was most likely post-transcriptional. Also, using cycloheximide to inhibit new protein synthesis, we found that the half-life of Rb2/p130 protein in cells treated with RA was greater than 60 h compared to a half life of 12 h in control-treated cells. These results suggest that RA increased the protein level of Rb2/p130 by increasing stability of Rb2/p130.

Many studies support the view that Rb2/p130 is regulated by a post-transcriptional mechanism. Rb2/p130 has been shown to undergo cell cycle-dependent changes in its phosphorylation status *(120–122)*. Also, it has been reported that only the hypophosphorylated form of Rb2/p130 associates in vivo with E2F4 while hyperphosphorylated forms do not *(123)*. Moreover, hyperphosphorylation of Rb2/p130 results in a dramatic degradation of the protein *(123,124)*. Ubiquitin-mediated protein degradation is thought to be involved in this process *(124)*. Using rat embryonic fibroblast cells (REF52) as a model, Smith et al. (1998) found that Rb2/p130 protein was only present in serum starved, quiescent cells but disappeared when the cells were stimulated to grow by addition of fresh serum. It took 24 h for Rb2/p130 protein to completely disappear. During this time the protein exhibited an alteration in the gel mobility, likely the consequence of G_1 cdk-mediated phosphorylation. However, Rb2/p130 RNA was relatively constant in growing and quiescent cells, consistent with a post-transcriptional mechanism for regulating Rb2/p130 expression and function. Finally, Smith et al. showed that addition of a 26S proteasome inhibitor early in the process of cell cycle reentry prevented the disappearance of Rb2/p130 and blocked the cell cycle at G_1. In contrast, later addition of the inhibitor allowed the cells to progress through G_1 and prevented the loss of the Rb2/p130 protein, resulting in an accumulation of phosphorylated form of Rb2/p130 *(124)*.

In our system, the effect of RA is opposite to that of serum stimulation. RA treatment caused actively growing cells to be arrested in G_1. The accumulation of Rb2/p130 is likely the result of decreased protein degradation. The traditional method to measure the rate of protein degradation would be a pulse chase experiment. However, because of the low level of Rb2/p130 expression in actively growing cells, it is not possible to obtain sufficient in vivo radioactively labeled Rb2/p130 to follow during the chase period. As an alternative, we used a method that did not require that the protein of interest become highly radioactively labeled. We used cycloheximide to inhibit new Rb2/p130 synthesis after the cells had been treated with RA or ethanol. The cells were harvested at different time points and the remaining Rb2/p130 was measured by Western blot assays. The results indicated that in RA treated cells the Rb2/p130 protein was degraded at a much slower rate compared to that of the ethanol-treated control. There are two possible mechanisms that could be responsible for the stabilization of Rb2/p130 protein by RA. First, Rb2/p130 protein could be targeted for degradation by phosphorylation. RA-mediated decrease in G_1 cyclin/CDK activity could lead to less Rb2/p130 phosphorylation. As a result, the unphosphorylated Rb2/p130 would no longer be a target for phosphorylation-dependent ubiquitination and proteasome degradation. Second, RA could target the components of the ubiquitination system or proteasome leading to inhibition of Rb2/p130 degradation. We have used Western blotting to examine many of the components of the ubiquitination and proteasome complexes. No change in the level of any of these components was observed following RA treatment of either CA-OV3 cells or SK-OV3 cells. Thus, we believe that the first explanation is more likely. Consistent with this is the fact that we observed a decrease in CDK2 kinase activity following RA treatment at the same time as the increase in Rb2/p130 expression. While we do not have direct evidence that the cyclinE/CDK2 complex phosphorylates Rb2/p130 in ovarian carcinoma cells during late G_1, other studies have shown that Rb2/p130 associates directly with cyclinA, cyclin E, and CDK2 *(99,100,125)*. In order to determine the precise mechanism of RA stablization of Rb2/p130, we would need to: 1) show that RA treament alters Rb2/p130 phosphorylation; 2) that Rb2/p130 protein is ubiquitinated during G_1 and that this ubiquitination is inhibited by RA treatment; and 3) that the half life of phosphorylated Rb2/p130 is shorter than that of unphosphorylated Rb2/p130 protein.

6. RB2/P130 MEDIATES RA INHIBITION OF CELL CYCLE PROGRESSION

As the newest member of the Rb family, the function of Rb2/p130 is not as thoroughly investigated as Rb protein. While the growth inhibitory effect of Rb is well-defined, the function of Rb2/p130 is not as well-understood. Surprisingly, mouse strains with mutations in the murine homologue of Rb, p107, and Rb2/p130 do not exhibit significant alteration in phenotype when carrying only the Rb2/p130 –/– mutation. A phenotype is observed only when the Rb2/p130 null is combined with a knock-out of either p107 or Rb *(126)*. Nevertheless, Rb2/p130 has been known to be the predominant form of the Rb family of proteins expressed in the quiescent stage of the cell cycle. A number of studies suggest that Rb2/p130 plays an important role in the resting status of the cells *(127–130)*. As cells progress through G_1, Rb2/p130 levels have been shown to decrease significantly *(124)*.

Is Rb2/p130 as equally important as Rb in mediating cell cycle regulation of ovarian carcinoma cells? Is Rb2/p130 alone able to inhibit cell cycle progression in this model? With these questions in mind, we investigated the importance of Rb2/p130 protein in RA-mediated growth inhibition. Since we observed a dramatic increase in Rb2/p130 protein level, we wanted to know whether this was the cause or result of RA-mediated cell cycle arrest. We reasoned that if this was the cause of growth arrest, preventing the increase in Rb2/p130 protein should abolish the growth inhibition. Conversely, over expression of Rb2/p130 protein in RA-resistant cells should lead to growth inhibition. If Rb2/p130 induction was simply the result of G_1 arrest caused by RA treatment, we would not expect any change in cell growth upon modulation of Rb2/p130 expression. We utilized a plasmid containing the Rb2/p130 cDNA cloned in the antisense direction to transfect the CA-OV3 cells. The RA-mediated induction of Rb2/p130 protein was blocked by expression of antisense transcripts from this construct.

Table 2
Correlation of RA mediated Inhibition of CA-OV3 Cell Growth and Induction
of Rb2/p130 Protein Expression[a]

Clone	% Growth inhibition (RA/control)	Rb2/p130 expression (RA/control)
CA-OV3	59 ± 5.7	5.0
AS-Rb2 Pool	25 ± 4.6	1.6
AS-1	14 ± 5.0	0.9
AS-8	20 ± 5.3	0.9
AS-15	27 ± 7.0	1.5
AS-20	15 ± 5.2	1.2
AS-25	26 ± 6.0	1.8
AS-28	19 ± 7.6	1.4
AS-32	12 ± 5.2	1.1

[a]Antisense Rb2 pool and seven antisense-Rb-2 clones were plated at 2×10^5 cells per 100-mm plate and treated with RA ($10^{-6} M$) or ethanol for 5 d. At the end of the treatment, the cells were trypsinized and the number of cells in each plate was counted using a hemocytometer. The percent of growth inhibition was determined by subtracting from 100 the number of cells in RA-treated plates divided by the number of cells in ethanol-treated plates × 100. Mean values ± standard deviation were calculated from triplicate samples. Rb2/p130 protein level was determined by measure of the density of bands in a Western blot using NIH Image. Rb2/p130 expression shown is fold induction upon RA treatment for 5 d.

Furthermore, these cells exhibited less growth inhibition upon RA treatment (Table 2). Likewise, in SK-OV3 cells where the Rb2/p130 protein level was not induced by RA, growth inhibition occurred when Rb2/p130 was overexpressed using a tetracycline-regulated expression system. Taken together, these results suggest that Rb2/p130 is truly a growth suppressor gene in ovarian carcinoma cells, which mediates G_1 arrest following RA treatment.

Our findings are consistent with those of other laboratories, which also suggest that overproduction of Rb2/p130 can interfere with cell cycle progression and tumor cell growth. In one study, the osteosarcoma cell line SAOS-2 was cotransfected with an Rb2/p130 expression plasmid and a cell surface protein CD19. Expression of Rb2/p130 reproducibly led to a significant increase in the fraction of cells with a G_0/G_1 DNA content (128). In another report, a tightly regulated Rb2/p130 gene was introduced into a hamster brain tumor cell line. When these tumor cells were injected subcutaneously into nude mice, expression of Rb2/p130 brought about a 3.2-fold reduction in tumor mass (131). In another study in nude mice, ectopic expression of pRb2/p130 suppressed the tumorigenicity of the erb-2-overexpressing SK-OV3 ovarian tumor cell line (132). The role of Rb2/p130 as a candidate for gene therapy in lung cancer is also under investigation (for review, see ref. 145).

It is significant that when we overexpressed Rb2/p130 in RA-resistant SK-OV3 cells, growth was inhibited. These results suggest that the growth inhibitory pathway downstream of Rb2/p130 accumulation is functional in SK-OV3 cells. Thus, the difference between CA-OV3 and SK-OV3 cells is that CA-OV3 cells are able to accumulate Rb2/p130 in response to RA treatment but the SK-OV3 cells fail to do so. Understanding why RA treatment of SK-OV3 cells fails to lead to Rb2/p130 accumulation will help us to further understand the mechanism of Rb2/p130-mediated growth inhibition.

7. RB2/P130 INHIBITS G1 PROGRESSION THROUGH INTERACTION WITH E2F4 AND REPRESSES THE TRANSCRIPTION OF THE GENES CONTAINING E2F BINDING SITES

As we have mentioned previously, Rb2/p130 only complexes with E2F4 and E2F5 but not with E2F1, 2 or 3. The Rb2/E2F complexes are only seen in G_0 and early G_1 and disappear gradually with cell cycle progression through the restriction point. We observed a significant increase of Rb2/p130 protein and E2F4 protein in response to RA treatment in CA-OV3 cells. The coincidental increase of Rb2/p130 and E2F4 suggests that they might form a complex and act together to cause growth inhibition. As we expected, when we performed co-immuno-precipitation assays using antibody to E2F4, we precipitated an increased amount of Rb2/p130 in RA-treated cells compared to vehicle-treated controls. This result suggests that as the Rb2/p130 protein level increased in response to RA treatment, the amount of Rb2/E2F4 complex also increased. We suspect that the accumulation of E2F4 is a consequence of the induction of Rb2/p130 since it has been reported that E2F4 can be protected from ubiquitin-mediated degradation by Rb2/p130 binding *(133)*.

Our immunoprecipitation assays also showed association between p27 and cyclinE. Although cyclin E protein level did not change with RA treatment, p27 bound to cyclin E did increase with RA treatment. This would predict that RA treatment would lead to decreased CDK2 activity, which we did in fact observe.

When we used a consensus E2F binding site as probe to perform electro-phoretic mobility shift assays, we found that RA treated CA-OV3 cells had much less free E2F1, 2, 3 binding to the probe in comparison to control treatment. In contrast, free E2F4 binding remained the same even after RA treatment. As a result, there was a change in the profile of EMSA probe binding by free E2Fs in control- vs RA-treated CA-OV3 cell nuclear extracts. In actively growing cells, all of the E2F family members bind equally to the E2F consensus oligonucle-otides. However, in nuclear extracts obtained from RA growth-arrested cells, E2F4 is the dominant E2F family member, which binds to the E2F consensus oligo probe. In addition to free E2F, we also attempted to identify the Rb/E2Fs complexes. Surprisingly, we found that the amount of Rb-containing complexes did not change significantly in actively growing vs RA-growth inhibited cells.

Unfortunately we were unable to identify Rb2/E2F4 complexes due to lack of good antibodies for supershift assays.

As for the functions of the free E2Fs, it is widely believed that free E2F1, 2, and 3 activate transcription of their target genes while free E2F4 and 5 is thought to repress target-gene expression. Some studies have provided evidence that various E2F family members may specifically activate the transcription of subsets of target genes *(134,135)*. On the other hand, E2F4 and 5 in conjunction with Rb2/p130 has been reported to control the expression of E2F1, 2, and 3 *(136)*.

When we examined the in vivo binding of the E2F transcription factors and Rb family proteins to representative E2F response genes using the chromatin immunoprecipitation (ChIPs) assay, we found that Rb2/p130 consistently exhibited increased binding to dihydrofolate reductase (DHFR), thymidine kinase (TK), and cdc2 promoters after RA treatment. We also found that the amount of acetylated histone H3 bound to the DHFR, TK, and cdc2 promoters decreased in response to RA treatment.

The ChIPs assay is a relatively new method to show in vivo binding of protein (can be either histone or transcription factors) to DNA. It has been used to examine the binding of c-Myc and USF to the cad promoter *(137,138)* and the binding of E2Fs and Rb protein family to the p107, E2F1, cdc25A, cdc6, B-myb, cyclin A, and cdc2 promoters (139). The beauty of the ChIPs assay is that it can distinguish among members of a family of DNA-binding proteins that regulate a specific promoter in live cells. We chose to study the binding of Rb, p107, Rb2/ p130, E2F1, E2F4, and acetylated histone H3 to DHFR, TK, and cdc2 promoters because these are cell cycle regulatory genes known to contain E2F binding sites in their promoter region *(140–142)*.

Our results show that in response to RA treatment Rb2/p130 protein was enriched at DHFR, TK, and cdc2 promoters, indicating the presence of Rb2/E2F complex at these promoters. The Rb2/E2F complexes have been known to exhibit transcription repression activity *(128,129)*. The mechanism of Rb2/p130-mediated transcription repression is thought to involve histone deacetylation. The three members of the Rb family share the ability to recruit histone deacetylase *(143,144)*. We observed a decreased amount of acetylated histone H3 bound to DHFR, TK, and cdc2 promoters. It should be noted, however, that we did not directly prove that decreased amount of acetylated histone H3 was caused by Rb2/p130. Also we have not proven that Rb2/E2F4 complex binding to these promoters is responsible for repressing the transcription from these promoters.

8. A MODEL OF RETINOIC ACID INDUCED OVARIAN CANCER CA-OV3 GROWTH ARREST

In summary, we showed that RA-mediated Rb2/p130 induction was a result of decreased protein degradation. The increased level of p27 following RA treatment might account for Rb2/p130 accumulation as well as hypophosphorylation of Rb through decreased activity of cyclinE/CDK 2 complex. Following RA treatment, Rb2/p130 was found to form a complex with E2F4. This complex was found to be associated with E2F sites of cell cycle regulatory genes and thus may be responsible for repressing the transcription of the genes necessary for entering S phase by recruitment of histone deacetylase. A plausible model for the action of RA in ovarian tumor cells is shown in Figs. 6 and 7.

In actively growing CA-OV3 cells, the kinase activity of cyclinD/CDK4 and cyclinE/CDK2 complexes increase during mid to late G_1, leading to phosphorylation of Rb, p107, and Rb2/p130. Phosphorylated Rb, p107, and Rb2/p130 dissociate from E2Fs, so that E2Fs could act as transcription activators and activate transcription of the genes required for S phase entry. The cells will progress through the cell cycle. However, in RA-treated CA-OV3 cells, p27 protein level increases, leading to decreased cyclinE/CDK2 kinase activity. This is the cause of Rb hypophosphorylation and Rb2/p130 accumulation (probably through decreased Rb2/p130 protein degradation). ChIPs assay and EMSA identify increased Rb2/p130/E2F4 binding to target genes. The transcription of the genes required for S phase entry is repressed by the Rb2/p130/E2F4 complex, leading to cell cycle arrest in G1.

ACKNOWLEDGMENTS

This work was supported by grants from the National Institutes of Health (CA64945 and DE13139) to K.J.S.

REFERENCES

1. Ross AC. Mutations in the gene encoding retinol binding protein and retinol deficiency: is there compensation by retinyl esters and retinoic acid? *Am J Clin Nutr* 1999;69(5):829–830.
2. Blomhoff R, et al. Vitamin A metabolism: new perspectives on absorption, transport, and storage. *Physiol Rev* 1991;71(4):951–990.
3. Napoli JL. Biochemical pathways of retinoid transport, metabolism, and signal transduction. *Clin Immunol Immunopathol* 1996;80(3 Pt 2):S52–S62.
4. Harrison EH, et al. Subcellular localization of retinoids, retinoid-binding proteins, and acyl-CoA:retinol acyltransferase in rat liver. *J Lipid Res* 1987;28(8):973–981.
5. Li E, et al. Fluorine nuclear magnetic resonance analysis of the ligand binding properties of two homologous rat cellular retinol-binding proteins expressed in *Escherichia coli*. *J Biol Chem* 1991;266(6):3622–3629.
6. Napoli JL, et al. Enzymes and binding proteins affecting retinoic acid concentrations. *J Steroid Biochem Mol Biol* 1995;53(1–6):497–502.
7. Kuppumbatti YS, et al. Cellular retinol-binding protein expression and breast cancer. *J Natl Cancer Inst* 2000;92(6):475–480.
8. Boylan JF, Gudas LJ. The level of CRABP-I expression influences the amounts and types of all-trans-retinoic acid metabolites in F9 teratocarcinoma stem cells. *J Biol Chem* 1992; 267(30):21486–21491.
9. Boylan JF, Gudas LJ. Overexpression of the cellular retinoic acid binding protein-I (CRABP-I) results in a reduction in differentiation-specific gene expression in F9 teratocarcinoma cells. *J Cell Biol* 1991;112(5):965–979.

10. Lampron C, et al. Mice deficient in cellular retinoic acid binding protein II (CRABPII) or in both CRABPI and CRABPII are essentially normal. *Development* 1995;121(2):539–548.
11. Chambon P. A decade of molecular biology of retinoic acid receptors. *FASEB J* 1996; 10(9):940–954.
12. Lohnes D, et al. Function of retinoic acid receptor gamma in the mouse. *Cell* 1993;73(4): 643–658.
13. Lufkin T, et al. High postnatal lethality and testis degeneration in retinoic acid receptor alpha mutant mice. *Proc Natl Acad Sci USA* 1993;90(15):7225–7229.
14. Mendelsohn C, et al. Function of the retinoic acid receptors (RARs) during development (II). Multiple abnormalities at various stages of organogenesis in RAR double mutants. *Development* 1994;120(10):2749–2771.
15. De Luca LM, et al. Retinoids in differentiation and neoplasia. *Scientific American* 1995;2:28–37.
16. Bannister AJ, Kouzarides T. The CBP co-activator is a histone acetyltransferase. *Nature* 1996;384(6610):641–643.
17. Chen H, et al. Nuclear receptor coactivator ACTR is a novel histone acetyltransferase and forms a multimeric activation complex with P/CAF and CBP/p300. *Cell* 1997;90(3):569–580.
18. Ogryzko VV, et al. The transcriptional coactivators p300 and CBP are histone acetyltransferases. *Cell* 1996;87(5):953–959.
19. Spencer TE, et al. Steroid receptor coactivator-1 is a histone acetyltransferase. *Nature* 1997;389(6647):194–198.
20. Yang XJ, et al. A p300/CBP-associated factor that competes with the adenoviral oncoprotein E1A. *Nature* 1996;382(6589):319–324.
21. Nakajima T, et al. RNA helicase A mediates association of CBP with RNA polymerase II. *Cell* 1997;90(6):1107–1112.
22. Kurokawa R, et al. Differential orientations of the DNA-binding domain and carboxy-terminal dimerization interface regulate binding site selection by nuclear receptor heterodimers. *Genes Dev* 1993;7(7B):1423–1435.
23. Hong WK, Itri LM. Retinoids and human cancer, in *The Retinoids*. Sporn MB, Roberts AB, Goodman DS, eds. Raven Press, New York, 1994, pp. 592–631.
24. Wolbach SB, Howe PR. Nutrition classics. The Journal of Experimental Medicine 1925;42:753-777. Tissue changes following deprivation of fat-soluble A vitamin. Wolbach, S Burt, Howe Percy, R. *Nutr Rev* 1978;36(1):16–19.
25. Lasnitzki I. The influence of a hyper-vitaminosis on the effect of 20-methylcholanthrene on mouse prostate glands growth in vitro. *Br J Cancer* 1955;9:434–441.
26. Lasnitzki I. Reversal of methylcholanthrene-induced changes in mouse prostates in vitro by retinoic acid and its analogues. *Br J Cancer* 1976;34(3):239–248.
27. Moon RC, Mehta RC, Rao KJVN. *Retinoids and Cancer in Experimental Animals*, Sporn MB, Roberts AB, Goodman DS, eds. Raven Press, New York, 1994, pp. 573–595.
28. Harisiadis L, et al. A vitamin A analogue inhibits radiation-induced oncogenic transformation. *Nature* 1978;274(5670):486–487.
29. Mordan LJ, Bertram JS. Retinoid effects on cell-cell interactions and growth characteristics of normal and carcinogen-treated C3H/1OT1/2 cells. *Cancer Res* 1983;43(2):567–571.
30. Lotan R. Retinoids in cancer chemoprevention. *FASEB J* 1996;10(9):1031–1039.
31. Creek KE, et al. Retinoic acid suppresses human papillomavirus type 16 (HPV16)-mediated transformation of human keratinocytes and inhibits the expression of the HPV16 oncogenes. *Adv Exp Med Biol* 1994;354:19–35.
32. Hong WK, et al. 13-cis-retinoic acid in the treatment of oral leukoplakia. *N Engl J Med* 1986;315(24):1501–1505.
33. Lippman SM, et al. Comparison of low-dose isotretinoin with beta carotene to prevent oral carcinogenesis. *N Engl J Med* 1993;328(1):15–20.
34. Hong WK, et al. Prevention of second primary tumors with isotretinoin in squamous-cell carcinoma of the head and neck. *N Engl J Med* 1990;323(12):795–801.

35. Lippman SM, et al. Retinoids and chemoprevention: clinical and basic studies. *J Cell Biochem Suppl* 1995;22:1–10.
36. Bjelke E. Dietary vitamin A and human lung cancer. *Int J Cancer* 1975;15(4):561–565.
37. Misset JL, et al. Regression of bronchial epidermoid metaplasia in heavy smokers with etretinate treatment. *Cancer Detect Prev* 1986;9(1–2):167–170.
38. Shekelle RB, et al. Dietary vitamin A and risk of cancer in the Western Electric study. *Lancet* 1981;2(8257):1185–1190.
39. Pastorino U, et al. Adjuvant treatment of stage I lung cancer with high-dose vitamin A. *J Clin Oncol* 1993;11(7):1216–1222.
40. Saffiotti U. et al. Experimental cancer of the lung. Inhibition by vitamin A of the induction of tracheobronchial squamous metaplasia and squamous cell tumors. *Cancer* 1967; 20(5):857–864.
41. Hislop TG, et al. Diet and histologic types of benign breast disease defined by subsequent risk of breast cancer. *Am J Epidemiol* 1990;131(2):263–270.
42. Moon RC, Mehta RG. Chemoprevention of experimental carcinogenesis in animals. *Prev Med* 1989;18(5):576–591.
43. Moon RC, et al. N-(4-Hydroxyphenyl)retinamide, a new retinoid for prevention of breast cancer in the rat. *Cancer Res* 1979;39(4):1339–1346.
44. Dowlatshahi K, et al. Therapeutic effect of N-(4-hydroxyphenyl)retinamide on N-methyl-N-nitrosourea-induced rat mammary cancer. *Cancer Lett* 1989;47(3):187–192.
45. McCormick DL, Moon RC. Retinoid-tamoxifen interaction in mammary cancer chemoprevention. *Carcinogenesis* 1986;7(2):193–196.
46. Ratko TA, et al. Chemopreventive efficacy of combined retinoid and tamoxifen treatment following surgical excision of a primary mammary cancer in female rats. *Cancer Res* 1989; 49(16):4472–4476.
47. Lippman SM, Benner SE, Hong WK. Cancer chemoprevention. *J Clin Oncol* 1994; 12(4):851–873.
48. Kraemer KH, et al. Prevention of skin cancer in xeroderma pigmentosum with the use of oral isotretinoin. *N Engl J Med* 1988;318(25):1633–1637.
49. Moore KG, Donadio AC, Sartorelli AC. Determination of type I transglutaminase in differentiating normal and neoplastic human keratinocytes by an in situ radioimmunoassay. *Biochem Biophys Res Commun* 1993;192(2):381–385.
50. Rowley JD, Golomb HM, Dougherty C. 15/17 translocation, a consistent chromosomal change in acute promyelocytic leukaemia. *Lancet* 1977;1(8010):549–550.
51. Zhong S, et al., Promyelocytic leukemia protein (PML) and Daxx participate in a novel nuclear pathway for apoptosis. *J Exp Med* 2000;191(4):631–640.
52. Flynn PJ, et al. Retinoic acid treatment of acute promyelocytic leukemia: in vitro and in vivo observations. *Blood* 1983;62(6):1211–1217.
53. Huang ME, et al. Use of all-trans retinoic acid in the treatment of acute promyelocytic leukemia. *Blood* 1988;72(2):567–572.
54. Huang ME, et al. All-trans retinoic acid with or without low dose cytosine arabinoside in acute promyelocytic leukemia. Report of 6 cases. *Chin Med J (Engl)* 1987;100(12):949–953.
55. de Palo G, Formelli F. Risks and benefits of retinoids in the chemoprevention of cancer. *Drug Safety* 1995;13(4):245–256.
56. Formelli F, Cleris L. Synthetic retinoid fenretinide is effective against a human ovarian carcinoma xenograft and potentiates cisplatin activity. *Cancer Res* 1993;53(22):5374–5376.
57. Harant H, et al. Retinoic acid receptors in retinoid responsive ovarian cancer cell lines detected by polymerase chain reaction following reverse transcription. *Br J Cancer* 1993;68(3):530–536.
58. Saunders DE, et al. Inhibition of c-myc in breast and ovarian carcinoma cells by 1,25-dihydroxyvitamin D3, retinoic acid and dexamethasone. *Anticancer Drugs* 1993;4(2): 201–208.

59. Chao WR, et al. Effects of receptor class- and subtype-selective retinoids and an apoptosis-inducing retinoid on the adherent growth of the NIH:OVCAR-3 ovarian cancer cell line in culture. *Cancer Lett* 1997;115(1):1–7.
60. Sabichi AL, et al. Retinoic acid receptor beta expression and growth inhibition of gynecologic cancer cells by the synthetic retinoid N-(4-hydroxyphenyl) retinamide. *J Natl Cancer Inst* 1998;90(8):597–605.
61. Pergolizzi R, et al. Role of retinoic acid receptor overexpression in sensitivity to fenretinide and tumorigenicity of human ovarian carcinoma cells. *Int J Cancer* 1999;81(5):829–834.
62. Grunt TW, et al. The effects of dimethyl sulfoxide and retinoic acid on the cell growth and the phenotype of ovarian cancer cells. *J Cell Sci* 1991;100(Pt 3):657–666.
63. Grunt TW, et al. Comparative analysis of the effects of dimethyl sulfoxide and retinoic acid on the antigenic pattern of human ovarian adenocarcinoma cells. *J Cell Sci* 1992;103(Pt 2):501–509.
64. Wu S, et al. All-trans-retinoic acid blocks cell cycle progression of human ovarian adenocarcinoma cells at late G1. *Exp Cell Res* 1997;232(2):277–286.
65. Wu S, et al. Critical role of both retinoid nuclear receptors and retinoid-X-receptors in mediating growth inhibition of ovarian cancer cells by all-trans retinoic acid. *Oncogene* 1998;17(22):2839–2849.
66. Li M, et al. Skin abnormalities generated by temporally controlled RXRalpha mutations in mouse epidermis. *Nature* 2000;407(6804):633–636.
67. Roberts AB, Lamb LC, Sporn MB. Metabolism of all-trans-retinoic acid in hamster liver microsomes: oxidation of 4-hydroxy- to 4-keto-retinoic acid. *Arch Biochem Biophys* 1980;199(2):374–383.
68. McCormick AM, et al. Isolation and identification of 5, 6-epoxyretinoic acid: a biologically active metabolite of retinoic acid. *Biochemistry* 1978;17(19):4085–4090.
69. Pijnappel WW, et al. The retinoid ligand 4-oxo-retinoic acid is a highly active modulator of positional specification. *Nature* 1993;366(6453):340–344.
70. Duell, E.A., et al., Human skin levels of retinoic acid and cytochrome P-450-derived 4-hydroxyretinoic acid after topical application of retinoic acid in vivo compared to concentrations required to stimulate retinoic acid receptor-mediated transcription in vitro. *J Clin Invest* 1992;90(4):1269–1274.
71. Van heusden J, et al. All-trans-retinoic acid metabolites significantly inhibit the proliferation of MCF-7 human breast cancer cells in vitro. *Br J Cancer* 1998;77(1):26–32.
72. Kok K, et al. Deletion of a DNA sequence at the chromosomal region 3p21 in all major types of lung cancer. *Nature* 1987;330(6148):578–581.
73. Gebert JF, et al. High frequency of retinoic acid receptor beta abnormalities in human lung cancer [published erratum appears in *Oncogene* 1992 Apr;7(4):821]. *Oncogene* 1991; 6(10):1859–1868.
74. Nervi C, et al. Expression of nuclear retinoic acid receptors in normal tracheobronchial cells and in lung carcinoma cells. *Exp Cell Res* 1991;195(1):163–170.
75. Xu XC, et al. Differential expression of nuclear retinoid receptors in normal, premalignant, and malignant head and neck tissues. *Cancer Res* 1994;54(13):3580–3587.
76. Xu XC, et al. Expression and up-regulation of retinoic acid receptor-beta is associated with retinoid sensitivity and colony formation in esophageal cancer cell lines. *Cancer Res* 1999;59(10):2477–2483.
77. Liu Y, et al. Retinoic acid receptor beta mediates the growth-inhibitory effect of retinoic acid by promoting apoptosis in human breast cancer cells. *Mol Cell Biol* 1996;16(3):1138–1149.
78. Lotan R. Retinoids and their receptors in modulation of differentiation, development, and prevention of head and neck cancers. *Anticancer Res* 1996;16(4C):2415–2419.
79. Wilcken NR, et al. Differential effects of retinoids and antiestrogens on cell cycle progression and cell cycle regulatory genes in human breast cancer cells. *Cell Growth Differ* 1996;7(1): 65–74.

80. Guilbaud, NF, et al. Effects of differentiation-inducing agents on maturation of human MCF-7 breast cancer cells. *J Cell Physiol* 1990;145(1):162–172.
81. Seewaldt VL, et al. Expression of retinoic acid receptor beta mediates retinoic acid-induced growth arrest and apoptosis in breast cancer cells. *Cell Growth Differ* 1995;6(9):1077–1088.
82. Zhou Q, Stetler-Stevenson M, Steeg PS. Inhibition of cyclin D expression in human breast carcinoma cells by retinoids in vitro. *Oncogene* 1997;15(1):107–115.
83. Turley JM, et al. Growth inhibition and apoptosis of RL human B lymphoma cells by vitamin E succinate and retinoic acid: role for transforming growth factor beta. *Cell Growth Differ* 1995;6(6):655–663.
84. Piacentini M, Fesus L, Melino G. Multiple cell cycle access to the apoptotic death programme in human neuroblastoma cells. *FEBS Lett* 1993;320(2):150–154.
85. Ewen ME, et al. Molecular cloning, chromosomal mapping, and expression of the cDNA for p107, a retinoblastoma gene product-related protein. *Cell* 1991;66(6):1155–1164.
86. Mayol X, et al. Cloning of a new member of the retinoblastoma gene family (pRb2) which binds to the E1A transforming domain. *Oncogene* 1993;8(9):2561–2566.
87. Whyte P, et al. Association between an oncogene and an anti-oncogene: the adenovirus E1A proteins bind to the retinoblastoma gene product. *Nature* 1988;334(6178):124–129.
88. Matsuo T, Thiele CJ. p27Kip1: a key mediator of retinoic acid induced growth arrest in the SMS-KCNR human neuroblastoma cell line. *Oncogene* 1998;16(25):3337–3343.
89. Naderi S., Blomhoff HK. Retinoic acid prevents phosphorylation of pRB in normal human B lymphocytes: regulation of cyclin E, cyclin A, and p21(Cip1). *Blood* 1999;94(4):1348–1358.
90. Seewaldt VL, et al. Dysregulated expression of cyclin D1 in normal human mammary epithelial cells inhibits all-trans-retinoic acid-mediated G0/G1-phase arrest and differentiation in vitro. *Exp Cell Res* 1999;249(1):70–85.
91. Spinella MJ, et al. Retinoic acid promotes ubiquitination and proteolysis of cyclin D1 during induced tumor cell differentiation. *J Biol Chem* 1999;274(31):22013–22018.
92. Sueoka N, et al. Posttranslational mechanisms contribute to the suppression of specific cyclin:CDK complexes by all-trans retinoic acid in human bronchial epithelial cells. *Cancer Res* 1999;59(15):3838–3844.
93. Teixeira, C, Pratt MA. CDK2 is a target for retinoic acid-mediated growth inhibition in MCF-7 human breast cancer cells. *Mol Endocrinol* 1997;11(9):1191–1202.
94. Watanabe Y, et al. pRb phosphorylation is regulated differentially by cyclin-dependent kinase (Cdk) 2 and Cdk4 in retinoic acid-induced neuronal differentiation of P19 cells. *Brain Res* 1999;842(2):342–350.
95. Zancai P, et al. Retinoic acid-mediated growth arrest of EBV-immortalized B lymphocytes is associated with multiple changes in G1 regulatory proteins: p27Kip1 up-regulation is a relevant early event. *Oncogene* 1998;17(14):1827–1836.
96. Caliaro MJ, et al. Response of four human ovarian carcinoma cell lines to all-trans retinoic acid: relationship with induction of differentiation and retinoic acid receptor expression. *Int J Cancer* 1994;56(5):743–748.
97. Marth C, et al. Effects of biological response modifiers on ovarian carcinoma cell lines. *Anticancer Res* 1989;9(2):461–467.
98. Soprano DR, et al. Overexpression of both RAR and RXR restores AP-1 repression in ovarian adenocarcinoma cells resistant to retinoic acid-dependent growth inhibition. *Oncogene* 1996;12(3):577–584.
99. Li Y, et al. The adenovirus E1A-associated 130-kD protein is encoded by a member of the retinoblastoma gene family and physically interacts with cyclins A and E. *Genes Dev* 1993;7(12A):2366–2377.
100. Hannon GJ, Demetrick D, Beach D. Isolation of the Rb-related p130 through its interaction with CDK2 and cyclins. *Genes Dev* 1993;7(12A):2378–2391.
101. Hsu SL, et al. Induction of p21(CIP1/Waf1) and activation of p34(cdc2) involved in retinoic acid-induced apoptosis in human hepatoma Hep3B cells. *Exp Cell Res* 1999;248(1):87–96.

102. Cariati R, et al. Retinoic acid induces persistent, RARalpha-mediated anti-proliferative responses in Epstein-Barr virus-immortalized b lymphoblasts carrying an activated C-MYC oncogene but not in Burkitt's lymphoma cell lines. *Int J Cancer* 2000;86(3):375–384.

103. Lee HY, et al. All-trans retinoic acid converts E2F into a transcriptional suppressor and inhibits the growth of normal human bronchial epithelial cells through a retinoic acid receptor- dependent signaling pathway. *J Clin Invest* 1998;101(5):1012–1019.

104. Mittnacht S. Control of pRB phosphorylation. *Curr Opin Genet Dev* 1998;8(1):21–27.

105. Paggi MG, et al. Retinoblastoma protein family in cell cycle and cancer: a review. *J Cell Biochem* 1996;62(3):418–430.

106. Liu M, Iavarone A, Freedman LP. Transcriptional activation of the human p21(WAF1/CIP1) gene by retinoic acid receptor. Correlation with retinoid induction of U937 cell differentiation. *J Biol Chem* 1996;271(49):31723–31728.

107. Chen YH, et al. Growth inhibition of a human myeloma cell line by all-trans retinoic acid is not mediated through downregulation of interleukin-6 receptors but through upregulation of p21(WAF1). *Blood* 1999;94(1):251–259.

108. Borriello A, et al. p27Kip1 accumulation is associated with retinoic-induced neuroblastoma differentiation: evidence of a decreased proteasome-dependent degradation. *Oncogene* 2000;19(1):51–60.

109. Weber E, et al. Retinoic acid-mediated growth inhibition of small cell lung cancer cells is associated with reduced myc and increased p27Kip1 expression. *Int J Cancer* 1999; 80(6):935–943.

110. Yaginuma Y, Westphal H. Abnormal structure and expression of the p53 gene in human ovarian carcinoma cell lines. *Cancer Res* 1992;52(15):4196–4199.

111. Langenfeld J, et al. Posttranslational regulation of cyclin D1 by retinoic acid: a chemoprevention mechanism. *Proc Natl Acad Sci USA* 1997;94(22):12070–12074.

112. Masciullo V, et al. Frequent loss of expression of the cyclin-dependent kinase inhibitor p27 in epithelial ovarian cancer. *Cancer Res* 1999;59(15):3790–3794.

113. Loda M, et al. Increased proteasome-dependent degradation of the cyclin-dependent kinase inhibitor p27 in aggressive colorectal carcinomas. *Nat Med* 1997;3(2):231–234.

114. Porter PL, et al. Expression of cell-cycle regulators p27Kip1 and cyclin E, alone and in combination, correlate with survival in young breast cancer patients. *Nat Med* 1997;3(2): 222–225.

115. Catzavelos C, et al. Decreased levels of the cell-cycle inhibitor p27Kip1 protein: prognostic implications in primary breast cancer. *Nat Med* 1997;3(2):227–230.

116. Esposito V, et al. Prognostic role of the cyclin-dependent kinase inhibitor p27 in non- small cell lung cancer. *Cancer Res* 1997;57(16):3381–3385.

117. Hsu SL, et al. Retinoic acid-mediated G1 arrest is associated with induction of p27(Kip1) and inhibition of cyclin-dependent kinase 3 in human lung squamous carcinoma CH27 cells. *Exp Cell Res* 2000;258(2):322–331.

118. Newcomb EW, et al. Expression of the cell cycle inhibitor p27KIP1 is a new prognostic marker associated with survival in epithelial ovarian tumors. *Am J Pathol* 1999;154(1):119–125.

119. Pagano M, et al. Role of the ubiquitin-proteasome pathway in regulating abundance of the cyclin-dependent kinase inhibitor p27. *Science* 1995;269(5224):682–685.

120. Cobrinik D, et al. Cell cycle-specific association of E2F with the p130 E1A-binding protein. *Genes Dev* 1993;7(12A):2392–2404.

121. Baldi A, et al. The RB2/p130 gene product is a nuclear protein whose phosphorylation is cell cycle regulated. *J Cell Biochem* 1995;59(3):402–408.

122. Mayol X, Garriga J, Grana X. Cell cycle-dependent phosphorylation of the retinoblastoma-related protein p130. *Oncogene* 1995;11(4):801–808.

123. Mayol X, Garriga J, Grana X. G1 cyclin/CDK-independent phosphorylation and accumulation of p130 during the transition from G1 to G0 lead to its association with E2F-4. *Oncogene* 1996;13(2):237–246.

124. Smith EJ, Leone G, Nevins JR. Distinct mechanisms control the accumulation of the Rb-related p107 and p130 proteins during cell growth. *Cell Growth Differ* 1998;9(4):297–303.
125. Claudio PP, et al. Functional analysis of pRb2/p130 interaction with cyclins. *Cancer Res* 1996;56(9):2003–2008.
126. Mulligan G., Jacks T. The retinoblastoma gene family: cousins with overlapping interests. *Trends Genet* 1998;14(6):223–229.
127. Chittenden T, Livingston DM, DeCaprio JA. Cell cycle analysis of E2F in primary human T cells reveals novel E2F complexes and biochemically distinct forms of free E2F. *Mol Cell Biol* 1993;13(7):3975–3983.
128. Vairo G, Livingston DM, Ginsberg D. Functional interaction between E2F-4 and p130: evidence for distinct mechanisms underlying growth suppression by different retinoblastoma protein family members. *Genes Dev* 1995;9(7):869–881.
129. Smith EJ, et al. The accumulation of an E2F-p130 transcriptional repressor distinguishes a G0 cell state from a G1 cell state. *Mol Cell Biol* 1996;16(12):6965–6976.
130. Dong F, et al. The role of cyclin D3-dependent kinase in the phosphorylation of p130 in mouse BALB/c 3T3 fibroblasts. *J Biol Chem* 1998;273(11):6190–6195.
131. Howard CM, et al. Retinoblastoma-related protein pRb2/p130 and suppression of tumor growth in vivo. *J Natl Cancer Inst* 1998;90(19):1451–1460.
132. Pupa SM, et al. Ectopic expression of pRb2/p130 suppresses the tumorigenicity of the c-erbB-2-overexpressing SKOV3 tumor cell line. *Oncogene* 1999;18(3):651–656.
133. Hateboer G, et al. Degradation of E2F by the ubiquitin-proteasome pathway: regulation by retinoblastoma family proteins and adenovirus transforming proteins. *Genes Dev* 1996; 10(23):2960–2970.
134. DeGregori J, et al. Distinct roles for E2F proteins in cell growth control and apoptosis. *Proc Natl Acad Sci USA* 1997;94(14):7245–7250.
135. Hurford RK, Jr, et al. pRB and p107/p130 are required for the regulated expression of different sets of E2F responsive genes. *Genes Dev* 1997;11(11):1447–1463.
136. Nevins JR. Toward an understanding of the functional complexity of the E2F and retinoblastoma families. *Cell Growth Differ* 1998;9(8):585–593.
137. Boyd KE, et al. c-Myc target gene specificity is determined by a post-DNAbinding mechanism. *Proc Natl Acad Sci USA* 1998;95(23):13887–13892.
138. Boyd KE, Farnham PJ. Coexamination of site-specific transcription factor binding and promoter activity in living cells. *Mol Cell Biol* 1999;19(12):8393–8399.
139. Takahashi Y, Rayman JB, Dynlacht BD. Analysis of promoter binding by the E2F and pRB families in vivo: distinct E2F proteins mediate activation and repression. *Genes Dev* 2000;14(7):804–816.
140. Furukawa Y, et al. The role of cellular transcription factor E2F in the regulation of cdc2 mRNA expression and cell cycle control of human hematopoietic cells. *J Biol Chem* 1994; 269(42):26249–26258.
141. Wade M, et al. An inverted repeat motif stabilizes binding of E2F and enhances transcription of the dihydrofolate reductase gene. *J Biol Chem* 1995;270(17):9783–9791.
142. Tommasi S, Pfeifer GP. Constitutive protection of E2F recognition sequences in the human thymidine kinase promoter during cell cycle progression. *J Biol Chem* 1997:272(48):30483–30490.
143. Brehm A, et al. Retinoblastoma protein recruits histone deacetylase to repress transcription. *Nature* 1998;391(6667):597–601.
144. Ferreira R, et al. The three members of the pocket proteins family share the ability to repress E2F activity through recruitment of a histone deacetylase. *Proc Natl Acad Sci USA* 1998;95(18):10493–10498.
145. Claudio PP, Caputi M, Giordano A. The RB2/p130 gene: the latest weapon in the war against lung cancer. *Clin Cancer Research* 2000; 6(3):754–764.

8 Modulators of Cyclin-Dependent Kinases

A Novel Therapeutic Approach for the Treatment of Neoplastic Diseases

Adrian M. Senderowicz, MD

1. REGULATION OF CELL CYCLE REGULATION AND ROLE OF CELL CYCLE IN CARCINOGENESIS

Upon activation of several growth factor/mitogenic signaling cascades, cells commit to entry into a series of regulated steps allowing traverse of the cell cycle. First, synthesis of DNA (genome duplication), also known as S phase, occurs followed by separation of two daughter cells (chromatid separation) or M phase.

From: *Cancer Drug Discovery and Development:*
Cell Cycle Inhibitors in Cancer Therapy: Current Strategies
Edited by: A. Giordano and K. J. Soprano © Humana Press Inc., Totowa, NJ

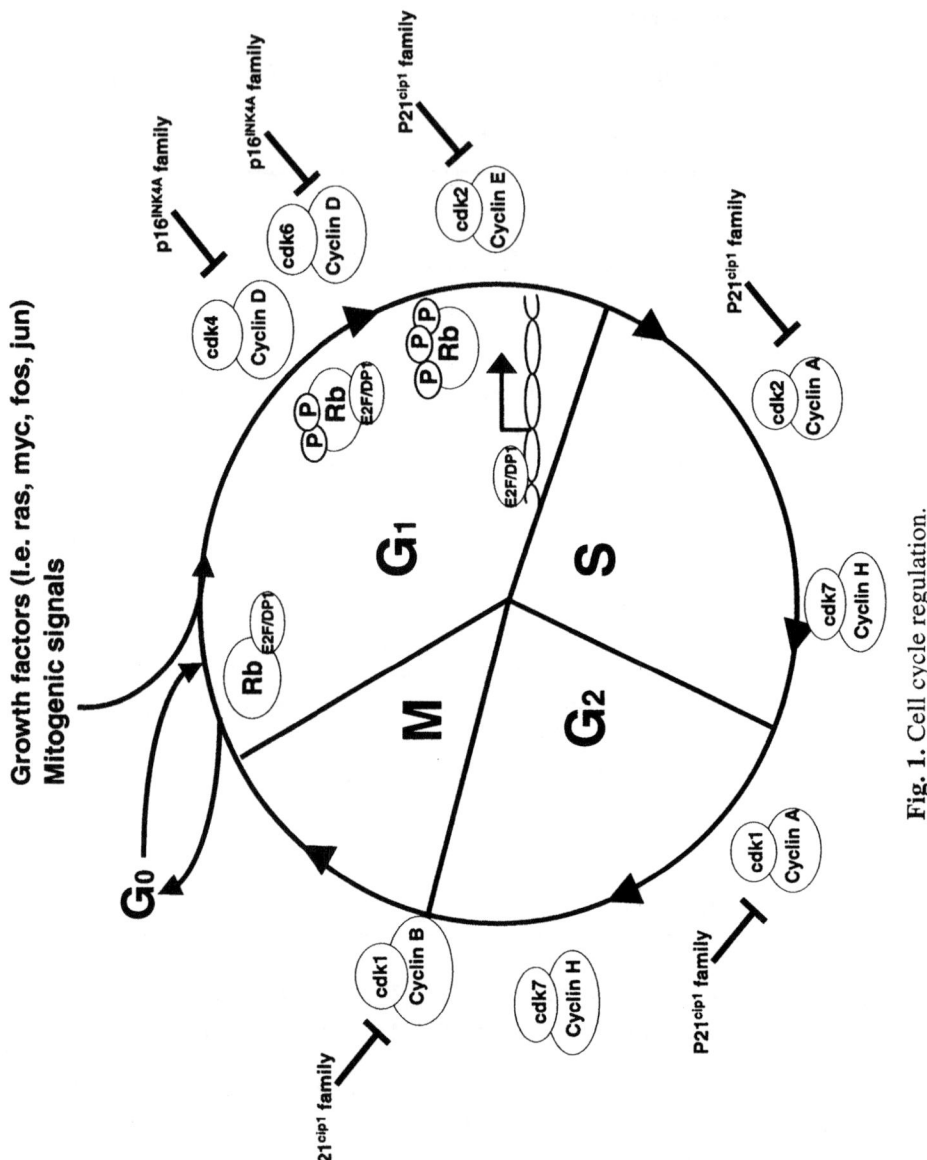

Fig. 1. Cell cycle regulation.

The time between the S and M phases is known as G_2 phase (*see* Fig. 1). This period is where cells can repair errors that occur during DNA duplication, preventing the propagation of these errors to daughter cells. In contrast, the G_1 phase represents the period of commitment to cell cycle progression that separates M and S phases as cells prepare for DNA duplication upon mitogenic signals *(1)*.

Over the past decade, it has been recognized that a universally utilized pathway allowing mitogenic signals to promote progression through G_1 to S phase utilizes phosphorylation and inactivation of the Retinoblastoma gene product (Rb), a tumor-suppressor gene product important for G_1 control (*see* Fig. 1) *(2,3)*. Rb inactivation is the result of its phosphorylation by the serine/threonine kinases, known as cyclin-dependent kinases (cdks) *(4)*. These key regulators of the cell cycle are enzymes that periodically form complexes with proteins known as cyclins (*see* Fig. 1). There are at least 9 different cdks (cdk1-cdk9) *(4–7)*. Cyclin-dependent kinases clearly involved in cell cycle control are cdk1 through 7. In contrast, cdk8 and cdk9, although structurally related to the cell cycle regulatory cdks, are important regulators of transcriptional control *(5,6)*. There are at least 15 different cyclins (cyclin A through T) *(7–10)*. Cyclin expression varies during the cell cycle and indeed their periodic expression forms the basis for defining the start and transition to succeeding cell cycle phases. When cyclins noncovalently form 1:1 complexes with their cognate cdk catalytic subunits to form the cdk holoenzyme, the complex becomes activated by phosphorylation in specific residues of the catalytic subunit of the cdk by cdk7/cyclin H, also known as "cdk-activating kinase" (CAK) *(11,12)*.

Different cdks operate during different phases of the cell cycle (*see* Fig. 1). For example, cdk4 and cdk6, in concert with their respective D-type cyclin partners, are responsible for progression through G_1, and cdk2 in combination with cyclin E is responsible for progression from G_1 into S phase. Cdk2/cyclin A is required for progression through S phase, and cdk1 (also known as cdc2) combined with cyclin B is necessary for mitosis to occur *(1)*. These complexes are in turn regulated by a stoichiometric combination with small inhibitory proteins, called endogenous cyclin-dependent kinase inhibitors (CKIs). The INK4 (inhibitor of cdk4) family members include p16^{ink4a}, p15^{ink4b}, p18^{ink4c}, p19^{ink4d}, and specifically inhibit cyclin D-associated kinases. The members of the kinase inhibitor protein (KIP) family, p21^{waf1}, and p27^{Kip1} and p57^{kip2}, bind and inhibit the activity of cyclin E/cdk2 and cyclin A/cdk2 complexes *(13)*. Although the KIP family members were initially thought to be exclusive G_1/S regulators, several reports demonstrated that these proteins could regulate G_2/M transition as well (*see* Fig. 1) *(14–16)*. Other investigators have clearly demonstrated that this family of proteins are specific cdk2 inhibitors while promoting assembly and activation of the cdk4/cdk6 holoenzymes *(17,18)*.

DNA synthesis (S phase) occurs when the retinoblastoma gene product (Rb) is phosphorylated by active cdk4 and/or cdk6 releasing the transcriptional factor

E2F from its complex with Rb (*see* Fig. 1). The released E2F promotes the transcription of several genes necessary for progression through S phase *(2,19,20)*. For further insight into cell cycle regulation, excellent reviews of cell cycle control have recently been published *(21–24)*.

Most human neoplasms have abnormalities in some component of the Rb pathway either due to hyperactivation of cdks as a result of amplification/overexpression of positive cofactors, cyclins/cdks, or downregulation of negative factors, endogenous CKIs, or mutation in the Rb gene product. These aberrations promote deregulated S phase progression in a way that ignores growth factor signals, with loss of G_1 checkpoints *(1,25)*. Therefore, development of pharmacologic cdk inhibitors (smCDKI) "mechanism-based therapy" would be of great interest as a treatment strategy for many neoplasms *(26)*. Furthermore, inappropriate, or deregulated activation of cdks might have adverse consequences for cells, and indeed cdk activation/inactivation has been reported to correlate with cellular response to apoptotic stimuli in several preclinical models *(27–30*; and *see* below). Two cdk modulators, flavopiridol and UCN-01, have recently completed initial human Phase I trials *(26,31–38)* and will be described below.

2. PERTURBATION OF CELL CYCLE COMPONENTS IN NEOPLASTIC DISEASES

In the last three decades, it became apparent that that neoplastic cells display alterations in the progression of the normal cell cycle *(1,39–42)*. Cancer cells become malignant as a consequence of activating (i.e., gain-of-function) mutations and/or increased expression of one or more cellular protooncogenes, and/or inactivating (i.e., loss-of-function) mutations and/or decreased expression of one or more tumor-suppressor genes. Most tumor-suppressor genes and oncogenes are components of signal-transduction pathways that control crucial cellular functions including cell cycle entry/exit. In contrast to normal cells, tumor cells are unable to stop at predetermined points of the cell cycle, so called "checkpoints." These pauses in the cell cycle are necessary to verify the integrity of the genome before cells advance to the next phase *(43,44)*. Interestingly, critical activities of tumor-suppressor genes ultimately regulate these "checkpoints."

Approximately 90% of human malignancies have an abnormality in some component of the Retinoblastoma gene product (Rb) pathway. As expected, specific inhibitors of cdks including inhibitors of cdk4 or cdk6, could prevent cells from entering S phase, promoting cell cycle arrest and perhaps propensity to apoptosis *(26,45,46)*. In cells where the Rb gene product is not present *(47)*, development of cdk2 inhibitors could alternatively efficiently act to prevent S phase progression/apoptosis *(48–50)*.

Table 1
Cellular Consequences of Loss in cdk Activity

- Cell cycle arrest
- Apoptosis
- Differentiation
- Transcription (cdk9-PTEFb)
- Neuronal physiology (cdk5)

3. THERAPEUTIC APPROACHES FOR THE MANIPULATION OF THE CELL CYCLE MACHINERY

Several strategies could be considered to modulate cdk activity. These strategies are divided into direct effects on the catalytic cdk subunit or indirect modulation of regulatory pathways that govern cdk activity *(26,51)*. The small molecular cdk inhibitors (SCDKI) are compounds that directly target the catalytic cdk subunit. Most of these compounds modulate cdk activity by interacting specifically with the ATP binding site of cdks *(26,51–53,54)*. The second class of cdk inhibitors are compounds that inhibit cdk activity by targeting the regulatory "upstream pathways" that modulate the activity of cdks: by altering the expression and synthesis of the cdk/cyclin subunits or the cdk inhibitory proteins; by modulating the phosphorylation of cdks; by targeting cdk-activating kinase, cdc25, and wee1/myt1; or by manipulating the proteolytic machinery that regulates the catabolism of cdk/cyclin complexes or their regulators (*see* Tables 1 and 2) *(26,51)*.

4. SMALL MOLECULE CDK MODULATORS

4.1. Purine Derivatives: Olomoucine, Roscovitine and Derivatives

The first cdk inhibitor discovered was dimethylaminopurine *(55)*. This compound was demonstrated clear evidence of inhibition of mitosis in sea urchin embryos without evidence of protein synthesis inhibition, due to inhibition of cdk1 activity (IC_{50}: 120 μM) *(52)*. Subsequent studies demonstrated that this molecule is relatively nonspecific. Isopentenyladenine, a derivative of this compound, was somewhat more potent and specific for the cdk's (IC_{50}: 55 μM) *(56)*, although not a very potent antiproliferative agent. Subsequent screening efforts yielded more specific and potent inhibitors. Olomucine (*see* Fig. 2) displayed potent ability to inhibit cdk1 and cdk2 (IC_{50}: 7 μM) *(52,56)*. Roscovitine (*see* Fig. 2), an even more potent cdk inhibitor (IC_{50}s for cdk1/cdk2 of 0.7 μM), was derived from the olomucine structure *(52)*, showing more potent effects on cellular proliferation assays in the 60-cell line anticancer screen panel. The crystal structure of cdk2 in complex with isopentenyladenine, olomucine, or roscovitine was resolved, confirming that that all three inhibitors can bind to the ATP site

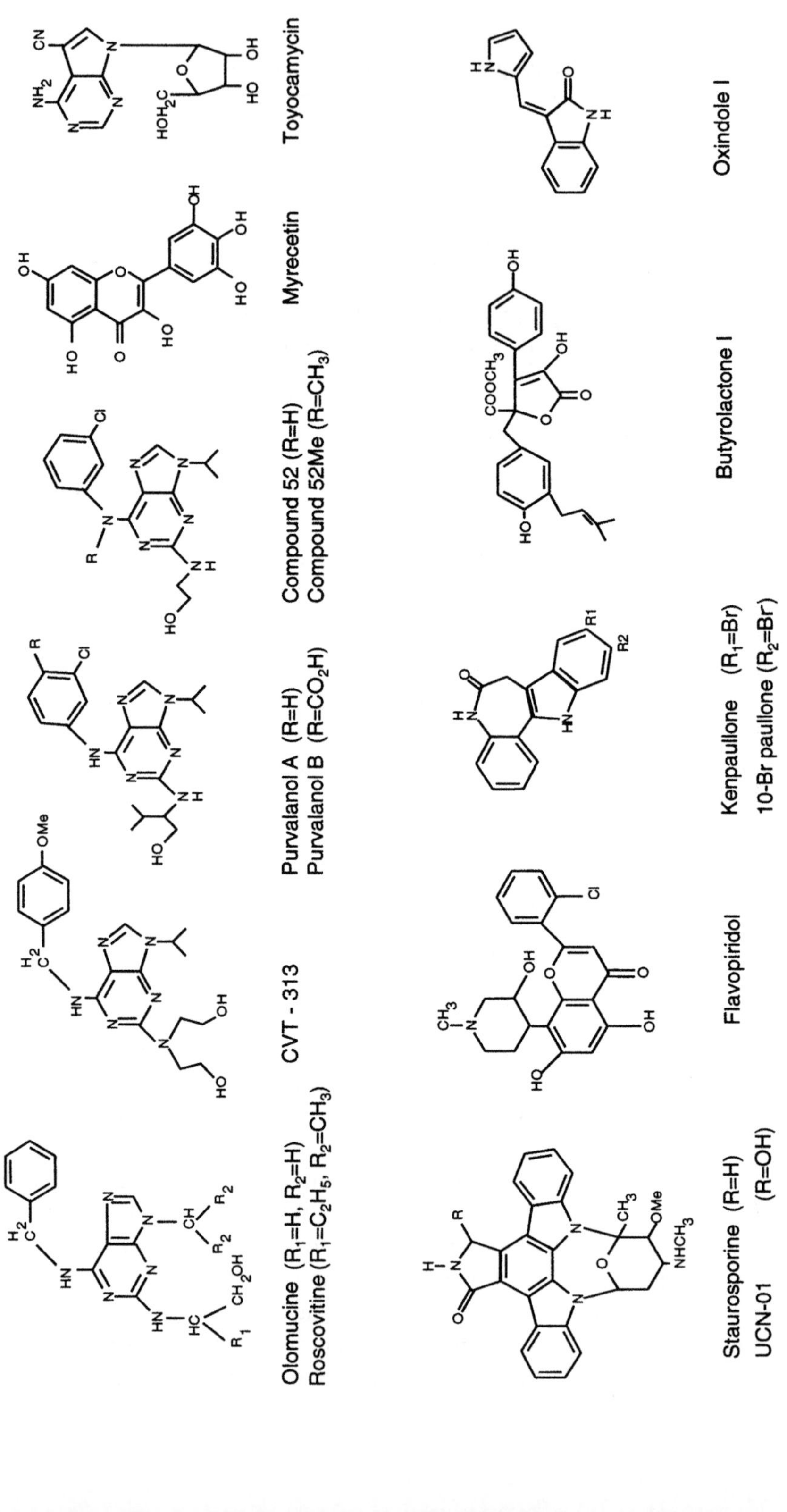

Fig. 2. Chemical structures of small molecular cdk inhibitors.

Toyocamycin

Myrecetin

Compound 52 (R=H)
Compound 52Me (R=CH₃)

Purvalanol A (R=H)
Purvalanol B (R=CO₂H)

CVT - 313

Olomucine (R₁=H, R₂=H)
Roscovitine (R₁=C₂H₅, R₂=CH₃)

Oxindole I

Butyrolactone I

Kenpaullone   (R₁=Br)
10-Br paullone (R₂=Br)

Flavopiridol

Staurosporine (R=H)
UCN-01   (R=OH)

(54,57). Another novel purine analogue, CVT-313, was obtained using a combinatorial library strategy and the knowledge of the crystal structure of cdk2 bound to chemical cdk inhibitors. Similar to the previous analogs, CVT-313 *(see* Fig. 2) was specific for cdk1 and cdk2 with an IC_{50} of 4.2 and 1.5 μM, respectively) *(58)*. Not only CVT-313 showed expected cell cycle arrest but also demonstrated potent inhibition in neointima revascularization after baloon angioplasty in in vivo preclinical models *(58)*. Although there are no clear plans to start clinical trials with these compounds, they clearly serve as important tools to dissect cellular effects due to cdk action.

Based on the knowledge of the binding properties of olomucine to the ATP binding site of cdk2, a combinatorial approach to modifying the purine scaffold revealed several compounds with very potent and specific inhibitory properties against cdc2 and cdk2. Four novel compounds, purvalanol A, purvalanol B, compound 52, and compound 52E were characterized in a battery of in vitro kinase experiments *(see* Fig. 2) *(59)*. Crystal structure studies of purvalanol B and cdk2 showed that this compound fits into the ATP-binding pocket, resembling the binding of olomucine to cdk2. Moreover, cell cycle studies with more membrane permeable, purvalanol A, in human fibroblasts exposed revealed a clear arrest in G_1/S and G_2/M, compatible with the putative inhibitory properties in cdk2 and cdc2, respectively *(59)*.

4.2. Paullones

Using flavopiridol's antiproliferative in vitro profile in the NCI anticancer drug screen, several compounds display similar antiproliferative pattern to flavopiridol, as determined by the COMPARE algorithm *(60)*. Kenpaullone (NSC 664704; *see* Fig. 2) displayed potent inhibitory properties against cdk1/cyclin B (IC_{50}, 0.4 μM), cdk2/cyclin A (IC_{50}, 0.68 μM), cdk2/cyclin E (IC_{50}, 7.5 μM), and cdk5/p25 (IC_{50}, 0.4 μM) with much less effect on other kinases *(53)*. Unfortunately, kenpaullone was not a very potent antiproliferative agent with $GI_{50}s \sim 42$ μM. Kenpaullone behaves as a competitor with respect to ATP with an apparent Ki of ~2.5 μM. Molecular modeling studies demonstrated that Kenpaullone may bind in the ATP binding site with residue contacts similar to other cdk2 inhibitors *(53)*. When kenpaullone was tested in serum-starved synchronized MCF10A breast epithelial cells, loss in S progression was observed in the presence of 30 μM kenpaullone. Thus, the G_1/S arrest observed underscores the cellular effects of kenpaullone on the activity of G_1 cdks and cell cycle progression. Alsterpaullone (9-nitro-paullone; 9NP) is an analogue of kenpaullone with more potent cdk inhibitory activity and lower $GI_{50}s$ for tumor growth *(61–63)*. The cell cycle effects of 9NP are not dependent on p53 or p21 expression *(63)*. Further preclinic studies with these compounds and novel analogues are being undertaken.

5. OTHER CDK INHIBITORS

Kent et al. discovered several new small molecule cdk inhibitors by high-throughput screening of small molecule compound libraries. They were able to discover 4 distinct cdk inhibitors, oxindole I (*see* Fig. 2), urea I, urea II, and benzoic acid *(64)*. Interestingly, the last 3 compounds show some selectivity against cdk4/cyclin D_1 with IC_{50}s ~ 1.2–6.7 μM *(64)*. In contrast, oxindole I, showed nonselective inhibitory activity against cdk4/cyclin D_1, cyclin E/cdk2, and cyclin B_1/cdc1 (4.9, 10, and 10.2 μM, respectively). The effects and specificity of these compounds with respect to other kinases are not known *(64)*. When these four compounds were tested against three different tumor cell lines, only the less potent albeit nonselective compound oxindole I was able to promote antiproliferative effects, suggesting that in order to have potent antiproliferative activity in vitro, small molecule cdk inhibitors need to target more than one cdk *(64)*. Interestingly, flavopiridol, also a nonspecific cdk inhibitor, has more potent in vitro antiproliferative activity compared with more selective ones such as olomucine and roscovitine. This potent antiproliferative property, again, may reflect the nonspecific inhibitory nature of flavopiridol with respect to different cdks.

A novel flavonoid, Myrecetin (*see* Fig. 2), was recently discovered by Lovejoy and Walker *(65)*. Preliminary studies demonstrated that this compound is a less potent cdk2 inhibitor (IC_{50} ~ 10 μM). Also, preliminary crystal structural efforts demonstrated that myrecetin binds in the ATP binding pocket of cdk2 in reverse orientation as compared to flavopiridol *(65)*. However, the specificity of this compound with respect to cdks or the effects of this compound in cellular systems are not known.

6. CELLULAR EFFECTS OF LOSS IN CDK ACTIVITY
(*SEE* TABLE 1)

Several possible approaches to assess the role of cdks in cellular models may involve the use of dominant negative (DN) forms of cdks, heterologous expression of CKIs such as p16[INK4a] or p27[kip1], use of chemical cdk inhibitors, or the use of CKI peptidomimetics *(26,51)*.

Several models could be studied in order to assess the functional role of cdks in cellular physiology. Initial studies in yeast cells were possible because only one cdk (cdc2) is responsible for the cell cycle progression. However, human cells are more complex: several cdks govern cell cycle progression and their inhibition leads to either cell cycle arrest at different periods and/or apoptosis (programmed cell death).

6.1. Cell Cycle Arrest

Initial studies by Van den Heuvel et al. *(66)* demonstrated that forced expression of cdc2 dominant-negative alleles (DN) was able to block cell cycle progression of U2OS osteosarcoma cell lines at the G_2/M boundary. In contrast, expression of either cdk2 or cdk3 DN prevented S phase progression *(66)*. Thus, this seminal observation helped to determine the role of most cdks in human cell cycle progression.

Forced expression of CKIs such as p16, p21, or p27 or peptidomimetics derived from p21, p16, or E2F1 *(26,51)* clearly demonstrates G_1/S cell cycle arrest.

Furthermore several smCDKI including roscovitine, olomucine, purvalanol, and flavopiridol arrest cells at either the G_1/S or G_2/M boundaries *(48,49,58,59,67)*. It is unclear why these agents provoke a G_1/S arrest phenotype in some cells and a G_2/M or combined arrest in others; as mentioned later, in the case of flavopiridol, the arrest is independent of functional p53 or Rb *(48,68)*. Interestingly, in some experimental models, the antiproliferative effect was accompanied, in the case of olomucine, flavopiridol, and roscovitine, by the induction of apoptosis *(49,69,70)*.

6.2. Apoptosis

As mentioned earlier, these smCDKI may induce apoptosis in some preclinical models. In one example, susceptibility to apoptosis by chemical cdk inhibitors (flavopiridol and olomucine) varied depending on the growth state of the cells. Thus, postmitotic nondividing PC-12 cells were protected from apoptosis-induced by NGF deprivation by the presence of flavopiridol or olomucine; on the other hand, cycling PC-12 cells were not protected from NGF withdrawal but actually were induced to undergo apoptosis after exposure to flavopiridol *(70)*. In a similar model of apoptosis only cdk4 and cdk6 DN but not cdk2 or cdk3 DN protected neurons against NGF deprivation *(71)*. Further evidence of the role of cdks in apoptosis is based on the protective role of DN-cdc2, cdk2, or cdk3 in the apoptosis in HeLa cells induced by staurosporine and tumor necrosis factor-α (TNF-α). However, only DN cdk2 block apoptosis induced by ectopic expression of topoisomerase II α *(30)*. Finally, it has become clear that certain apoptotic stimuli provoke the induction of cleavage in CKI's (p21^{wafl}/p27^{kip1}) or CDK inhibitory proteins (wee1 and cdc27) by caspases leading to activation of cdks *(72–74)*. Clearly, the final outcome of loss of cdk activity to promote cell cycle arrest/apoptosis depends on several factors including the mechanism of inhibition, cell type, and proliferation status. Thus, some cell types cannot tolerate loss of cdk activity and/or cell cycle arrest leading to cell death.

6.3. Differentiation

It became clear recently that cells become differentiated when exit of the cell cycle (G_0) and loss of cdk2 activity occurs. Based on this information, Lee and coworkers tested flavopiridol and roscovitine, both known cdk2 inhibitors, to determine if they induce a differentiated phenotype. For this purpose, NCI-H358 lung carcinoma cell lines were exposed to either cdk2 antisense construct, flavopiridol, or roscovitine. Clear evidence of mucinous differentiation along with loss in cdk2 activity was observed. However, each cdk2-antagonist therapy had different cell cycle regulatory expression despite a similar differentiated phenotype (75).

In another effort to study the differentiating effects of aminopurvalanol, U937 myelomonocytic leukemia cell lines were treated with this compound. These cells acquired a phenotype characteristic of differentiated macrophages. Moreover, this potent cdk1 and cdk2 inhibitor displayed evidence of G_2/M arrest with subsequent apoptosis (76). Thus, it is possible for a cell to become differentiated with 4N DNA content as observed in experiments where ectopic expression of p21^{wafl} or p27^{kip1} results in a differentiated phenotype as cells arrest in G_1/S or G_2/M phases (77).

6.4. Transcriptional Effects

To compare the effects of several cdk inhibitors on mRNA expression from yeast cells, Gray et al. exposed *Sacchonomyces cerevisae* to compound 52 and flavopiridol (25 μ*M*) for 2 h and quantified mRNA by oligonucleotide array methods (59). It became clear that 2–3% of a total of 6200 yeast genes showed significant (greater than twofold) changes in transcript level when treated with these agents. Interestingly, almost 50% of affected transcripts were shared by compound 52 and flavopiridol. These genes belong to genes that regulate progression of cell cycle, phosphate, and cellular energy metabolism; and GTP or ATP binding proteins. However, more than 40% of mRNA changes are not concordant between flavopiridol and compound 52. These discrepant behaviors could be explained by the universal cdk inhibitory activity of flavopiridol compared with the selective cdk2/cdk1 effects of compound 52, by the different intracellular concentrations achieved of these inhibitors, their distinctive molecular structures, or from their putative effects on other cellular targets. When the compound 52E (inactive analogue to compound 52) or a yeast strain (cdc28p) that is mutant for the putative target for both flavopiridol and compound 52 were studied, very few mRNA alterations were noted with 52E, implying that the net effect of these agents is due to the inhibition of cdks and not due to chemical structural motifs of the compound. Moreover, the mutant cdc28p revealed some overlap-ping effects with compound 52 and flavopiridol (59). Modulation in transcription (cyclin D_1 and vascular endothelial growth factor [VEGF]) was also observed in human cells (*see* below, flavopiridol section).

7. CYCLIN-DEPENDENT KINASE MODULATORS
IN CLINICAL TRIALS: FLAVOPIRIDOL

7.1. Mechanism of Antiproliferative Effects

Flavopiridol (L86-8275 or HMR 1275) is a semisynthetic flavonoid derived from rohitukine, an indigenous plant from India (see Fig. 2). Initial studies with flavopiridol demonstrated modest in vitro inhibitory activity with respect to epidermal growth factor receptor (EGFR) and protein kinase A (PKA)(IC_{50} = 21 and 122 μM, respectively) (46). However, when this compound was tested in the National Cancer Institute (NCI) 60 cell line anti-cancer drug screen panel, this compound demonstrated a very potent growth inhibition (IC_{50} 66 nM), a concentration that is about 1000 times lower than the concentration required to inhibit PKA and EGFR (46). Initial studies with this flavonoid revealed clear evidence of G_1/S or G_2/M arrest, due to loss in cdk1 and cdk2 (78–80). Studies using purified cdks showed that the inhibition observed is reversible and competitively blocked by ATP, with a K_i of 41 nM (45,48,78–80). Furthermore, the crystal structure of the complex of deschloroflavopiridol and cdk2 showed that flavopiridol binds to the ATP binding pocket, with the benzopyran occupying the same region as the purine ring of ATP (81), confirming the earlier biochemical studies with flavopiridol (79). Flavopiridol inhibits all cdks thus far examined (IC_{50} ~ 100 nM), but it inhibits cdk7 (cdk-activating kinase) less potently (IC_{50} ~ 300 nM) (45,48,79).

In addition to inhibiting cdks directly, flavopiridol promotes a decrease in the level of cyclin D_1, an oncogene that is overexpressed in many human neoplasias. Of note, neoplasms that overexpress cyclin D_1 have a poor prognosis (82–84). When MCF-7 human breast carcinoma cells were incubated with flavopiridol, levels of cyclin D_1 protein decreased within 3 h (85). This effect was followed by a decline in the levels of cyclin D_3 with no alteration in the levels of cyclin D_2 and cyclin E, the remaining G_1 cyclins, leading to loss in the activity of cdk4. Thus, depletion of cyclin D_1 appears to lead to the loss of cdk activity (85). The depletion of cyclin D_1 is caused by depletion of cyclin D_1 mRNA and was associated with a specific decline in cyclin D_1 promoter, measured by a luciferase reporter assay (85). The transcriptional repression of cyclin D_1 observed after treatment with flavopiridol is consistent with the effects of flavopiridol on yeast cells (see above) and underscores the conserved effect of flavopiridol on eukaryotic cyclin transcription (59). In summary, flavopiridol can induce cell cycle arrest by at least three mechanisms: 1) by direct inhibition of cdk activities by binding to the ATP binding site; 2) by prevention of the phosphorylation of cdks at threonine-160/161 by inhibition of cdk7/cyclin H (45,80); and 3) for G_1/S phase arrest, by a decrease in the amount of cyclin D_1, an important cofactor for cdk4 and cdk6 activation.

Another effect of flavopiridol effects on transcription is attenuation on the induction of VEGF mRNA in monocytes after hypoxia (*see* below, antiangiogenic properties of flavopiridol). This effect is due to alterations in the stability of VEGF mRNA *(86)*.

Recently, Chao et al. demonstrated that flavopiridol potently inhibits P-TEFb (also known as cdk9/cyclin T), with a Ki of 3 nM, leading to inhibition of transcription by RNA polymerase II by blocking the transition into productive elongation. Interestingly, in contrast with all cdks tested so far, flavopiridol was not competitive with ATP in this reaction. P-TEFb is a required cellular cofactor for the human immunodeficiency virus (HIV-1) transactivator, Tat. Consistent with its ability to inhibit P-TEFb, flavopiridol blocked Tat transactivation of the viral promoter in vitro. Furthermore, flavopiridol blocked HIV-1 replication in both single-round and viral-spread assays with an IC$_{50}$ of less than 10 nM *(87)*. With this novel knowledge, it is reasonable to test flavopiridol in clinical trials of patients with HIV-related malignancies.

An important biochemical effect involved in the antiproliferative of flavopiridol is the induction of apoptotic cell death. Hematopoietic cell lines are often quite sensitive to flavopiridol-induced apoptotic cell death *(69,88–90)*, but the mechanism(s) by which flavopiridol induces apoptosis have not yet been elucidated. Flavopiridol does not modulate topoisomerase I/II activity *(69)*. In certain hematopoietic cell lines, neither BCL-2/BAX nor p53 appeared to be affected *(69,91)*, whereas, in other systems, BCL-2 may be inhibited *(90)*. Preliminary evidence from one laboratory demonstrated that flavopiridol-induced apoptosis in leukemia cells is associated with early activation of the MAPK protein kinase family of proteins (MEK, p38, and JNK) *(92)*. This activation may lead to activation of caspases *(92)*. As seen in this and other models, caspase inhibitors prevent flavopiridol-induced apoptosis *(89,92)*. It is unclear whether the putative flavopiridol-induced inhibition of cdk activity is required for induction of apoptosis.

Clear evidence of cell cycle arrest along with apoptosis was observed in a panel of squamous head and neck cell lines, including a cell line (HN30) that is refractory to several DNA damaging agents, such as γ-irradiation and bleomycin *(93)*. Again, the apoptotic effect was independent of p53 status and was associated with the depletion of cyclin D$_1$ *(93)*. These findings have been corroborated in other preclinical models *(68,91,94,95)*. Efforts to understand flavopiridol-induced apoptosis are under intense investigation.

Not only flavopiridol targets tumor cells but also targets angiogenesis pathways. Brusselbach et al. *(96)* incubated primary human umbilical vein endothelial cells (HUVECs) with flavopiridol and observed apoptotic cell death even in cells that were not cycling, leading to the notion that flavopiridol may have antiangiogenic properties due to endothelial cytotoxicity. In other model systems, Kerr et al. *(97)* tested flavopiridol in an in vivo Matrigel model of angiogenesis and found that flavopiridol decreased blood vessel formation, a surrogate marker for antiangiogenic effect of this compound. Furthermore, as mentioned earlier, Melillo et al. *(86)* demonstrated that, at low nanomolar concentrations, flavopiridol prevented the induction of vascular endothelial growth factor (VEGF) by hypoxic conditions in human monocytes. This effect was caused by a decreased stability of VEGF mRNA, which paralleled the decline in VEGF protein. Thus, the antitumor activity of flavopiridol observed may be in part due to antiangiogenic effects. Whether the various antiangiogenic actions of flavopiridol result from its interaction with a cdk target or other targets requires further study.

Several investigators have attempted to determine if flavopiridol has synergistic effects with standard chemotherapeutic agents. For example, synergistic effects in A549 lung carcinoma cells were demonstrated when treatment with flavopiridol followed treatment with paclitaxel, cytarabine, topotecan, doxorubicin, or etoposide *(98,99)*. In contrast, a synergistic effect was observed with 5-fluorouracil only when cells were treated with flavopiridol for 24 h before addition of 5-fluorouracil. Furthermore, synergistic effects with cisplatin were not schedule-dependent *(99)*. However, Chien et al. *(68)* failed to demonstrate a synergistic effect between flavopiridol and cisplatin and/or γ-irradiation in bladder carcinoma models. One important issue to mention is that most of these studies were performed in in vitro models. Thus, confirmatory studies in in vivo animal models are needed.

Experiments using colorectal (Colo205) and prostate (LnCap/DU-145) carcinoma xenograft models in which flavopiridol was administered frequently over a protracted period demonstrated that flavopiridol is cytostatic *(46,100)*. This demonstration lead to human clinical trials of flavopiridol administered as a 72-h continuous infusion every 2 wk *(101)* *(see* below). Subsequent studies in human leukemia/lymphoma xenografts demonstrated that flavopiridol administered intravenously as a bolus rendered animals tumor-free, whereas flavopiridol administered as an infusion only delayed tumor growth *(88)*. Moreover, in head and neck (HN-12) xenografts flavopiridol administered as an intraperitoneal bolus daily at 5 mg/kg for 5 d demonstrated a substantial growth delay *(93)*. Again, apoptotic cell death and cyclin D_1 depletion were observed in tissues from xenografts treated with flavopiridol *(88)*. Based on these results, a Phase I trial of 1 h infusional flavopiridol for 5 consecutive days every 3 wk is currently being conducted at the NCI *(see* below).

8. CLINICAL EXPERIENCE WITH FLAVOPIRIDOL

Two Phase I clinical trials of flavopiridol administered as a 72-h continuous infusion every 2 wk have been completed *(35,101)*. In the NCI Phase I trial of infusional flavopiridol, 76 patients were treated. Dose-limiting toxicity (DLT) was secretory diarrhea with a maximal-tolerated dose (MTD) of 50 mg per m^2 per day for 3 d. In the presence of antidiarrheal prophylaxis (a combination of cholestyramine and loperamide), patients tolerated higher doses, defining a second maximal-tolerated dose, 78 mg per m^2 per day for 3 d. The dose-limiting toxicity observed at the higher-dose level was a substantial proinflammatory syndrome (fever, fatigue, local tumor pain, and modulation of acute-phase reactants) and reversible hypotension *(101)*. Minor responses were observed in patients with non-Hodgkin's lymphoma (NHL), colon, and kidney cancer for more than 6 mo. Moreover, one patient with refractory renal cancer achieved a partial response for more than 8 mo *(101)*. Of 14 patients who received flavopiridol for more than 6 mo, five patients received flavopiridol for more than 1 yr and one patient received flavopiridol for more than 2 yr *(101)*. Plasma concentrations of 300–500 nM flavopiridol, which inhibit cdk activity in vitro, were safely achieved during this trial *(101)*.

In a complementary Phase I trial also exploring the same schedule (72-h continuous infusion every 2 wk) Thomas et al. *(35)* found that the dose-limiting toxicity was diarrhea, corroborating the NCI experience. Moreover, plasma concentrations of 300–500 nM flavopiridol were also observed. Interestingly, there was one patient in this trial with refractory metastatic gastric cancer that progressed after a treatment regimen containing 5-fluorouracil. When treated with flavopiridol, this patient achieved a sustained complete response without any evidence of disease for more than 2 yr after treatment was completed.

The first Phase I trial of a daily 1-h infusion of flavopiridol for 5 consecutive days every 3 wk was recently completed *(32,32a)*. This schedule was based on antitumor results observed in leukemia/lymphoma and head and neck xenografts treated with flavopiridol *(88,93)*. A total of 48 patients were treated in this trial. The recommended Phase II dose is 37.5 mg per m^2 per day for 5 consecutive days. Dose-limiting toxicities observed at 52.5 mg per m^2 per day are nausea/vomiting, neutropenia, fatigue, and diarrhea *(32,32a)*. Other (nondose-limiting) side effects are "local tumor pain" and anorexia. To reach higher flavopiridol concentrations, the protocol was amended to administer flavopiridol for 3 d (initially) and then for 1 d only. These protocol modifications allowed to achievement of higher flavopiridol concentrations (~4 μM) *(32,32a)*. Unfortunately, the half-life observed in this trial is much shorter (~3 h) than the infusional trial (~10 h). Thus, high micromolar concentrations in the 1-h infusional trial will be maintained for very short periods of time *(32,32a)*. Several Phase II trials in patients with refractory head and neck cancer, chronic lymphocytic leukemia (CLL), and mantle cell lymphoma (MCL) are currently being tested using this schedule (*see* below).

A Phase I trial testing the combination of paclitaxel and infusional (24 h) flavopiridol demonstrated good tolerability with a dose-limiting pulmonary toxicity *(34)*.

Phase II trials of flavopiridol given as a 72-h continuous infusion with the MTD in the absence of anti-diarrheal prophylaxis (50 mg/m^2/d) to patients with CLL, non-small cell lung cancer (NSCLC), NHL, and colon, prostate, gastric, head and neck, and kidney cancer, and Phase I trials of flavopiridol administered on novel schedules and in combination with standard chemotherapeutic agents are being performed (102–106). In a recently published Phase II trial of flavopiridol in metastatic renal cancer, two objective responses (response rate = 6%, 95% confidence interval, 1–20%) were observed. Most patients developed Grade 1–2 diarrhea and asthenia (106). In this trial, patients that demonstrated glucuronide flavopiridol metabolites in plasma, as measured by high performance liquid chromatography (HPLC) methodology, have less pronounced diarrhea in comparison to nonmetabolizers (107). Thus, it may be possible that patients with higher metabolic rates may tolerated higher doses of flavopiridol.

Phase II trials of shorter (1 h) infusional flavopiridol are being conducted in MCL, CLL, and HNSCC. Of interest, several refractory CLL and MCL patients demonstrated clear evidence of responses (partial responses) in these trials (J. R. Suarez, personal communications).

Although the initial studies of flavopiridol in humans are encouraging, the best schedule of administration of flavopiridol needs to be determined. Furthermore, Phase III studies in patients with non-small cell lung cancer in combination with standard chemotherapy, such as docetaxel, are being planned (J. R. Suarez, personal communications).

9. UCN-01

9.1. Mechanism of Antiproliferative Activity

Staurosporine is a potent nonspecific protein and tyrosine kinase inhibitor, with a very low therapeutic index in animals (108). Thus, efforts to find staruosporine analogues have identified compounds that specifically inhibit protein kinases. One staurosporine analogue, UCN-01 (7-hydroxystaurosporine; Fig. 2), has potent activity against several protein kinase C isoenzymes, particularly the Ca^{2+}-dependent protein kinase C (PKC) with an IC$_{50}$ ~ 30 nM (109–111). In addition to its effects on PKC, UCN-01 has antiproliferative activity in several human tumor cell lines (112–116). In contrast, another highly selective potent PKC inhibitor, GF 109203X, has minimal antiproliferative activity, despite a similar capacity to inhibit PKC in vitro (113). These results suggest that the antiproliferative activity of UCN-01 can not be explained solely by inhibition of PKC. Although UCN-01 moderately inhibited the activity of immunoprecipitated cdk1(cdc2) and cdk2 (IC$_{50}$ = 300–600 nM), exposure of UCN-01 to intact cells leads to "inappropriate activation" of the same kinases (113). This phenomenon correlates with the G$_2$ abrogation checkpoint observed with this agent (see below).

Experimental evidence suggests DNA damage leads to cell cycle arrest to allow DNA repair. In cells where the G_1 phase checkpoint is not active because of p53 inactivation, irradiated cells accumulate in G_2 phase due to activation of the G_2 checkpoint (inhibition of cdc2). In contrast, Wang et al. exposed CA46 cell lines to radiation followed by UCN-01 promoting the inappropriate activation of cdc2/cyclin B and early mitosis with the onset of apoptotic cell death (117). These effects could be partially explained by the inactivation of Wee1, the kinase that negatively regulates the G_2/M-phase transition (118). Moreover, UCN-01 can have a direct effect on chk1, protein kinase that regulates the G_2 checkpoint (119–121). Thus, although UCN-01 at high concentrations can directly inhibit cdks in vitro, UCN-01 can modulate cellular "upstream" regulators at much lower concentration, leading to inappropriate cdc2 activation. Studies from other groups suggest that not only is UCN-01 able to abrogate the G_2 checkpoint induced by DNA damaging agents but also, in some circumstances, UCN-01 is able to abrogate the DNA damage-induced S-phase checkpoint (122,123).

Another interesting property of UCN-01 is its ability to arrest cells in G_1 phase of the cell cycle (112,115,116,124–128). For example, when human epidermoid carcinoma A431 cells (mutated p53) are incubated with UCN-01, these cells were arrested in G_1 phase with Rb hypophosphorylation and p21^{waf1}/p27^{kip1} accumulation (116). In another report, E6- and E7-derived strains of normal cells revealed that pRb and not p53 function is essential for UCN-01-mediated G_1 arrest (127). However, Shimuzu et al. demonstrated lung carcinoma cell lines with either absent (N417 small cell lung cancer cells), mutant (H209 small cell lung cancer cells), and wild-type Rb (Ma-31 NSCLC cells) exposed to UCN-01, G_1 arrest and antiproliferative effect occurred in all three cell lines independent of the functional Rb status, leading to the conclusion that the antiproliferative effect of UCN-01 in tumor cells was not dependent on the functional status of Rb (126). Thus, the G_1 arrest observed with UCN-01 is not clearly dependent on the status of p53 or Rb. However, further studies on the putative target(s) for UCN-01 in the G_1-phase arrest of cells need to be conducted.

Another interesting pharmacological feature of UCN-01 is the observed increased cytotoxicity in cells that harbor mutated p53 (117). In CA-46 and HT-29 tumor cell lines carrying mutated p53 genes, potent cytotoxicity results following exposure to UCN-01. To further extend these observations, the MCF-7 cell line with no endogenous p53 because of the ectopic expression of E6, a human papillomavirus type-16 protein, showed enhanced cytotoxicity when treated with a DNA-damaging agent, such as cisplatin, and UCN-01, compared with the isogenic wild-type MCF-7 cell line. Thus, a common feature observed in more than 50% of human neoplasias, associated with poor outcome and refractoriness to standard chemotherapies (129,130) may render tumor cells more sensitive to UCN-01.

As mentioned earlier, synergistic effects of UCN-01 have been observed with many chemotherapeutic agents, including mitomycin C, 5-fluorouracil, carmustine, and camptothecin, among others *(122,131–138)*. Therefore, it is possible that combining UCN-01 with these or other agents could improve its therapeutic index. Clinical trials exploring these possibilities are being developed. Studies of UNC-01 in preclinical animal models revealed a beta half-life approx 4–12 hr *(26,51)*. Although concentrations ~330 nM were obtained safely in dogs, concentrations ~1000 nM (1µM) were lethal *(26,51)*.

UCN-01 administered by an intravenous or intraperitoneal route displayed antitumor activity in xenograft model systems with breast carcinoma (MCF-7 cells), renal carcinoma (A498 cells), and leukemia (MOLT-4 and HL-60) cells (A. Senderowicz, unpublished results). The antitumor effect was greater when UCN-01 was given over a longer period. This requirement for a longer period of treatment was also observed in in vitro models, with greatest antitumor activity observed when UCN-01 was present for 72 h *(112)*. Thus, a clinical trial using a 72-h continuous infusion every 2 wk was conducted (described below).

10. CLINICAL TRIALS OF UCN-01

The first Phase I trial of UCN-01 was recently completed *(33,38)*. UCN-01 was initially administered as a 72 h-continuous infusion every 2 wk based on data from in vitro and xenograft preclinical models. However, it became apparent in the first few patients that the drug had an unexpectedly long half-life (~30 d). This half-life was 100 times longer than the half-life observed in preclinical models (*see* above), most likely due to the avid binding of UCN-01 to α_1-acid glycoprotein *(139,140)*. Thus, the protocol was modified to administer UCN-01 every 4 wk (one half-life) and subsequent courses, the duration of infusion was decreased by half (total 36 h). Thus, it was possible to reach similar peak plasma concentrations in subsequent courses with no evidence of drug accumulation. There was no evidence of myelotoxicity or gastrointestinal toxicity (prominent side effects observed in animal models), despite very high plasma concentrations achieved (35–50 µM) *(33,38,139,140)*. Dose-limiting toxicities were nausea/vomiting (amenable to standard antiemetic treatments), symptomatic hyperglycemia associated with an insulin-resistance state (increase in insulin and c-peptide levels while receiving UCN-01), and pulmonary toxicity characterized by substantial hypoxemia without obvious radiologic changes. The recommended Phase II dose of UCN-01 given on a 72-h continuous infusion schedule was 42.5 mg per m^2 per d *(38)*. One patient with refractory metastatic melanoma developed a partial response that lasted 8 mo. Another patient with refractory anaplastic large cell lymphoma that had failed multiple chemotherapeutic regimens including high-dose chemotherapy has no evidence of disease 4 yr after the initiation of

UCN-01. Moreover, a few patients with leiomyosarcoma, NHL, and lung cancer demonstrated stable disease for ≥6 mo *(38,141)*. Of note, one patient with refractory large cell lymphoma that failed prior high-dose combination chemotherapy protocol-EPOCH-2 combination chemotherapy had rapidly progressive disease after one cycle of UCN-01. He required immediate systemic chemotherapy due to hepatic and bone marrow failure (thrombocytopenia) due to progression of disease. Based on the poor status of this patient, a dose-reduced EPOCH combination chemotherapy was administered. His liver function and thrombocytopenia resolved completely with significant improvement in performance status within 2 wk after combination chemotherapy. Unfortunately, he developed Candida *kruzei* septicemia and expired. His postmortem examination revealed a pathological complete response after only one cycle of chemotherapy *(142)*. Thus, this refractory large cell lymphoma patient became "chemotherapy-sensitive" after only one dose of UCN-01. This phenomenon recapitulates the synergistic effect observed in preclinical models with several chemotherapeutic agents. Several combination trials are being developed based on this observation.

In order to estimate "free UCN-01 concentrations" in body fluids, several efforts were considered. Plasma ultracentrifugation and salivary determination of UCN-01 revealed similar results. At the recommended Phase II dose (37.5 mg/m^2/d over 72 h), concentrations of "free-salivary" UCN-01 (~110 nM) that may cause G_2 checkpoint abrogation can be achieved. As mentioned earlier, UCN-01 is a potent PKC inhibitor. In order to determine the putative signaling effects of UCN-01 in tissues, bone marrow aspirates and tumor cells were obtained from patients before and during the first cycle of UCN-01 administration. Western blot studies were performed in those samples against phosphorylated adducin, a cytoskeletal membrane protein, an specific substrate phos-phorylated by PKC *(143)*. Clear loss in phospho-adducin content in the post-treatment samples was observed in all tumor and bone marrow samples tested, concluding that UCN-01 can modulate PKC activity in tissues from patients in this trial *(38,141)*.

Several groups are conducting shorter (3 h) infusional trials of UCN-01. Interestingly, the toxicity profile of shorter infusions is similar to the toxicities observed with the 72 h infusion trial *(36,37)*. However, with shorter infusions, more pronounced hypotension was observed *(36,37)*. Determination of free UCN-01 in these trials is of utmost importance as higher free concentrations for shorter periods may be more or less beneficial compared with the free-concentrations observed in the 72-h infusion trial.

Based on the unique pharmacological features and anecdotal clinical evidence of synergistic effects in one patient with refractory disease *(142)*, several combination trials with standard chemotherapeutic agents recently commenced. A Phase I/II trial of gemcitabine followed by 72-h infusional UCN-01 in chronic lymphocytic leukemia started at the NCI. Other studies in combination with cisplatin, and 5-fluorouracil, among others, also commenced recently.

11. SUMMARY

Based on the frequent aberration in cell cycle regulatory pathways in human cancer by "cdk hyperactivation," novel ATP competitive cdk inhibitors are being developed. The first two tested in clinical trials, flavopiridol and UCN-01, showed promising results with evidence of antitumor activity and plasma concentrations sufficient to inhibit cdk-related functions. Best schedule to be administered, combination with standard chemotherapeutic agents, and demonstration of cdk modulation from tumor samples from patients in these trials are important issues that need to be answered in order to advance these agents to the clinic.

REFERENCES

1. Sherr CJ. Cancer cell cycles, *Science* 1996;274:1672–1677.
2. Hatakeyama M, Weinberg RA. The role of RB in cell cycle control. *Prog Cell Cycle Res* 1995;1:9–19.
3. Sellers WR, Kaelin, WG, Jr. Role of the retinoblastoma protein in the pathogenesis of human cancer. *J Clin Oncol* 1997;15:3301–3312.
4. Morgan DO. Cyclin-dependent kinases: engines, clocks, and microprocessors. *Annu Rev Cell Dev Biol* 1997;13:261–291.
5. Rickert P, Seghezzi W, Shanahan F, Cho H, Lees E. Cyclin C/CDK8 is a novel CTD kinase associated with RNA polymerase II. *Oncogene* 1996;12:2631–2640.
6. Wei P, Garber ME, Fang SM, Fischer WH, Jones KA. A novel CDK9-associated C-type cyclin interacts directly with HIV-1 Tat and mediates its high-affinity, loop-specific binding to TAR RNA. *Cell* 1998;92:451–462.
7. Grana X, De Luca A, Sang N, Fu Y, Claudio PP, Rosenblatt J, et al. PITALRE, a nuclear CDC2-related protein kinase that phosphorylates the retinoblastoma protein in vitro. *Proc Natl Acad Sci USA* 1994;91:3834–3838.
8. MacLachlan TK, Sang N, Giordano A. Cyclins, cyclin-dependent kinases and cdk inhibitors: implications in cell cycle control and cancer. *Crit Rev Eukaryot Gene Expr* 1995;5:127–156.
9. Edwards MC, Wong C, Elledge SJ. Human cyclin K, a novel RNA polymerase II-associated cyclin possessing both carboxy-terminal domain kinase and Cdk-activating kinase activity. *Mol Cell Biol* 1998;18:4291–4300.
10. Peng J, Zhu Y, Milton JT, Price DH. Identification of multiple cyclin subunits of human P-TEFb. *Genes Dev* 1998;12:755–762.
11. Kaldis P, Russo AA, Chou HS, Pavletich NP, Solomon MJ. Human and yeast Cdk-activating kinases (CAKs) display distinct substrate specificities. *Mol Biol Cell* 1998;9:2545–2560.
12. Tassan JP, Schultz SJ, Bartek J, Nigg EA. Cell cycle analysis of the activity, subcellular localization, and subunit composition of human CAK (CDK-activating kinase). *J Cell Biol* 1994;127:467–478.
13. Sherr CJ, Roberts JM. CDK inhibitors: positive and negative regulators of G1-phase progression. *Genes Dev* 1999;13:1501–1512.
14. Bates S, Ryan KM, Phillips AC, Vousden KH. Cell cycle arrest and DNA endoreduplication following p21Waf1/Cip1 expression. *Oncogene* 1998;17:1691–1703.
15. Dulic V, Stein GH, Far DF, Reed SI. Nuclear accumulation of p21Cip1 at the onset of mitosis: a role at the G2/M-phase transition. *Mol Cell Biol* 1998;18:546–557.

16. Niculescu AB, 3rd, Chen X, Smeets M, Hengst L, Prives C, Reed SI. Effects of p21(Cip1/Waf1) at both the G1/S and the G2/M cell cycle transitions: pRb is a critical determinant in blocking DNA replication and in preventing endoreduplication [published erratum appears in *Mol Cell Biol* 1998 Mar;18(3):1763]. *Mol Cell Biol* 1998;18:629–643.

17. LaBaer J, Garrett MD, Stevenson LF, Slingerland JM, Sandhu C, Chou HS, et al. New functional activities for the p21 family of CDK inhibitors. *Genes Dev* 1997;11:847–862.

18. Cheng M, Olivier P, Diehl JA, Fero M, Roussel MF, Roberts JM, Sherr CJ. The p21(Cip1) and p27(Kip1) CDK 'inhibitors' are essential activators of cyclin D-dependent kinases in murine fibroblasts. *EMBO J* 1999;18:1571–1583.

19. Zhang HS, Postigo AA, Dean DC. Active transcriptional repression by the Rb-E2F complex mediates G1 arrest triggered by p16INK4a, TGFbeta, and contact inhibition. *Cell* 1999;97:53–61.

20. Dyson N. The regulation of E2F by pRB-family proteins. Genes Dev 1998;12:2245–2262.

21. DelSal G, Loda M, Pagano M. Cell cycle and cancer: critical events at the G1 restriction point. *Crit Rev Oncol* 1996;7:127–142.

22. Grana X, Reddy EP. Cell cycle control in mammalian cells: role of cyclins, cyclin dependent kinases (CDKs), growth suppressor genes and cyclin-dependent kinase inhibitors (CKIs). *Oncogene* 1995;11:211–219.

23. Pardee AB. Multiple molecular levels of cell cycle regulation. *J Cell Biochem* 1994; 54:375–378.

24. Pines J. Cyclins and cyclin-dependent kinases: theme and variations. *Adv Cancer Res* 1995;66:181–212.

25. Weinberg RA. The retinoblastoma protein and cell cycle control. *Cell* 1995;81:323–330.

26. Senderowicz AM, Sausville EA. Preclinical and clinical development of cyclin-dependent kinase modulators. *J Natl Cancer Inst* 2000;92:376–387.

27. Kasten MM, Giordano A. pRb and the cdks in apoptosis and the cell cycle. *Cell Death Differ* 1998;5:132–140.

28. Chiarugi V, Magnelli L, Cinelli M, Basi G. Apoptosis and the cell cycle. *Cell Mol Biol Res* 1994;40:603–612.

29. Shimizu T, O'Connor P, Kohn KW, Pommier Y. Unscheduled activation of cyclin B1/Cdc2 kinase in human promyelocytic leukemia cell line HL60 cells undergoing apoptosis induced by DNA damage. *Cancer Res* 1995;55:228–231.

30. Meikrantz W, Schlegel R. Suppression of apoptosis by dominant negative mutants of cyclin-dependent protein kinases. *J Biol Chem* 1996;271,10205–10209.

31. Senderowicz AM, Headlee D, Stinson S, Lush RM, Tompkins A, Brawley O, et al. Phase I trial of a novel cyclin-dependent kinase inhibitor flavopiridol in patients with refractory neoplasms, in 9th National Cancer Institute-European Organization for Research on Treatment of Cancer Symposium Proceedings, Amsterdam, Holland, 1996, p. 77.

32. Senderowicz AM, Messmann R, Arbuck S, Headlee D, Zhai S, Murgo A, et al. A Phase I trial of 1 hour infusion of flavopiridol (Fla), a novel cyclin-dependent kinase inhibitor, in patients with advanced neoplasms, in Proceedings of the Annual Meeting of the American Society of Clinical Oncology, New Orleans, May, 2000.

32a. Tan A, Messmann R., Sausville E, et al. Phase I clinical and pharmacokinetic study of Flavopiridol administered as a daily 1-hour infusion in patients with advanced neoplasms. *J Clin Oncol* (in press).

33. Senderowicz AM, Headlee D, Lush R, Bauer K, Figg W, Murgo A, et al. Phase I trial of infusional UCN-01, a novel protein kinase inhibitor, in patients with refractory neoplasms, in 10th National Cancer Institute-European Organization for Research on Treatment of Cancer Symposium Proceedings, Amsterdam, Holland, June, 1998.

34. Schwartz G, Kaubisch A, Saltz L, Ilson D, O'Reilly E, Barazzuol J, et al. Phase I trial of sequential paclitaxel and the cyclin-dependent kinase inhibitor flavopiridol, in Proceedings of the American Society of Clinical Oncology, Atlanta, GA, 1999, p. 160.

35. Thomas J, Cleary J, Tutsch K, Arzoomanian R, Alberti D, Simon K, et al. Phase I clinical and pharmacokinetic trial of flavopiridol, in Proceedings of the Eighty-Eightieth Annual Meeting of the American Association of Cancer Research, San Diego, CA, 1997.

36. Dees E, O'Reilly S, Figg W, Elza-Brown K, Aylesworth C, Carducci M, et al. A Phase I and pharmacologic study of UCN-01, a protein kinase C inhibitor, in Proceedings of the American Society of Clinical Oncology, New Orleans, 2000.

37. Tamura T, Sasaki Y, Minami H, Fujii H, Ito K, Igarashi T, et al. Phase I study of UCN-01 by 3-hour infusion, in Proceedings of the American Society of Clinical Oncology, Atlanta, GA, 1999, p. 159.

38. Sausville EA, Arbuck SG, Messmann R, Headlee D, Bauer KS, Lush RM, et al. Phase I trial of 72-hour continuous infusion UCN-01 in patients with refractory neoplasms. *J Clin Oncol* 2001;19:2319–2333.

39. Hartwell LH, Kastan MB. Cell cycle control and cancer. *Science* 1994;266:1821–1828.

40. Pardee S. A restriction point for control of normal animal cell proliferation. *Proc Nat Acad Sci USA* 1974;71:1286–1290.

41. Harper J, Elledge S. Cdk inhibitors in development and cancer. *Curr Opin Genet Dev* 1996; 6:56–64.

42. Cordon-Cardo C. Mutations of cell cycle regulators. Biological and clinical implications for human neoplasia. *Am J Pathol* 1995;147:545–560.

43. Elledge SJ. Cell cycle checkpoints: preventing an identity crisis. *Science* 1996;274: 1664–1672.

44. Paulovich A, Toczyski D, Hartwell L. When checkpoints fail. *Cell* 1997;88:315–321.

45. Carlson B, Pearlstein R, Naik R, Sedlacek H, Sausville E, Worland P. Inhibition of CDK2, CDK4 and CDK7 by flavopiridol and structural analogs, in Proceedings of the American Association for Cancer Research, San Francisco, CA, 1996, p. 424.

46. Sedlacek HH, Czech J, Naik R, Kaur G, Worland P, Losiewicz M, et al. Flavopiridol (L86-8275, NSC-649890), a new kinase inhibitor for tumor therapy. Intl J Oncol 1996; 9:1143–1168.

47. Bartek J, Bartkova J, Lukas J. The retinoblastoma protein pathway and the restriction point. *Curr Opin Cell Biol* 1996;8:805–814.

48. Carlson BA, Dubay MM, Sausville EA, Brizuela L, Worland PJ. Flavopiridol induces G1 arrest with inhibition of cyclin-dependent kinase (CDK) 2 and CDK4 in human breast carcinoma cells. *Cancer Res* 1996;56:2973–2978.

49. Meijer L, Borgne A, Mulner O, Chong JP, Blow JJ, Inagaki N, et al. Biochemical and cellular effects of roscovitine, a potent and selective inhibitor of the cyclin-dependent kinases cdc2, cdk2 and cdk5. *Eur J Biochem* 1997;243:527–536.

50. Chen YN, Sharma SK, Ramsey TM, Jiang L, Martin MS, Baker K, et al. Selective killing of transformed cells by cyclin/cyclin-dependent kinase 2 antagonists [see comments]. *Proc Natl Acad Sci USA* 1999;96:4325–4329.

51. Senderowicz A. Small molecule modulators of cyclin-dependent kinases for cancer therapy. *Oncogene* 2000;19:6600–6606.

52. Meijer L, Kim SH. Chemical inhibitors of cyclin-dependent kinases. *Methods Enzymol* 1997;283:113–128.

53. Zaharevitz DW, Gussio R, Leost M, Senderowicz AM, Lahusen T, Kunick C, et al. Discovery and initial characterization of the paullones, a novel class of small-molecule inhibitors of cyclin-dependent kinases [in process citation]. *Cancer Res* 1999;59:2566–2569.

54. De Azevedo WF, Leclerc S, Meijer L, Havlicek L, Strnad M, Kim SH. Inhibition of cyclin-dependent kinases by purine analogues: crystal structure of human cdk2 complexed with roscovitine. *Eur J Biochem* 1997;243:518–526.

55. Meijer L, Pondaven, P. Cyclic activation of histone H1 kinase during sea urchin egg mitotic divisions. *Exp Cell Res* 1988;174:116–129.

56. Rialet V, Meijer L. A new screening test for antimitotic compounds using the universal M phase-specific protein kinase, p34cdc2/cyclin Bcdc13, affinity-immobilized on p13suc1-coated microtitration plates. *Anticancer Res* 1991;11:1581–1590.

57. Schulze-Gahmen U, Brandsen J, Jones HD, Morgan DO, Meijer L, Vesely J, Kim SH. Multiple modes of ligand recognition: crystal structures of cyclin-dependent protein kinase 2 in complex with ATP and two inhibitors, olomoucine and isopentenyladenine. *Proteins* 1995;22:378–391.

58. Brooks EE, Gray NS, Joly A, Kerwar SS, Lum R, Mackman RL, et al. CVT-313, a specific and potent inhibitor of CDK2 that prevents neointimal proliferation. *J Biol Chem* 1997; 272:29,207–29,211.

59. Gray NS, Wodicka L, Thunnissen AM, Norman TC, Kwon S, Espinoza FH, et al. Exploiting chemical libraries, structure, and genomics in the search for kinase inhibitors. *Science* 1998;281:533–538.

60. Paull KD, Shoemaker RH, Hodes L, Monks A, Scudiero DA, Rubinstein L, et al. Display and analysis of patterns of differential activity of drugs against human tumor cell lines: development of mean graph and COMPARE algorithm. *J Natl Cancer Inst* 1989;81:1088–1092.

61. Schultz C, Link A, Leost M, Zaharevitz DW, Gussio R, Sausville EA, et al. Paullones, a series of cyclin-dependent kinase inhibitors: synthesis, evaluation of CDK1/cyclin B inhibition, and in vitro antitumor activity. *J Med Chem* 1999;42:2909–2919.

62. Lahusen J, Singh S, Sausville EA, Senderowicz AM. Alsterpaullone (Alp) blocks cell cycle progression at G1/S and G2/M with altered expression of G1 and G2 cyclins, in Proceedings of the Twentieth Annual Meeting of the American Association of Cancer Research, San Francisco, CA, 2000.

63. Lahusen T, Singh SS, Sausville E, Senderowicz AM. Cell cycle arrest at G1/S and G2/M by alsterpaullone (alp) is independent of p53 function or p21WAF1 expression, in Proceedings of the AACR, New Orleans, 2001.

64. Kent LL, Hull-Campbell NE, Lau T, Wu JC, Thompson SA, Nori M. Characterization of novel inhibitors of cyclin-dependent kinases. *Biochem Biophys Res Commun* 1999;260:768–774.

65. Walker DH. Small-molecule inhibitors of cyclin-dependent kinases: molecular tools and potential therapeutics. *Curr Top Microbiol Immunol* 1998;227:149–165.

66. van den Heuvel S, Harlow E. Distinct roles for cyclin-dependent kinases in cell cycle control. *Science* 1993;262:2050–2054.

67. Buquet-Fagot C, Lallemand F, Montagne M, Mester J. Effects of olomucine, a selective inhibitor of cyclin-dependent kinases, on cell cycle progression in human cancer cell lines. *Anti-Cancer Drugs* 1997;8:623–631.

68. Chien M, Astumian M, Liebowitz D, Rinker-Schaeffer, C, Stadler W. In vitro evaluation of flavopiridol, a novel cell cycle inhibitor, in bladder cancer. *Cancer Chemother Pharmacol* 1999;44:81–87.

69. Parker B, Kaur G, Nieves-Neira W, Taimi M, Kolhagen G, Shimizu T, et al. Early induction of apoptosis in hematopoietic cell lines after exposure to flavopiridol. *Blood* 1998; 91:458–465.

70. Park DS, Farinelli SE, Greene LA. Inhibitors of cyclin-dependent kinases promote survival of post-mitotic neuronally differentiated PC12 cells and sympathetic neurons. *J Biol Chem* 1996;271:8161–8169.

71. Park DS, Morris EJ, Greene LA, Geller HM. G1/S cell cycle blockers and inhibitors of cyclin-dependent kinases suppress camptothecin-induced neuronal apoptosis. *J Neurosci* 1997; 17:1256–1270.

72. Gervais JL, Seth P, Zhang H. Cleavage of CDK inhibitor p21(Cip1/Waf1) by caspases is an early event during DNA damage-induced apoptosis. *J Biol Chem* 1998;273:19207–19212.

73. Levkau B, Koyama H, Raines EW, Clurman BE, Herren B, Orth K, et al. Cleavage of p21Cip1/Waf1 and p27Kip1 mediates apoptosis in endothelial cells through activation of Cdk2: role of a caspase cascade. *Mol Cell* 1998;1:553–563.

74. Zhou BB, Li H, Yuan J, Kirschner MW. Caspase-dependent activation of cyclin-dependent kinases during Fas-induced apoptosis in Jurkat cells. *Proc Natl Acad Sci USA* 1998;95: 6785–6790.

75. Lee HR, Chang TH, Tebalt MJ, 3rd, Senderowicz AM, Szabo E. Induction of differentiation accompanies inhibition of cdk2 in a non-small cell lung cancer cell line. *Int J Oncol* 1999; 15:161–166.

76. Rosania GR, Merlie J, Jr, Gray N, Chang YT, Schultz PG, Heald R. A cyclin-dependent kinase inhibitor inducing cancer cell differentiation: biochemical identification using Xenopus egg extracts. *Proc Natl Acad Sci USA* 1999;96:4797–4802.

77. Liu M, Subramanyam YV, Baskaran N. Preparation and analysis of cDNA from a small number of hematopoietic cells [in process citation]. *Methods Enzymol* 1999;303:45–55.

78. Kaur G, Stetler-Stevenson M, Sebers S, Worland P, Sedlacek H, Myers C, et al. Growth inhibition with reversible cell cycle arrest of carcinoma cells by flavone L86-8275. *J Natl Cancer Inst* 1992;84:1736–1740.

79. Losiewicz MD, Carlson BA, Kaur G, Sausville EA, Worland PJ. Potent inhibition of CDC2 kinase activity by the flavonoid L86-8275. *Biochem Biophys Res Commun* 1994;201:589–595.

80. Worland PJ, Kaur G, Stetler-Stevenson M, Sebers S, Sartor O, Sausville EA. Alteration of the phosphorylation state of p34cdc2 kinase by the flavone L86-8275 in breast carcinoma cells. Correlation with decreased H1 kinase activity. *Biochem Pharmacol* 1993;46:1831–1840.

81. De Azevedo WF, Jr, Mueller-Dieckmann HJ, Schulze-Gahmen U, Worland PJ, Sausville E, Kim SH. Structural basis for specificity and potency of a flavonoid inhibitor of human CDK2, a cell cycle kinase. *Proc Natl Acad Sci USA* 1996;93,2735–2740.

82. Michalides R, van Veelen N, Hart A, Loftus B, Wientjens E, Balm A. Overexpression of cyclin D1 correlates with recurrence in a group of forty-seven operable squamous cell carcinomas of the head and neck. *Cancer Res* 1995;55:975–978.

83. Gansauge S, Gansauge F, Ramadani M, Stobbe H, Rau B, Harada N, Beger HG. Overexpression of cyclin D1 in human pancreatic carcinoma is associated with poor prognosis. *Cancer Res* 1997;57:1634–1637.

84. Fredersdorf S, Burns J, Milne AM, Packham G, Fallis L, Gillett CE, et al. High level expression of p27(kip1) and cyclin D1 in some human breast cancer cells: inverse correlation between the expression of p27(kip1) and degree of malignancy in human breast and colorectal cancers. *Proc Natl Acad Sci USA* 1997;94:6380–6385.

85. Carlson B, Lahusen T, Singh S, Loaiza-Perez A, Worland PJ, Pestell R, et al. Downregulation of cyclin D1 by transcriptional repression in MCF-7 human breast carcinoma cells induced by flavopiridol. *Cancer Res* 1999;59:4634–4641.

86. Melillo G, Sausville EA, Cloud K, Lahusen T, Varesio L, Senderowicz AM. Flavopiridol, a protein kinase inhibitor, down-regulates hypoxic induction of vascular endothelial growth factor expression in human monocytes. *Cancer Res* 1999;59:5433–5437.

87. Chao SH, Fujinaga K, Marion JE, Taube R, Sausville EA, Senderowicz AM, et al. Flavopiridol inhibits P-TEFb and blocks HIV-1 replication. *J Biol Chem* 2000;275:28345–28348.

88. Arguello F, Alexander M, Sterry J, Tudor G, Smith E, Kalavar N, et al. Flavopiridol induces apoptosis of normal lymphoid cells, causes immunosuppresion, and has potent antitumor activity in vivo against human and leukemia xenografts. *Blood* 1998;91:2482–2490.

89. Byrd JC, Shinn C, Waselenko JK, Fuchs EJ, Lehman TA, Nguyen PL, et al. Flavopiridol induces apoptosis in chronic lymphocytic leukemia cells via activation of caspase-3 without evidence of bcl-2 modulation or dependence on functional p53. *Blood* 1998;92:3804–3816.

90. Konig A, Schwartz GK, Mohammad RM, Al-Katib A, Gabrilove JL. The novel cyclin-dependent kinase inhibitor flavopiridol downregulates Bcl-2 and induces growth arrest and apoptosis in chronic B-cell leukemia lines. *Blood* 1997;90:4307–4312.
91. Shapiro GI, Koestner DA, Matranga CB, Rollins BJ. Flavopiridol induces cell cycle arrest and p53-independent apoptosis in non-small cell lung cancer cell lines. *Clin Cancer Res* 1999;5:2925–2938.
92. Lahusen J, Loaiza-Perez A, Sausville EA, Senderowicz AM. Flavopiridol-induced apoptosis is associated with p38 and MEK activation and is prevented by caspase and MAPK inhibitors, in Proceedings of the Twentieth Annual Meeting of the American Association of Cancer Research, San Francisco, CA, 2000.
93. Patel V, Senderowicz AM, Pinto D, Igishi T, Raffeld M, Quintanilla-Martinez L, et al. Flavopiridol, a novel cyclin-dependent kinase inhibitor, suppresses the growth of head and neck squamous cell carcinomas by inducing apoptosis. *J Clin Invest* 1998;102:1674–1681.
94. Schrump DS, Matthews W, Chen GA, Mixon A, Altorki NK. Flavopiridol mediates cell cycle arrest and apoptosis in esophageal cancer cells. *Clin Cancer Res* 1998;4:2885–2890.
95. Bible KC, Kaufmann SH. Flavopiridol: a cytotoxic flavone that induces cell death in noncycling A549 human lung carcinoma cells. *Cancer Res* 1996;56:4856–4861.
96. Brusselbach S, Nettelbeck DM, Sedlacek HH, Muller, R. Cell cycle-independent induction of apoptosis by the anti-tumor drug Flavopiridol in endothelial cells. *Int J Cancer* 1998;77:146–152.
97. Kerr JS, Wexler RS, Mousa SA, Robinson CS, Wexler EJ, Mohamed S, et al. Novel small molecule alpha v integrin antagonists: comparative anti-cancer efficacy with known angio-genesis inhibitors [in process citation]. *Anticancer Res* 1999;19:959–968.
98. Schwartz G, Farsi K, Maslak P, Kelsen D, Spriggs D. Potentiation of apoptosis by flavopiridol in mitomycin-C-treated gastric and breast cancer cells. *Clin Cancer Res* 1997;3:1467–1472.
99. Bible KC, Kaufmann SH. Cytotoxic synergy between flavopiridol (NSC 649890, L86-8275) and various antineoplastic agents: the importance of sequence of administration. *Cancer Res* 1997;57:3375–3380.
100. Drees M, Dengler W, Roth T, Labonte H, Mayo J, Malspeis L, et al. Flavopiridol (L86-8275): Selective antitumor activity in vitro and activity in vivo for prostate carcinoma cells. *Clin Cancer Res* 1997;32:273–279.
101. Senderowicz AM, Headlee D, Stinson SF, Lush RM, Kalil N, Villalba L, et al. Phase I trial of continuous infusion flavopiridol, a novel cyclin-dependent kinase inhibitor, in patients with refractory neoplasms. *J Clin Oncol* 1998;16:2986–2999.
102. Wright J, Blatner GL, Cheson BD. Clinical trials referral resource. Clinical trials of flavopiridol. *Oncology (Huntingt)* 1998;12:1018,1023–1024.
103. Werner J, Kelsen D, Karpeh M, Inzeo D, Barazzuol J, Sugarman A, Schwartz GK. The cyclin-dependent kinase inhibitor flavopiridol is an active and unexpectedly toxic agent in advanced gastric cancer, in Proceedings of the American Society of Clinical Oncology, Los Angeles, CA, 1998.
104. Shapiro G, Patterson A, Lynch C, Lucca J, Anderson I, Boral A, et al. A Phase II trial of flavopiridol in patients with stage IV non-small cell lung cancer, in Proceedings of the American Society of Clinical Oncology, Atlanta, GA, 1999.
105. Bennett S, Mani S, O'Reilly S, Wright J, Schilsky R, Vokes E, Grochow L. Phase II trial of flavopiridol in metastatic colorectal cancer: preliminary results, in Proceedings of the American Society of Clinical Oncology, Atlanta, GA, 1999.
106. Stadler WM, Vogelzang NJ, Amato R, Sosman J, Taber D, Liebowitz D, Vokes EE. Flavopiridol, a novel cyclin-dependent kinase inhibitor, in metastatic renal cancer: a University of Chicago Phase II Consortium study. *J Clin Oncol* 2000;18:371–375.

107. Innocenti F, Stadler W, Iyer L, Vokes E, Ratain M. Flavopiridol-induced diarrhea is related to the systemic metabolism of flavopiridol to its glucuronide, in Proceedings of the American Society of Clinical Oncology, New Orleans, 2000.

108. Tamaoki T. Use and specificity of staurosporine, UCN-01, and calphostin C as protein kinase inhibitors. *Methods Enzymol* 1991;201:340–347.

109. Takahashi I, Kobayashi E, Asano K, Yoshida M, Nakano H. UCN-01, a selective inhibitor of protein kinase C from Streptomyces. *J Antibiot (Tokyo)* 1987;40:1782–1784.

110. Takahashi I, Saitoh Y, Yoshida M, Sano H, Nakano H, Morimoto M, Tamaoki T. UCN-01 and UCN-02, new selective inhibitors of protein kinase C. II. Purification, physico-chemical properties, structural determination and biological activities. *J Antibiot (Tokyo)* 1989; 42:571–576.

111. Seynaeve CM, Kazanietz MG, Blumberg PM, Sausville EA, Worland PJ. Differential inhibition of protein kinase C isozymes by UCN-01, a staurosporine analogue. *Mol Pharmacol* 1994;45:1207–1214.

112. Seynaeve CM, Stetler-Stevenson M, Sebers S, Kaur G, Sausville EA, Worland PJ. Cell cycle arrest and growth inhibition by the protein kinase antagonist UCN-01 in human breast carcinoma cells. *Cancer Res* 1993;53:2081–2086.

113. Wang Q, Worland PJ, Clark JL, Carlson BA, Sausville EA. Apoptosis in 7-hydroxystaurosporine-treated T lymphoblasts correlates with activation of cyclin-dependent kinases 1 and 2. *Cell Growth Differ* 1995;6:927–936.

114. Akinaga S, Gomi K, Morimoto M, Tamaoki T, Okabe M. Antitumor activity of UCN-01, a selective inhibitor of protein kinase C, in murine and human tumor models. *Cancer Res* 1991;51:4888–4892.

115. Akinaga S, Nomura K, Gomi K, Okabe M. Effect of UCN-01, a selective inhibitor of protein kinase C, on the cell-cycle distribution of human epidermoid carcinoma, A431 cells. *Cancer Chemother Pharmacol* 1994;33:273–280.

116. Akiyama T, Yoshida T, Tsujita T, Shimizu M, Mizukami T, Okabe M, Akinaga S. G1 phase accumulation induced by UCN-01 is associated with dephosphorylation of Rb and CDK2 proteins as well as induction of CDK inhibitor p21/Cip1/WAF1/Sdi1 in p53-mutated human epidermoid carcinoma A431 cells. *Cancer Res* 1997;57:1495–1501.

117. Wang Q, Fan S, Eastman A, Worland PJ, Sausville EA, O'Connor P. UCN-01: a potent abrogator of G2 checkpoint function in cancer cells with disrupted p53. *J Natl Cancer Inst* 1996;88:956–965.

118. Yu L, Orlandi L, Wang P, Orr M, Senderowicz AM, Sausville EA, et al. UCN-01 abrogates G2 arrest through a cdc2-dependent pathway that involves inactivation of the Wee1Hu kinase. *J Biol Chem* 1998;273:33455–33464.

119. Sarkaria JN, Busby EC, Tibbetts RS, Roos P, Taya Y, Karnitz LM, Abraham RT. Inhibition of ATM and ATR kinase activities by the radiosensitizing agent, caffeine. *Cancer Res* 1999;59:4375–4382.

120. Graves PR, Yu L, Schwarz JK, Gales J, Sausville EA, O'Connor PM, Piwnica-Worms H. The Chk1 protein kinase and the Cdc25C regulatory pathways are targets of the anticancer agent UCN-01. *J Biol Chem* 2000;275:5600–5605.

121. Busby EC, Leistritz DF, Abraham RT, Karnitz LM, Sarkaria JN. The radiosensitizing agent 7-hydroxystaurosporine (UCN-01) inhibits the DNA damage checkpoint kinase hChk1. *Cancer Res* 2000;60:2108–2112.

122. Shao RG, Cao CX, Shimizu T, O'Connor PM, Kohn KW, Pommier Y. Abrogation of an S-phase checkpoint and potentiation of camptothecin cytotoxicity by 7-hydroxystaurosporine (UCN-01) in human cancer cell lines, possibly influenced by p53 function. *Cancer Res* 1997;57:4029–4035.

123. Bunch RT, Eastman A. 7-Hydroxystaurosporine (UCN-01) causes redistribution of prolif-erating cell nuclear antigen and abrogates cisplatin-induced S-phase arrest in Chinese hamster ovary cells. *Cell Growth Differ* 1997;8:779–788.
124. Akiyama T, Shimizu M, Okabe M, Tamaoki T, Akinaga S. Differential effects of UCN-01, staurosporine and CGP 41 251 on cell cycle progression and CDC2/cyclin B1 regulation in A431 cells synchronized at M phase by nocodazole [in process citation]. *Anticancer Drugs* 1999;10:67–78.
125. Kawakami K, Futami H, Takahara J, Yamaguchi K. UCN-01, 7-hydroxyl-staurosporine, inhibits kinase activity of cyclin-dependent kinases and reduces the phosphorylation of the retinoblastoma susceptibility gene product in A549 human lung cancer cell line. *Biochem Biophys Res Commun* 1996;219:778–783.
126. Shimizu E, Zhao MR, Nakanishi H, Yamamoto A, Yoshida S, Takada M, et al. Differing effects of staurosporine and UCN-01 on RB protein phosphorylation and expression of lung cancer cell lines. *Oncology* 1996;53:494–504.
127. Chen X, Lowe M, Keyomarsi K. UCN-01-mediated G1 arrest in normal but not tumor breast cells is pRb-dependent and p53-independent. *Oncogene* 1999;18:5691–5702.
128. Usuda J, Saijo N, Fukuoka K, Fukumoto H, Kuh HJ, Nakamura T, et al. Molecular determinants of UCN-01-induced growth inhibition in human lung cancer cells. *Int J Cancer* 2000;85:275–280.
129. Marchetti A, Buttitta F, Merlo G, Diella F, Pellegrini S, Pepe S, et al. p53 alterations in non-small cell lung cancers correlate with metastatic involvement of hilar and mediastinal lymph nodes. *Cancer Res* 1993;53:2846–2851.
130. Lowe SW, Bodis S, Bardeesy N, McClatchey A, Remington L, Ruley HE, et al. Apoptosis and the prognostic significance of p53 mutation. *Cold Spring Harb Symp Quant Biol* 1994;59:419–426.
131. Akinaga S, Nomura K, Gomi K, Okabe M. Enhancement of antitumor activity of mitomycin C in vitro and in vivo by UCN-01, a selective inhibitor of protein kinase C. *Cancer Chemother Pharmacol* 1993;32:183–189.
132. Bunch RT, Eastman A. Enhancement of cisplatin-induced cytotoxicity by 7-hydroxystaurosporine (UCN-01), a new G2-checkpoint inhibitor. *Clin Cancer Res* 1996;2:791–797.
133. Hsueh CT, Kelsen D, Schwartz GK. UCN-01 suppresses thymidylate synthase gene expression and enhances 5-fluorouracil-induced apoptosis in a sequence-dependent manner [in process citation]. *Clin Cancer Res* 1998;4:2201–2206.
134. Husain A, Yan XJ, Rosales N, Aghajanian C, Schwartz GK, Spriggs DR. UCN-01 in ovary cancer cells: effective as a single agent and in combination with cis-diamminedichloro-platinum(II)independent of p53 status. *Clin Cancer Res* 1997;3:2089–2097.
135. Pollack IF, Kawecki S, Lazo JS. Blocking of glioma proliferation in vitro and in vivo and potentiating the effects of BCNU and cisplatin: UCN-01, a selective protein kinase C inhibitor. *J Neurosurg* 1996;84:1024–1032.
136. Tsuchida E, Urano M. The effect of UCN-01 (7-hydroxystaurosporine), a potent inhibitor of protein kinase C, on fractionated radiotherapy or daily chemotherapy of a murine fibrosarcoma. *Int J Radiat Oncol Biol Phys* 1997;39:1153–1161.
137. Sugiyama K, Shimizu M, Akiyama T, Tamaoki T, Yamaguchi K, Takahashi R, et al. UCN-01 selectively enhances mitomycin C cytotoxicity in p53 defective cells which is mediated through S and/or G(2) checkpoint abrogation. *Int J Cancer* 2000;85:703–709.
138. Jones CB, Clements MK, Wasi S, Daoud SS. Enhancement of camptothecin-induced cytotoxicity with UCN-01 in breast cancer cells: abrogation of S/G(2) arrest. *Cancer Chemother Pharmacol* 2000;45:252–258.
139. Sausville EA, Lush RD, Headlee D, Smith AC, Figg WD, Arbuck SG, et al. Clinical pharmacology of UCN-01: initial observations and comparison to preclinical models. *Cancer Chemother Pharmacol* 1998;42 Suppl:S54–S59.

140. Fuse E, Tanii H, Kurata N, Kobayashi H, Shimada Y, Tamura T, et al. Unpredicted clinical pharmacology of UCN-01 caused by specific binding to human alpha1-acid glycoprotein. *Cancer Res* 1998;58:3248–3253.

141. Senderowicz AM, Headlee D, Lush R, Bauer K, Figg W, Murgo A, et al. Phase I trial of infusional UCN-01, a novel protein kinase inhibitor, in patients with refractory neoplasms, in Proceedings of the Thirty-fifth Annual Meeting of the American Society of Clinical Oncology, Atlanta, GA, May 15–18, 1999.

142. Wilson WH, Sorbara L, Figg WD, Mont EK, Sausville E, Warren KE, et al. Modulation of clinical drug resistance in a B cell lymphoma patient by the protein kinase inhibitor 7-hydroxystaurosporine: presentation of a novel therapeutic paradigm. *Clin Cancer Res* 2000;6:415–421.

143. Fowler L, Dong L, Bowes RC, 3rd, van de Water B, Stevens JL, Jaken S. Transformation-sensitive changes in expression, localization, and phosphorylation of adducins in renal proximal tubule epithelial cells. *Cell Growth Differ* 1998;9:177–184.

9 Cell Cycle Regulators

Interactions and Their Role in Diagnosis, Prognosis, and Treatment of Cancer

Paul J. van Diest, MD, PhD
and Rob J. A. M. Michalides, PhD

CONTENTS

1. INTRODUCTION

Tumors develop gradually as a result of a multistep acquisition of genetic alterations where cells ultimately emerge as selfish, intruding, and metastatic cells. The genetic defects associated with the process of tumor progression affect control of proliferation, programmed cell death (or apoptosis), cell-aging, angiogenesis, escape from immune response, and invasion and metastasis *(1)*. These characteristics of tumor cells are to be considered as interactive control boxes

From: *Cancer Drug Discovery and Development:*
Cell Cycle Inhibitors in Cancer Therapy: Current Strategies
Edited by: A. Giordano and K. J. Soprano © Humana Press Inc., Totowa, NJ

that are well taken care of in normal cells, but in which one or more failures have occurred during tumor development. The multistep nature of tumor development is evident from pathological examination of various tumor progression systems, indicating a continuous morphological progression from normal cells to premalignant stages to invasive tumors. The multistep process in tumorigenesis is responsible for the age-dependent appearance of tumors in humans; four to seven major genetic alterations that accumulate over time are responsible for the development of the ultimate tumor cell.

Fundamental cancer research over the last 30 years has revealed a multitude of genetic alterations that specify more or less separate steps in tumor development and that are collectively responsible for the process of tumor progression. However, the large number of genetic alterations, the complexity of the interactions between the different affected genes, and the unpredictability of the functional effect of disturbances in individual markers renders it difficult to devise a strategy for diagnosis-making, assessment of prognosis, and prediction of response to treatment that is based on individual alterations, unless these alterations would end up in a central control system, which ultimately determines the fate of the cell. Also for practical reasons, it is essential to distinguish either common themes amid the numerous genetic alterations or to recognize the most relevant ones.

What could we expect from a survey of genetic alterations in cancer in order to predict course of disease or to specify modality of treatment? Is the malignant phenotype associated with a particular genetic defect, or with a set of defects? Should one look for combinations of defects in all the hallmarks of cancer mentioned earlier, rather than for an accumulation of defects within one control box in order to indicate degree of malignancy? How are functional endpoints of each control box affected by genetic alterations within one particular control box, and how by alterations outside the control box? How do the findings generated in in vitro model systems relate to clinical findings in vivo? These questions pose a major challenge for pathology of cancer in its quest for markers of diagnosis, prognosis, and treatment.

Despite the vast literature on this topic, this issue is still at its infancy because of several reasons: the complexity of interactions between the genetic defects in cancer, problems in standardization and reproducibility of the read-out of the genetic defects, tumor heterogeneity, and the apparent arbitrariness of genetic lesions in a particular tissue. The process of growth control can especially demonstrate this where cell cycle regulators, DNA damage control genes, cyclin dependent kinases (CDKs), and cyclin dependent kinase inhibitors (CKIs) show complex interactions. Several of these issues have been dealt with in other chapters, so here we focus especially on interactions between cell cycle regulators that are important for the assessment of clinical usefulness of different genetic alterations.

2. CONTROL OF CELLULAR PROLIFERATION

Growth of cells is the net-result of cell proliferation, differentiation, and death of cells, which are mutually regulated. Cells enter the cell cycle and commit to DNA synthesis in response to external factors, including growth factors and cellular adhesion. During the first phase of the cell cycle, G_1, cells are responsive to these mitogenic stimuli and are depending on them in order to reach a critical restriction point, termed R, at the end of G_1 *(2)*. Beyond the restriction point R, cell cycle transition becomes more or less autonomous. The activities of CDKs, and their inhibitors, CKIs, regulate transition through the cell cycle. A CDK is active as a serine/threonine kinase when it becomes associated with a cyclin protein and becomes activated by phosphorylation and dephosphorylation via CAK (cyclin activated kinase), wee1-kinase, and cdc25 phosphatase *(3,4)*. This complex activation mechanism of a CDK provides multiple levels of control. Cyclin proteins are only present during specific phases of the cell cycle. This is the result of specific induction and elimination of these proteins in the cell cycle. Induction of cyclins starts when cells enter into the cell cycle from a quiescent state and requires growth factors and adherence of cells onto extracellular matrix (ECM) components. Binding of growth factors to receptors, either at the surface of the cells (for instance for the epidermal growth factor [EGF]), or in the cytoplasm (in case of steroids), triggers a cascade of events by which the signal of ligand binding to the receptor (or the ligand/receptor itself) is transmitted to the nucleus and which finally results in activation of transcription factors. The number of intermediates in each of these signal-transduction pathways varies, and mutations in their genes provide ample opportunities for continuous stimulation. All these signal-transduction pathways finally activate transcription factors, which are responsible for transcription of, among others, the cyclin D gene, coding for the first cyclin protein acting in G_1. Three D type cycling proteins, D_1-3, have been identified. Their distribution is somewhat cell type specific with cyclin D_1 being expressed in most epithelial and mesenchymal cells and cyclin D_3 in lymphoid cells *(5)*. The promoter of the cyclin D_1 gene contains multiple DNA binding sites for transcription factors that are either induced or activated by growth factors to regulate its expression *(6–12)*. Adhesion of cells onto ECM components also induces transcription of cyclin D_1, most likely via the Mitogen Actived Protein Kinase (MAPK)-pathway, which becomes activated when integrin receptors bind to ECM components *(13–16)*. D-type cyclins are rate-limiting for cell cycle progression, since enforced overexpression of cyclin D_1 accelerates G_1 transition, whereas, conversely, inactivation of cyclin D_1 by microinjection of antibodies or antisense DNA constructs induces a G_1 arrest *(17–19)*. Cyclin D_1 protein associates with CDK4 or -6, and this complex is then positively regulated by CAK and cdc25 and negatively by wee1/mik kinase and cyclin kinase inhibitors (*see* below). The final target of an activated cyclin

D:CDK4 or -6 kinase complex is the retinoblastoma protein, pRb *(20)*. Its phosphorylation releases E2F transcription factors that are required for transcription of E2F responsive genes, including those whose proteins are involved in DNA synthesis and are mandatory for S-phase progression *(20)*. E2F represents a family of at least five different transcription factors, which bind to hypophosphorylated pRb or to related p107 and p130 proteins *(21)*. pRb appears unique among these E2F binding proteins, since elimination of pRb alone is sufficient to liberate abundant E2F activity to render growth of cells growth factor-independent *(22)*. Once activated, each of these E2Fs acts as a transactivator and mediates transcription of E2F responsive genes, among which cyclins D_1, E, and A. The promoters of cyclins D_1, E, and A contain E2F binding sites *(12,23)*. Thus, once cyclin D_1:CDK4 is active, it generates more cyclin D_1 by a positive feedback mechanism. Further progression through G_1 to restriction point R requires activity of cyclin E (the second important G_1 cyclin), and passage through S phase demands cyclin A activity, each in a complex with CDK2. Induction of these two cyclins depends on E2F *(24,25)*, implying that once cyclin D_1:CDK4 activity has set the G_1 regulatory system into motion, cyclin E- and cyclin A-CDK activities are induced and cell cycle transition may occur. Each of these G_1 cyclin:CDK complexes phosphorylates pRb, however, at different sites *(26)* and with different effects *(27,28)*. The different effects may be due to the release of different E2F members from pRb or pRb family members *(29–31)* and/or to specific activities of each of the cyclins (*see* below). Activity of G_1 cyclins is directly linked to DNA synthesis, since cdc6 protein, which is essential for DNA replication in S-phase, is induced by E2F that is released by cyclin D or cyclin E:CDK activity, but not by cyclin A kinase activity *(32–34)*. The latter is more likely involved in the release of restrictive component(s) from the DNA replication complex during S-phase *(35)*. Activation of G_1 cyclins results in induction of cyclin B during G_2, which becomes associated with CDK1 that also binds to cyclin A. Their combined activities mediate transition through G_2/M phase of the cell cycle *(36,37)*.

Degradation of cyclin D is either due to specific degradation of its mRNA *(38)* or to degradation of the protein by proteases after recognition of degradation-specific sequences at the C-terminus or via ubiquitin-dependent proteosomal degradation. Cyclins E and A serve as a substrate of their own cyclin: CDK complex, cyclin D_1 becomes phosphorylated by a yet unknown kinase *(39)*. Phosphorylation of cyclins creates a target for ubiquitin-dependent, protease-mediated degradation of cyclins D_1, E, A, and B *(39–41)*. This degradation of cyclins terminates its action and provides a one-way direction to the cell cycle.

Stimulation of growth is mediated by the action of the cyclin:CDK complexes, whereas inhibition of growth is imposed by the CKI suppressor proteins *(42–44)*. The CKIs include two families: the INK4 family that encompasses p16/INK4A, p15/INK4B, p18/INK4C, and p19/INK4D. All of these inhibit cyclin D:CDK4 kinase activity by binding to the CDK4 site that associates with cyclin D *(45)*. The CIP/Kip family members, including p21, p27, and p57, bind to all cyclin:CDK complexes and inhibit their activity. CKIs are subject to regulation at various levels, by transcription, by post-translational modulation, and by a shift in their cyclin:CDK targets. When cells enter the cell cycle from quiescence, growth factors induce cyclin D_1 expression and formation of cyclin D:CDK4 complexes. This increased complex formation will absorb CKI-p27 until a point is reached where excess cyclin D:CDK4/6 complex has titrated out all available p27. From this point on, cyclin D:CDK4/6 will function as an active kinase and generate free E2F, which induces transcription of cyclin E. The story is now reiterated: increasing cyclin E:CDK2 levels titrate out p27 by which unbound, active cyclin E:CDK2 is generated *(46,47)*. Moreover, Cip-CKIs inhibit cyclin:CDKs with different efficiency and affinity: p27 inhibits cyclin A:CDK2 more efficiently than cyclin D:CDK *(48)*, whereas p21 inhibits both with equal efficacy *(49)*. In addition, cellular levels of CKIs affect inhibition: p21 and p27 in low concentrations stabilize cyclin D:CDK complexes, whereas they inhibit its kinase activity when present in high concentrations *(50)*. These data suggest that cyclin D:CDK complexes may function as a catcher for p27 or p21. When cyclin D_1 levels increase, cyclin D:CDK complexes absorb more p27/p21 at the expense of its binding to cyclin E or A:CDK2 complexes. This results in G_1 transit. Such a shift in targets of CKIs is the basis of action of transforming growth factor-β (TGF-β), anti-estrogens or of rapamycin: TGF-β stabilizes CKI-p15 *(51)*, which preferentially binds to cyclin D:CDK. This causes a displacement of CKI-p27 from cyclin D_1:CDK4, which now becomes associated with cyclin E:CDK2, causing a G_1 arrest in epithelial cells. In addition, arrest of estrogen-receptor positive cells by anti-estrogens reduces protein levels of cyclin D_1, whereby CKI-p27 is released from cyclin D_1:CDK4 complexes and now becomes associated with cyclin E:CDK2, thereby causing a G_1 arrest *(52,53)*. Also, rapamycin delays accumulation of cyclin D_1 mRNA, which leads to impaired formation of cyclin D_1:CDK4 complexes. This results in a retargeting of CKI-p27 to cyclin E:CDK2, thereby causing a rapamycin-induced G_1 arrest *(54)*.

Cki p21 influences not only G_1/S, but also G_2/M transition, depending on the status of Rb. In Rb +/+ cells, p21 expression causes a G_1/S arrest, whereas a G_2 arrest by p21 is more prominent in Rb–/– cells *(55,56)*. p21 is induced in a p53-dependent and in a p53-independent manner, where the p53 protein is a transcription factor induced upon DNA damage. p53 promotes expression of genes involved in growth arrest (Cki-p21) or apoptosis (bax) *(57,58)*. The specific response of p53 is depending on Rb status: in Rb-wt cells, p53 induction leads to cell cycle arrest by induction of p21, whereas Rb-deficient cells bypass the G_1 checkpoint and undergo apoptosis.

3. ESSENTIAL DERAILMENTS IN CANCER

The aforementioned makes clear that there are complex physiological inter-actions and control mechanisms for cell cycle progression. All of the genes noted may be a target of genetic changes during carcinogenesis and tumor progression, as well genes involved in control over apoptosis and aging. The essential dis-turbed pathways in carcinogenesis are, respectively, the Rb-pathway, p53, and telomerase (re)activation. Derailments in these pathways provide to tumor cells increasing autonomy and selective advantage over other cells. For example, overexpression of cyclin D_1 protein in MCF7 breast cancer cells renders that these cells now can proliferate under reduced serum concentrations by affecting the proportion of cells being in G_0, quiescence state (59). Overexpression of cyclin D_1 prevents cells to enter quiescence and therefore enhances the prolifera-tive fraction of tumor cells. Since tumor cells in vivo will encounter various growth factor conditions, overexpression of cyclin D_1 most likely allows tumor cells to continue to proliferate in low growth factor conditions in vivo as well.

Distortion of the Rb-pathway is a common phenomenon in cancer (see below), and is achieved by either disruption of Rb, overexpression of cyclin D_1 or CDK4, or downregulation of CKI-p16 (1,60). Various mechanisms may account for these deregulations. For Rb, this includes point mutation, deletion and functional inactivation by the binding of viral proteins (e.g., HPV E8) at the site of interac-tion with cyclin:CDKs. For cyclin D_1, there may be amplification of the gene, inter- and intrachromosomal recombination (61), loss of destabilizing sequences in the mRNA by deletion (62) or alternative splicing (63,64), and overexpression as result of aberrant growth factor stimulation. For p16 this includes most fre-quently deletion and infrequently point mutation and methylation of promoter sequences. CDK4 may be subject to amplification (65) and mutation of its inter-action site with p16 (66,67). When one adds up to all these possibilities and examines series of breast, lung, head and neck, or melanoma cancers for either of these alterations, one is likely to find that all tumors have undergone some distortion in the Rb pathway (68). The same accounts for disruption of the p19[ARF]-p53 pathway, which prevents apoptosis to occur, whereas most advanced carci-nomas also show telomerase activation in order to become immortal (1,69,70).

4. WHAT DOES DISTORTION OF THE RB PATHWAY DO TO CELLS?

The idea that progression of the cell cycle through G_1 to S requires only phosphorylation of pRb and thereby releases E2F turns out to be too simple. Cyclin E can overcome a p16-induced arrest of the cell cycle without phospho-rylation of pRb (71), indicating that other targets of cyclin E:CDK2 activity determine the full transit through G_1. It is not (yet) clear which other target this may be. In general, overexpression of cyclins D_1 or E leads to accelerated transition through G_1, and overexpression of cyclin D_1 to reduced growth factor dependency and a reduced entry into G_0 (quiescence). Activation of E2F by overexpression of cyclin D_1 or cyclin E leads to p53 dependent apoptosis under reduced serum conditions *(72)*. In transformation assays, overexpression of cyclin D_1 by itself does not induce transformation, but it does so together with adenovirus E1A *(73)*. In transgenic mouse models, the effect of cyclin D_1 overexpression depends on the promoter that is used in the transgene: use of the Epstein-Barr virus (EBV) promoter yields squamous cell carcinomas *(74)*, that of immunoglobulin enhancer stimulates lymphoma development in conjunction with myc *(75)*, that of keratin in epidermal hyperproliferation *(76)* and that of mouse mammary tumor virus (MMTV) causes hyperplasia, ultimately leading to carcinoma development *(77)*. However, cyclin E in a transgene under control of the promoter of β-lactoglobulin also yields hyperplasia in the mammary gland *(78)*. These data show that overexpression of cyclin D_1 and of cyclin E alleviates growth restriction, but does not lead to transformation itself. Additional genetic alterations are mandatory for full transformation.

Knock-out mice for cyclin D illustrate the side-jobs that D-type cyclins fulfill in addition to activating CDK4 or –6. Mice lacking cyclin D_1 have reduced body size, and show symptoms of retina deformation and fail to undergo proliferation of breast cells upon steroid stimulation in pregnancy *(79,80)*. The latter correlates with the ability of cyclin D_1 to activate the estrogen receptor independently of estrogen itself *(81,82)*. Female mice lacking cyclin D_2 are sterile owing to the inability of ovarian granulosa cells to proliferate in response to follicle stimulating hormone, whereas mutant males display hypoplastic testes *(83)*. These data show that individual D-type cyclin are dispensable (mice lacking these D-type cyclins are still alive), and that other D-type cyclins most likely take over the role of the missing one. Furthermore, their side-jobs are not dispensable: for cyclin D_1 this is activation of ER in mammary gland development, for cyclin D_2 activation of a still to be determined pathway that is involved in testes development.

The crucial role of Rb is underlined by the nonviability of Rb homozygous knock-out mice, whereas heterozygotes display increased apoptosis and sensitivity to tumor development *(84)*. A peculiar, and a bit overlooked, aspect of overexpression of cyclin D_1 is its ability to enhance gene amplification *(85)*, which may well contribute to genomic instability.

5. INTERACTIONS BETWEEN GENETIC EVENTS IN GROWTH CONTROL

The complexity of interactions between genetic lesions found in cancer may well be illustrated from distortions in the control genes affecting proliferation and apoptosis. Essential pathways in these are the pRb proliferation pathway and the p53 apoptotic pathway. Key element in the overall control of the cell cycle is the transcription factor E2F as described earlier. The balance between positive and negative regulators of E2F determines progression through the cell cycle *(1,60,86)*. To analyze any disturbance in cell cycle progression, it is essential to determine any interaction between cell cycle regulators. This may also lead to unexpected, sometimes confusing results, such as: 1) increased expression of the CKI p21 results in cell cycle arrest in G_1, but this has no effect in cells with a nonfunctioning pRb. 2) Overexpression of cyclin D_1 (which may be estrogen receptor regulated) results also in elevated levels of CKIs p21 and p27. 3) Mutation of Rb leads to reduced levels of cyclin D_1 protein. These apparent contradictions are the result of disturbance of the delicate balance between positive and negative regulators of E2F activity in cancer cells.

Approximately all cancer cells carry alterations in the proliferation controlling cyclin D_1/CDK4/p16/Rb pathway *(1,60)*. These mutations all have the same end result, i.e., uncontrolled activation of E2F transcription factor. This can be generated by substituting events such as overexpression of cyclin D_1 or of CDK4, or by functional inactivation of pRb or of p16. Each of these alterations can be due to various mechanisms, either affecting the gene directly such as deletion and mutation (e.g., in p16 and Rb), or chromosomal rearrangement (e.g., cyclin D_1 and CDK4 amplification), or affecting gene expression (e.g., methylation of the p16 promotor). In case of cyclin D_1, overexpression may also result from constitutive activation by signaling pathways, among others by altered growth factor receptors.

The expression of the negative regulator of cyclin D:CDK4, CKI p16 is also under control of its end result, E2F. This is a feedback mechanism ensuring the turning off of cyclin D_1-CDK activity at the end of early G_1. p16 inhibits cyclin D_1-CDK4 activity by competing with cyclin D_1 in binding to CDK4. As a net result, overstimulation of E2F (for instance by mutation of Rb) results in enhanced p16, which replaces cyclin D_1 in the complex with CDK4. The released cyclin D_1 is now a target for proteosomal degradation, which explains why tumor cells with mutations in Rb have a low expression level of cyclin D_1 protein *(86)*.

Another example of apparent confusion is the induction of CKIs p21 and p27 by cyclin D_1 activity. These are frequently co-overexpressed in differentiated squamous cell carcinomas. Here, the effect of overexpression of cyclin D_1 does not lead to growth advantage, but instead, via elevated p21 and p27, to proliferation arrest and differentiation *(87)*.

These experimental findings illustrate that measuring only one or just a few cell cycle parameters in early developmental stages in sporadic cancer is of limited value in assessing distortion of the cell cycle machinery and effect thereof on progression, prognosis, and treatment. When all genetic alterations affecting cell cycle control have been elucidated (and this is not expected to take too much longer), the ultimate challenge will be to put these puzzle pieces together to unravel the biocomplexity of their interactions in tumors.

The biocomplexity of genetic alterations and gene and protein interactions is especially relevant in sporadic tumors that arise as a consequence of a multistep accumulation of genetic alterations. In sporadic cancer, there is a prevalence of particular alterations to occur in certain tissues, which may well have to do with hormonal regulation, accessibility, and processing of carcinogens or with type of natural rearrangements that occur during tissue development. A unique example of the latter is the overexpression of cyclin D_1 due to chromosomal 14:22 translocation that occurs in most parathyroid adenomas and all B cell-derived mantle cell lymphomas. Cyclin D_1 overexpression therefore has become a biochemical marker for the latter type of tumor (88). For most of the gene alterations in sporadic cancers, however, it remains an enigma why just those rearrangements occur. On the other hand, in hereditary cancer distortion of a particular gene in all body cells is already indicative of increased risk of tumor development. This is either a consequence of expression of the mutated form in a particular tissue during early development or due to less time needed for the build-up of other gene mutations required for tumor development. In hereditary cancer, particular genes are involved, and those are therefore directly useful for diagnosis and risk evaluation. Good examples of hereditary cancer genes implicated in cell cycle control are pRb in retinoblastoma, p53 in the Li Fraumeni syndrome, and the BRCA 1/2 genes (that have a cell cycle repressing function [89]) in the hereditary breast/ovarian cancer syndrome.

The genetic alterations in growth control also affect response to DNA damage that is monitored by expression of p53, a transcription factor involved in the induction of cki p21 and of the apoptosis promoting protein bax. Expression of p53 is elevated upon damage of DNA (90). Under normal conditions, p53 protein is rapidly degraded upon binding to mdm2, a protein that is induced by p53 itself. P19-Arf that is induced by E2F prevents the binding of p53 to mdm2. A connection between the growth stimulatory pathway (E2F regulation) and the DNA damage control pathway (p53 pathway) is provided by p19-Arf. P19-Arf expression causes a stabilization of p53 resulting in cell cycle arrest and/or apoptosis, and functions as a safety guard against excessive growth factor stimulation (91). Inactivation of p19-arf as well as overexpression of mdm2 (via amplification of the gene) promotes degradation of p53 protein. Both have a similar effect as mutation of p53. These three ways of disrupting the p53-DNA damage control pathway are frequently observed in human cancer and contribute all to poor prognosis (90).

p53 protein becomes also stabilized by modification after DNA damage, resulting in cell cycle arrest and/or apoptosis. Elevated p53 levels therefore, reflect a cellular response to DNA damage as well as to excessive growth stimulation. Overexpression of cyclin D_1 results via E2F release in elevated expression of p53 and consequently, of p21. Overexpression of cyclin D_1 enhances by this mechanism the response of cells to X-irradiation, in vitro as well as in vivo

(92,93). Cyclin D_1 is also involved in a more rapid response to DNA damage. DNA damage causes a rapid p53-independent G_1 arrest caused by the degradation of cyclin D_1 protein. This degradation is mediated via an N-terminally located destruction box in the cyclin D_1 protein. Degradation of cyclin D_1 protein leads to the release of p21 that now will bind to cyclin E-cdk2, leading to a G_1 arrest. Binding of p21 to cyclin D_1-cdk4 hardly hampers its kinase activity, whereas binding of p21 to cyclin E-cdk2 results in inactivation of cdk2 activity leading to cell cycle arrest *(50).*

p53 is a crucial monitor of DNA damage, so when p53 is mutated, this results in replication of cells with an accumulation of genetic mistakes that are associated with tumor progression and poor prognosis *(90).* Since cells with a mutated p53 do not undergo growth arrest or apoptosis upon DNA damage, p53 mutation is also associated with resistance to chemotherapy and radiotherapy, whose efficacy is based on DNA damage. Introduction of wild-type p53 in tumor cells carrying p53 mutations reverses this sensitivity in vitro and in vivo *(94).* Tumors with a p53 mutation have therefore, in general, a worse prognosis, but respond worse to chemotherapy or X-irradiation treatment.

Furthermore, enforced activity of transcription factor E2F stimulates expression of the E2F dependent genes thymidilate synthetase and dihydrofolate reductase, and renders those cells more resistant to treatment with chemotherapeutic agents, such as 5-fluorouracil and methotrexate *(95).*

Several reviews have recently appeared describing distortions of the Rb and p19[ARF]-p53 pathway in different types of tumors *(1,60,86,90).* The studies quoted below complement these and illustrate novel tendencies, and especially focus on the possible clinical relevance of alterations in cell cycle regulators.

6. CLINICAL RELEVANCE OF ALTERATIONS IN CELL CYCLE REGULATORS: GENERAL CONSIDERATIONS

Are the particular aberrations in the cell regulation pathways described earlier relevant for the process of tumor progression, diagnosis, assessment of prognosis, and for prediction of response to treatment? Examination of different stages of tumor progression in individual colon cancers indicated that tumor progression by morphological criteria is paralleled by a stepwise accumulation of genetic alterations in the different control pathways *(96).* Similar tendencies have been seen for other tumors that arise through clearly definable pre-invasive stages such as head and neck squamous cell cancer *(97,98)* and breast cancer *(99–101).* Certain mutations occur more frequently in earlier stages than others do, however the order of events is far from an absolute one. For most cancers, therefore, it can be stated that progression is rather the result of accumulation of an arbitrary number of major and minor genetic alterations in any order than the stepwise-ordered accumulation of specific events (the "bingo" principle).

As genetic alterations in tumors will usually occur in multiple pathways during tumor progression leading to progressive disturbances in growth control, accumulation of errors in different pathways may in fact be more indicative of a worse prognosis than a defect in one pathway *(102)*. Therefore, one might wonder what the value is the many published studies on a single or just a few markers that have revealed associations with disease-free or overall survival for tumors (without obvious dissemination). Some effects may however be rather dominant over others. Within the cyclinD$_1$/CDK4/ p16/pRb pathway controlling G$_1$/S transition, effects of inactivation of p16 and of overexpression of cyclin D$_1$ or CDK4 amplification are less severe than inactivation of pRb. An example for this can be found in squamous carcinomas of the head and neck. In these cancers, cyclin D$_1$ overexpression is a frequent finding *(60)*, but one hardly finds Rb mutation *(103)* and rather frequently p16 mutations *(104)*. Furthermore, most of these tumors lack a functional p53. Overexpression of cyclin D$_1$ would only provide a selective advantage to cells when they are normal for Rb and lack expression of p16. At the other hand, expression of p16 would have no effect on cyclin D$_1$ in Rb mutated cells. If one presumes that all squamous carcinomas of the head and neck originate from smoking and/or alcohol abuse, and that these neoplasms have circumvented p53-mediated arrest/or apoptosis by mutation of p53, then growth advantage would be acquired either in Rb mutant cells, or in cyclin D$_1$ overexpressing cells with a mutation or reduced expression of p16. These tumor cells would be less dependent on growth factor stimulation or on adhesion onto ECM components. Why this reduced dependency in head and neck cancer is mainly achieved by overexpression of cyclin D$_1$, and not by direct deregulation of Rb, remains an enigma. This may explain, however, that overexpression of cyclin D$_1$ is consistently associated with poor prognosis.

Nevertheless, the aim to discern different stages of tumor progression according to genetic alterations is in general not likely to be fulfilled by examination of a single or just a few of these alterations, but this approach has frequently been used as is clear from the overview of many published studies below. The studies suffer further from lack of standardization of methodology, and reproducibility of the read out and intra-tumor heterogeneity have largely been neglected. However, despite these shortcomings, some promising results can be presented anyway. It becomes evident from these studies that derailments leading to increased proliferation will in general be associated with poor prognosis.

7. CELL CYCLE-RELATED GENETIC EVENTS IN DIAGNOSIS AND PROGNOSIS OF CANCER

7.1. Cyclin A

Cyclin A is expressed in the late S, G$_2$, and M phases of the cell cycle, thus shortly before mitosis. As the mitosis is the end stage of the successfully completed cell cycle, cyclin A positivity is therefore the functional end results of growth regulation, and consequently among the most indicative markers of tumor proliferation. Indeed, expression of cyclin A correlates strongly with Ki67 expression *(105–107)* and expression in a high percentage of cells will in general indicate poor prognosis. Cyclin A staining is usually confined to the nucleus, but cytoplasmic staining is often found in late G_2 and mitotic cells.

As rate of proliferation is an important diagnostic feature to discriminate between benign and malignant tumors *(108)*, cyclin A could help here. An example of this is leimyomatous tumours of the soft tissue, where cyclin A was expressed in leiomyoma with much lower labeling indexes than in leiomyosarcoma *(109)*. It is expected that many more such diagnostic applications of cyclin A will emerge in the upcoming years.

Examples of high cyclin A labeling indices indicating poor prognosis can be found in adenocarcinomas such as breast cancer *(390)*, colorectal cancer *(110)*, and prostate cancer *(111,112)*, but a gastric cancer study failed to show significance *(113)*. In hepatocellular carcinoma, cyclin A was associated with advanced stage, portal invasion, intrahepatic metastasis, poor differentiation, and high Ki67 labeling index, and predicted prognosis although not indendently *(106)*. In esophageal SCC, cyclin A was a significant prognosticator *(114)* also in patients treated with neoadjuvant chemotherapy *(115)*. In a heterogenous group of lung cancers *(116)*, patients with high cyclin A labeling had significantly shorter survival times. This was confirmed in another study on non-small cell lung cancer (NSCLC) *(117)* and squamous-cell lung carcinomas *(118,119)*.

In patients with transitional cell carcinoma of the renal pelvis and ureter, the prevalence of cases exhibiting cyclin A staining was higher in the high-grade and invasive tumors than in the other types of tumors. Patients whose tumors expressed a high level of cyclin A protein had a significantly poorer prognosis than those without cyclin A expression *(120)*.

The prognostic value of cyclin A holds in a similar way also in sarcomas such as leiomyosarcoma of the soft tissue *(109)*, osteosarcoma *(121)*, and non-metastatic *(122)* and metastatic soft tissue sarcoma *(123)*, although the latter was not always confirmed *(124)*. In B-cell NHL, cyclin A showed lowest expression in low-grade NHL, and the highest in high-grade NHL, and showed a significant prognostic value for both disease free and overall survival *(107)*.

In summary, cyclin A labeling index can be viewed as a good marker of proliferation, and is expected to develop as an important diagnostic and prognostic feature for tumors at different sites.

7.2. Cyclin B

Cyclin B, like cyclin A, is expressed in the late S, G_2, and M phases of the cell cycle, and is potentially an important proliferation marker. There have however been few studies yet on cyclin B. Cyclin B was found in increasing percentages of positive cells from normal breast tissue to atypical ductal hyperplasia (ADH), ductal carcinoma *in situ* (DCIS), and invasive carcinoma *(125)*. In hepatocellular carcinoma *(106)*, cyclin B was associated with advanced stage, portal invasion, intrahepatic metastasis, poor differentiation, and high Ki67 labeling index, and predicted prognosis although not indendently. In esophageal squamous cell carcinoma, prevalence of cyclin B_1 expression was significantly higher in cases with invasion deeper than the muscularis propria and with venous invasion than in other cases. Patients having high levels of cyclin B_1 protein expression had a significantly poorer prognosis *(126)*.

In summary, although cyclin B has potential as a proliferation marker, studies are too scarce as yet to have realistic expectations on its value as a diagnostic or prognostic feature.

7.3. Cyclin D

Cyclin D_1 is expressed mainly in the G_1 phase of the cell cycle, where it is required for cell cycle transition to S-phase. As explained earlier, cyclin D_1 acivation may have various effects, depending on the mechanism (amplification or hormone sensitivity). Overexpression of cyclin D_1 may force cells into the S-phase, thereby increasing proliferation, which will in general be associated with more aggressive tumors and poor prognosis. However, overexpression of cyclin D_1 (especially when due to hormone effects) may also result in feedback mechanisms resulting in elevated levels of p21 and p27 leading to cell cycle arrest, thereby being prognostically favorable. These various effects have indeed been found in the different clinical studies on cyclin D_1.

On the diagnostic side, overexpression of cyclin D_1 (due to chromosomal 14:22 translocation) is quite specific for parathyroid adenomas *(127)* and B cell-derived mantle cell lymphomas (due to t(11;14) chromosomal translocations). Cyclin D_1 overexpression therefore has become a biochemical marker for the latter type of tumor *(88,128,129)*. Mantle-cell lymphoma comprises approx 10% of all non-Hodgkin lymphomas (NHL) and represents a generalized disease with poor prognosis. More than 90% of these mantle cell lymphomas show overexpression of cyclin D_1 *(88,128,130,131)*. This is a remarkable example of a sporadic tumor type in which almost 100% of all cases is consistently associated with a particular genetic aberration, namely overexpression of cyclin D_1. This unique association permits the use of overexpression of cyclin D_1 in the rather difficult morphological diagnosis of diffuse small cell B-type NHL. Consequently, in diffuse B-cell lymphomas, cyclin D_1 positivity is associated with poor prognosis, probably due to the fact the most of these are mantle cell lymphomas *(131)*.

Prognostically, quite a number of studies on cyclin D_1 have been published. In breast cancer, no clear prognostic value of cyclin D_1 seems to be present. In breast carcinogenesis, cyclin D_1 seems to play a role as mRNA and protein overexpression is quite often found in ductal hyperplasia and *in situ* carcinoma

(132,133), especially in high-grade ductal carcinomas *in situ*, which show a more frequent recurrence than low-grade ones *(134,135)*. Overexpression of cyclin D_1 protein or mRNA occurs in the vast majority of invasive lobular carcinomas, but not in lobular carcinoma *in situ (136)*. Overexpression of cyclin D_1 in invasive breast cancers occurs in 40–50% of all cases *(61,137,138)*, of which about half is due to amplification of cyclin D_1 on chromosome 11q13. This amplification, and corresponding overexpression, is associated with a more aggressive tumor phenotype and/or worse prognosis *(139–143)*. However, overexpression of cyclin D_1 protein by itself was not indicative of prognosis in large series of patients with stage I/II breast cancer *(137,138,144–146)*, whereas the mRNA studies gave contradictory results *(147,148)*. This apparent contradiction between the clinical impact of amplification and protein overexpression may be explained by the fact that approximately only half of all cases with overexpression of cyclin D_1 protein can be accounted for by amplification of cyclin D_1 gene, which is the most frequent genetic aberration and which is linked with poor prognosis. Since overexpression of cyclin D_1 protein is highly significantly linked with ER positivity *(137,138,145,149)*, and since cyclin D_1 is turned on by activated ER, the other half of cases with overexpression of cyclin D_1 protein in breast cancer may be due to "normal" stimulation by estradiol. The strong association between cyclin D_1 and ER may explain the fact that cyclin D_1-positive patients respond better to adjuvant therapy *(150)*. Also p21 and p27 may play a role in these apparently contradictory results, as immunohistochemical studies also confirm the experimental findings that overexpression of cyclin D_1 is associated with increased expression of p27 *(151)* and may induce p21 *(87)* in a p53-independent manner *(152)*. Activation of these cell cycle inhibitors, which may well depend on the level of cyclin D_1 protein, results in cell cycle arrest. Co-overexpression of cyclin D_1 together with epidermal growth factor receptor (EGFR) or pRb is more indicative of poor prognosis than expression of cyclin D_1 alone *(153)*.

Overexpression of cyclin D_1 is an independent prognostic factor in colonic cancer *(154,155)*, and overexpression of cyclin D_1 is more prevalent in advanced stages *(110,156)* and is associated with intestinal adenomas of familial adenomatous polyposis patients *(157)*. Not all studies, however, could confirm the prognostic results *(158)*. Overexpression of cyclin D_1 was also associated with poor prognosis in a few studies on other adenocarcinomas like pancreatic cancer *(159–161)*, prostate adenocarcinoma *(162)*, and extrahepatic duct carcinoma *(163)*. In hepatocellular carcinoma, cases with cyclin D_1 overexpression showed poorer outcomes for disease-free survival in one study *(164)*, whereas in another, hepatocellular carcinomas with both downregulation of cyclin D_1 and overexpression of cyclin E had worse survival *(165)*. In gastric carcinogenesis, cyclin D_1 did not appear to be relevant *(166)* and in gastric cancer, cyclin D_1 also seems to be prognostically irrelevant *(167–170)*.

In nonpapillary renal cell cancer, high cyclin-D_1 expression was significantly associated with a better prognosis as compared with highly aggressive tumours with low cyclin-D_1 levels *(171)*. Prognostic results of cyclin D_1 overexpression in superficial bladder cancer *(172–175)* and ovarian tumors *(176)* have been contradictory.

The most consistent adverse effect of cyclin D_1 overexpression is seen in head and neck squamous cell cancers (SCC) *(177–181)* where overexpression is usually the result of gene amplification. There have been several studies in laryngeal SCC, most of them showing that cyclin D_1 overexpression or amplification is strongly correlated to poor prognosis *(181–184)* and radio-resistance of tumors *(93)*. In hypopharyngeal and esophageal SCC, cyclin D_1 overexpression is similarly an adverse prognostic factor *(185–197)* and related to chemoradioresistance *(194,198)*, although some studies could not confirm this *(199–202)*. Only in oral SCC, contradictory results have been published on the prognostic value of cyclin D_1 overexpression *(203–204)*.

In SCC and other non-small cell types of lung cancer, results are contradictory. In some studies cyclin D_1 overexpression appeared to be an adverse prognostic factor *(205,206)*; two other studies showed the opposite *(207,208)*, and several studies showed no prognostic value at all *(118,209–211)*.

In extremity soft-tissue sarcomas *(124)*, cyclin D_1 was significantly associated with worse overall survival. In osteosarcoma patients, cyclin D_1 positivity was a favorable prognostic factor *(121)*. In astrocytomas, cyclin D_1 overexpression was an adverse prognostic factor *(212)*. Patients with ALL who were strongly positive for cyclin D_1 had a lower probability of remaining in first continuous remission than ALL patients who were negative or weakly positive *(213)*, and these prognostic results were confirmed by others. Sauerbery et al. showed that ALL patients with high cyclin D_1-mRNA levels had a poorer prognosis *(214)*.

In summary, cyclin D_1 is an important diagnostic marker of mantle cell lymphomas in the differential diagnosis of small cell B-type NHL, and an important prognostic factor in SCC of the head and neck. For other tumors, results at present are preliminary or contradictory.

Only few studies have been published on cyclin D_2. In gastric cancer, however cyclin D_2 appeared to be prognostically important *(169)*. Few further clinical results have been described for cyclin D_2. One problem in such studies is the cross-reactivity of currently available cyclin D_2 antibodies with other D-type cyclins. Aberrant expression of cyclin D_2 is associated with testis tumor development *(215)*.

7.4. Cyclin E

Cyclin E, like cyclin D_1, is expressed mainly in the G_1 phase of the cell cycle, where it plays a role in cell cycle progression. Therefore, high levels of cyclin E in general correlate with increased proliferation and thereby with less favorable prognosis, although few clinical studies have been performed on cyclin E.

Diagnostically, cyclin E was expressed exclusively in leiomyosarcoma and predicted a poor prognosis in recurrence- or metastasis-free survival and overall survival *(109)*. In localized synovial sarcoma, cyclin E was correlated with survival, although not in an independent way *(216)*. In extremity soft-tissue sarcomas *(124)*, cyclin E was of no significance for prediction of outcome.

In breast cancer, cyclin E overexpression is correlated with a more aggressive phenotype *(217,218)* and reduced survival *(218–224)*. Also in colorectal adenocarcinomas, cyclin E overexpression is related to poor prognosis *(155,221,225)*. In gastric cancer, contradictory results have been reported *(167–169,226)*. Similar contradictory results have been reported for NSCLC *(116,227,228)*.

Hepatocellular carcinoma cases with cyclin E overexpression showed poorer outcomes for disease-free survival *(164,165)*, especially in combination with low cyclin D_1 expression *(165)*. Patients with TCC of the renal pelvis and ureter coexpressing cyclin E and p53 had a significantly poorer prognosis than those expressing neither cyclin E nor p53 *(229)*. In malignant lymphomas, high cyclin E was also associated with a poor prognosis *(230)*. No significance for cyclin E could be demonstrated in acute myeloid leukemia (AML) *(231)*, esophageal squamous cell cancer *(185,191)*, and cervical cancer *(232–234)*.

In summary, cyclin E has potential as a prognostic feature in some adenocarcinomas, especially in combination with other cell cycle markers, but studies are too scarce at present to draw firm conclusions.

7.5. The KIP Family of Cyclin Dependent Kinase Inhibitors

7.5.1. P21

p21 binds to cyclin E- and A:CDK2 and cyclin D:CDK complexes to inhibit their activity, with higher affinity to cyclin D2:CDK4 than to cyclin E:CDK2, thereby blocking the cell cycle. Basically, high p21 levels should therefore lead arrest in cellular proliferation, and to low proliferation and thereby good prognosis in tumors with many p21-positive cells. However, this effect is not so clearly present in various tumors as pointed out hereafter.

Diagnostically, p21 is expressed in a remarkable number of cells in clear cell cancers of different sites *(235)*. This indicates that p21 may play a role in the typical morphology of the cells in these cancers. This fits well with the fact that p21 has been implicated in differentiation *(87,236)*. p21 may therefore be used in the diagnosis of clear cell cancers. Prognostically, p21 has not provided unequivocal results. p21 expression may not be sufficient to result in cell cycle arrest in cells with severely disrupted proliferation pathways, and even cell cycle arrest in half of the tumor cells may not have a high impact on tumor growth if the other half keep on dividing rapidly. p21may also be the result of cyclin D_1 overexpression *(87)*, which is an unfavorable event in several cancers. Indeed, p21 overexpression has been associated with both favorable and unfavorable prognosis, depending on the site of the primary cancer.

p21 was a good prognosticator in a mixed group of squamous cell cancers of the head and neck region, high expression being unfavorable *(181)*. In esophageal squamous cell cancer, however, overexpression of p21 was an indicator of favorable prognosis in most studies *(115,189,199,237,238)*, but in one study high p21 was unfavorable *(239)*. In other specific subgroups of oral *(240)*, hypopharyngeal *(201)*, and laryngeal *(183,241)* SCC, no prognostic value of p21 was found.

In adenocarcinomas, high p21 expression was a marker of tumor radio-sensitivity in patients with rectal cancer *(242)*, and also an indicator of good prognosis in surgically treated colorectal cancer *(243,244)*. In invasive breast cancer patients, overexpression of p21 was correlated with reduced disease-free survival in several studies *(245,246)*, but not in all *(146)*. In advanced ovarian cancer, high p21 expression appeared to be a favorable prognosticator *(247–250)* except for one study *(251)*.

In gastric cancer, results have been contradictory *(168,252,253)*, and there have been scarce studies on cervical *(234)* adenocarcinoma where low p21 was unfavorable, on prostate cancer where high expression of p21 was unfavorable *(111,254)*, and on pancreatic cancer where p53(+)p21(–) patients had a poor prognosis *(255)*, but as a single factor p21 failed *(160)*.

In NSCLC, risk of relapse was associated with p21 status, with no relapse in patients with normal p21 *(256)*. A next study in lung cancer *(257)*, however, revealed no prognostic value. In cutaneous melanoma, high p21 was favorable although not in an independent way *(258)*. In Hodgkin's disease, high expression of p21 protein correlated independently with poor response to the first-line treatment, especially in combination with p53 positivity *(259)*.

p21 failed to reveal prognostic value in occasional studies on diffuse small cell B-cell NHL *(260)*, TCC bladder *(261,262)*, and high-grade astrocytomas *(263)*.

These data hint towards a model where inactivation of p53 (and consequently downregulation of p21) leads to poor prognosis, most likely by generating increased genomic instability, and to poor response to treatment since the ability of those cells to undergo cell cycle arrest or apoptosis has been eradicated. Elevated p21 levels indicate either a functioning, wild-type p53, or a p53-independent expression of p21 leading to cell cycle arrest and differentiation. These complex effects and interactions prevent p21 from being a useful prognostic feature in various tumors.

7.5.2. P27

p27, also a member of the KIP family, inhibits cyclin A:CDK2 more efficiently than cyclin D:CDK. Cki-p27 binds to cyclin A:CDK2 with an approx 10-fold higher affinity than to cyclin D2:CDK4. As for p21, high p27 levels could therefore lead to arrest in cellular proliferation, and to low tumor proliferation and thereby good prognosis in tumors with many p27 positive cells. Also p27 becomes increased in cells with overexpression of cyclin D_1 (87,264). Clinical studies on p27 have provided much more unequivocal results than p21. High p27 is found in many benign tissues and in well-differentiated cancers, and p27 is progressively lost when tumors become less differentiated and more rapidly proliferating, lack or loss of p27 thereby usually indicating poor prognosis. For instance, this is the case in breast cancer (218–222,265–268), especially when p27 is lost in combination with overexpression of cyclin E (222). Not all studies have confirmed the adverse prognostic effect of loss of p27 (146), and in one study (269) high p27 expression interestingly indicated poor prognosis in node-negative cases. In other types of adenocarcinomas, similarly good p27 results have been reported. In colorectal cancer, all studies showed that low p27 is unfavorable (221,225,270–274), in gastric cancer most (169,275–277) but not all (167), and in prostate cancer also most (278–281) but not all (282). In a group of ovarian cancers of different stages (283) low p27 indicated bad prognosis, but in the subgroup of advanced ovarian cancers no prognostic value was found (251). No significant results could be demonstrated for cervical adenocarcinoma (234). In single studies on Barrett esophagus-associated adenocarcinoma (284), extrahepatic duct carcinoma (163), hepatocellular carcinoma (164), and gall-bladder carcinoma patients who had undergone radical surgery (285), p27 was again a good prognosticator.

In SCC of the esophagus, low p27 was associated with poor prognosis in most studies (115,185,286), but not in all (188,238). Also in SCC of the larynx (183,287), hypopharyx (202), and oral cavity (288) p27 had prognostic value for survival. In cervical SCC, a high p27 labeling index before RT was associated significantly with good disease-free and metastasis-free survival (289). The results are confusing of Dellas et al. (232), who showed in stage IB invasive cervical carcinomas that high levels of p27 were associated with poor overall survival. In NSCLC p27 status is a significant prognostic factor, the lack of expression of associated with poor prognosis (265,290–295). In scarce studies on acute myeloid leukemia (231), NHL (128,296), and brain tumors (297,298), patients with high p27 expression had a significantly better prognosis.

In summary, low p27 is in various cancers associated with poor prognosis, especially in combination with high cyclin E, and is therefore among the most promising cell cycle markers for clinical application.

7.6. The CIP Family of Cyclin Dependent Kinase Inhibitors
7.6.1. P16/P19

The INK4A/ARF locus on 9p21 contains two tumor suppressors, p16[INK4A] and p19[ARF] (sometimes called p14[ARF]), and is frequently deleted in human tumors with loss of expression of both p19 and p16 (299). These proteins block cells at the G_1 restriction point, but by a different mechanism, p16 by inhibition of cyclin D:cdk4 activity, and p19 by eliminating mdm2-mediated degradation of p53. Inactivation of p19 results therefore in a rapid breakdown of p53 and is similar to inactivation of p53 (*see* above). Loss or mutation of these can consequently result in an increase in proliferation and an expected poorer survival in most tumors. Hypermethylation of the promoter provides an alternative mechanism of inactivation.

Mutations in p16 are the cause of the familial atypical mole-melanoma syndrome (*300*), which also predisposes to pancreatic cancer. In different types of melanoma, loss of nuclear p16 protein expression was associated with increased tumor cell proliferation and decreased patient survival (*301–303*). p16 is a marker of dysplastic cells in cervical smears (*303a*).

In different types of adenocarcinomas, loss of p16 expression was associated with poor prognosis such as endometrial cancer (*304*), ovarian cancer (*305,306*), pancreatic cancer (*159,161,307*), and lung adenocarcinomas (*308*). In breast cancer, p16 loss seems to have no impact: varying frequencies of p16 loss have been described (*309,310*) without prognostic impact (*310*). p16 was of no prognostic impact in cervical and gastric adenocarcinomas (*311*).

In SCC of the esophagus (*197*) and lung (*312*), loss of p16 expression was associated with poor prognosis. In NSCLC in general, a similar observation was done in several studies (*290,292–295,313–315*) although not in all (*316,317*).

The results in ALL have been confusing. High p16 was shown to be unfavorable in childhood ALL (*318*), but in another study, the presence of a homozygous p16 deletion was an important risk factor for both relapse and death (*319*). In relapse T-ALL, patients with p16 deletion experienced a significantly shorter duration of postrelapse survival (*320*). In adult T-cell ALL, the deletion of p16 emerged as an independent prognostic indicator in one study (*321*) but not in another (*331*). In B cell NHLs, p16 was unfavorable (*322,323*), but no clinical correlations were found in Hodgkin's disease (*324*).

In neuroblastomas, lack of p16 expression significantly correlated with poor prognosis of patients and advanced stage of the disease. There was no correlation between loss of p16 expression and N-myc amplification in these tumors, indicating that inactivation of the p16 gene is involved in the progression of neuroblastoma independently of N-myc amplification (*325*). In oligodendrogliomas, p16 homozygous deletion indicated poor survival (*326*), but p16 had no impact in as astrocytic gliomas (*327*).

In soft tissue sarcomas, there has been a single study demonstrating the bad prognostic impact of loss of p16 (*328*). Conflicting results have been described in astrocytoma (*263,329*), and no value of p16 could be established in TCC of the urinary bladder (*173,262*).

In follicular lymphoma high p19 expression was associated with a significantly shorter survival time (*299*), indicating that also activation may have clinical significance. In superficial bladder TCC, patients bearing tumors with INK4A deletions affecting p19 had a lower recurrence free survival than those with wild-type INK4A *(330)*. In adult ALL *(331)*, p19 had no clinical value.

The apparent anomalies could be due to inappropriate evaluation of the pathways involved: p16 is only effective in the presence of a functional cyclin D_1, whereas cyclin D_1 is ineffective in tumors with a mutated Rb. p19 is only effective in tumors with a functional p53 *(see* above). However, tumors are either defective for p53 or for p19, and rarely for both *(86)*.

7.6.2. P15

p15^{INK4b} is an inhibitor of CDK4 and CDK6, also located on 9p21, and therefore often co-deleted with p19/p16 *(331)*. p15 inactivation by promoter methylation or deletion will in general have a similar effect as loss of p16/p19. p15 methylation was found in bone marrow or peripheral blood cells from 58% of patients with AML, ALL, or acute biphenotypic leukemia. An identical alteration was detected in blood plasma from 92% of these patients. Concomitant p16 and p15 methylation was present in 22% of adults with AML or ALL. Eighty-two percent of those with unmethylated p15 alleles had normal karyotypes or hyperdiploidies associated with a favorable prognosis. Conversely, 44% of patients with p15 methylation had chromosomal translocations, inversions, or deletions, suggesting an interplay of these abnormalities with p15 methylation. As a prognostic marker for disease monitoring, p15 methylation therefore appears to be more widely applicable than BCR-ABL, AF4-MLL, and AML1-ETO transcripts *(332)*. These results were confirmed in childhood ALL patients, where the 5-yr disease-free survival rate was 68% for patients without p16/p15 deletions and 35% for those with p16/p15 deletions *(333)*. In adult ALL, the results have been contradictory. The presence of a homozygous p16 deletion has emerged as an important risk factor in two studies *(321,333)* but not in all *(331)*. There has been a single study in myelodysplastic syndrome patients where p15 methylation indicated a bad prognosis *(334)*.

In summary, p16 shows promise as a marker of dysplastic epithelial cells and as a prognostic marker in SCC of the esophagus and lung, in NSCLC and NHL, and p15 in acute leukemias. The latter in particular may be useful for clinical application in the forseeable future.

7.7. The Retinoblastoma Family of Proteins

7.7.1. Rb

pRb (pRb1) is one of the most important human tumor-suppressor genes, and is involved in carcinogenesis of tumors at many sites. Since inactivation of pRb renders release of E2F insensitive to cyclin:cdk activity, one might presume that Rb mutations are in general, associated with increased and uncontrolled proliferation *(see* above). However, inactivation of Rb is difficult to evaluate from immunohistochemical analysis; only reduced intensity of staining or loss of staining is indicative of this. Only recently, antibodies have become available that distinguish the inactive (nonphosphorylated) pRb from active (phosphorylated) pRb. They have been used infrequently in clinical studies, and most older studies have provided unclear or conflicting results.

In breast cancer, pRb expression does not seem to be of prognostic significance (335–337). In ovarian cancer, however, lack of pRb was reported to be a marker of poor prognosis (305,306). In colorectal cancer (338), hepatocellular carcinoma (339), and adrenocortical neoplasms (340), pRb had no impact. In other epithelial neoplasms such as head and neck SCC (341–343), esophageal SCC (237,344–346), bladder cancer (173,262,347–352) and NSCLC (102,210, 314,317,361), results on pRb have been conflicting.

In soft-tissue sarcomas, pRb appeared to be prognostically relevant in several studies, but in one study high pRb was bad (358) and in another study low pRb was bad (359). In osteoblastic osteosarcoma, the probability of relapse was significantly higher in pRb-negative than in the pRb-positive patients in a single study (360).

In hematological malignancies, a similar situation is found. In AML (361,362) and Hodgkin's disease (363), low Rb was bad, but in diffuse large B-cell lymphoma, high pRb was favorable (364). In ALL (365,366), results have been conflicting.

A few studies on brain tumors revealed no clinical usefulness of pRb (263,327) for choroidal melanoma (367).

7.7.2. Rb2

Rb2 is a relatively newly discovered member of the Rb family. Low immunohistochemical levels of pRb2/p130 detected in untreated patients with NHLs of various histiotypes inversely correlated with a large fraction of cells expressing high levels of p107 and proliferation-associated proteins. Such a pattern of protein expression is normally observed in continuously cycling cells. Interestingly, such cases showed the highest survival percentage (82.5%) after the observation period of 10 yr (368). In choroidal melanoma, Rb2 had independent prognostic value (367), and in endometrial carcinoma, low Rb2 was unfavorable (369).

In summary, results on pRb1 have been disappointing. In many tumors, results are conflicting, probably because the methodology for detection of pRb functionality clearly is influencing its clinical evaluation. Rb2 is perhaps more promising, but at present too few studies have been performed to draw firm conclusions.

7.8. p53

p53 is probably the most important tumor-suppressor gene in humans, and p53 mutations are probably the most frequent genetic events in human cancer.

The crucial role of p53 in cell cycle arrest in case of DNA damage means that in case of a mutation, cells can rapidly accumulate genetic alterations leading to progressive disturbance in the cell cycle with consequently increased proliferation. The wild-type p53 protein has a short half life, but the half life increases in case of a mutation, usually leading to p53 accumulation making the p53 immunohistochemically detectable. p53 accumulation has indeed prognostic value in many tumors, although usually not all studies agree on this due to the varying protocols for staining and interpretation of the results.

At the time of finalizing the writing of this chapter (December 2000), approx 26000 references on studies involving p53 in cancer can be found in PubMed, some 2700 addressing prognostic value of p53. The large number of studies underscores the expectations of p53 as a prognostic tumor marker, but makes it at the same time impossible to review this within the scope of this chapter. Therefore, only some general considerations and a few examples of diagnostic and prognostic applications will be given.

There is hardly a tumor in which p53 has not been studied by either immunohistochemistry or mutation analysis. In general, one can say that strong p53 immunohistochemical positivity in a high percentage of cells is highly indicative of a mutation, but clearly there are exceptions. Mutations can be accompanied by negative staining, and staining in case of wild-type overexpression can be extensive. In addition, one must not forget the problems associated with both staining and scoring of immunohistochemistry (*see* below), and also that usually only the exons where p53 mutations are generally found are subjected to mutation analysis. Nevertheless, mutation detection still must be considered the best way of analyzing p53, although it is laborious. For most studied organs and sites, it has been found that p53 accumulation or mutation does not occur in benign lesions, may be present in dysplastic lesions, and often occurs in cancers, especially in high-grade cancers. Therefore, p53 was often found to have diagnostic and/or prognostic value. A few examples are given here.

On the diagnostic side, serous papillary cancer of uterine corpus shows high accumulation of p53, which may help to discriminate it from other types of cancer, which is relevant in view of the very aggressive nature of this tumor, despite limited infiltrative behavior *(370)*. Another example is pleural lesions that are often difficult to diagnose, but malignancy is quite likely when p53 accumulation is demonstrated *(371)*. In Barrett's esophagus, p53 accumulation helps to identify and grade dysplasia *(372,373)*.

Prognostically, breast cancer in particular has been studied. Most studies indicate that p53 accumulation *(374,375)* or mutation *(141)* is associated with poor prognosis. Other examples of frequently occurring carcinomas where p53 has prognostic value are ovarian cancer *(247,305,306)*, colonic cancer *(154,155, 244,273,376)*, gastric carcinoma *(226)*, and different SCC of the head and neck region *(189,200,239,240,377)*. Examples of noncarcinomatous malignancies where p53 is prognostically relevant are localized synovial sarcoma *(216)* and small cell lymphomas *(260,378)*.

In summary, many studies have been performed on p53 showing in general that p53 accumulation is associated with malignancy and bad prognosis. Therefore, p53 is among the markers that is closest to clinical application in tumors from some sites. However, even for p53 some important hurdles remain, which will be further addressed in the conclusion.

7.9. Cyclin-Dependent Kinases

This family concerns CDK1, CDK2, CDK4, and CDK6 *(44)*. CDK2, 4, and 6 phosphorylate pRB when complexed with cyclins, leading to release of E2F and thereby proliferation, whereas CDK1 is active in mitosis. In normal cell, the CDK proteins are present in excess concentration over their cyclin partners. Overexpression of CDKs, therefore, would only be advantageous to tumor cells in conjunction with a coinciding increase of their cyclin partners, or by binding to, and thereby reducing the effect of cycin kinase inhibitors such as p21. Increase in CDKs 2, 4, or 6 potentially leads to increased proliferation and thereby poor prognosis, whereas overexpression of CDK1 may lead to disturbed transit through mitosis leading to genetic instability.

Overexpression of CDK1 was related to advanced stage, portal invasion, intrahepatic metastasis, poor differentiation, high Ki-67 labeling index, and was an independent predictor of poor prognosis in hepatocellular carcinoma *(106)*. In B-cell NHL, CDK1 showed lowest expression in low-grade NHL, and the highest in high-grade NHL. CDK1 showed a significant prognostic value for achievement of complete remission and overall survival *(107)*.

CDK2 was not prognostically relevant in esophageal SCC *(191)*. In NSCLC, patients with high CDK2 *(117,118)* and CDK4 *(117)* labeling had significantly shorter survival times, although not all studies could confirm the positive CDK4 results *(118)*. Overexpression of CDK2 can be found in increasing percentages of positive cells from normal breast tissue to ADH, DCIS, and invasive carcinoma.

CDK4 has been considered to play a role in tumorigenesis from the finding that erythroleukemia cells terminally differentiate when CDK4 is suppressed, while its overexpression causes uncontrolled cell growth and eventual malignant transformation *(379)*. Recently, it was suggested that gene amplification and overexpression of CDK4 is associated with high proliferative activity of breast cancers, with CDK4 amplification also appearing to be of importance in the pathogenesis of subset of sporadic mammary tumors *(144)*. Zhang et al. reported that CDK4 overexpression is associated with significant increase in the proliferating cell number in colonic adenomas on the basis of BrdU incorporation and immunohistochemistry for PCNA *(157)*. CDK4 overexpression was associated with a poor prognosis in gastric cancer *(169)*. CDK4 protein overexpression as well as CDK4 gene amplification can also be found in invasive breast carcinomas but was not correlated with prognosis *(144)*. In squamous cell esophageal carcinoma, CDK4 immuno-reactivity was an independent risk factors *(191)*, especially in combination with cyclin D_1 positivity. In epithelial ovarian cancers, CDK4 had no prognostic value as a single feature, but patients with a CDK4-positive/p16-negative profile had a reduced overall survival than other phenotypes of cdk4/p16 *(380)*.

Children with CDK4-positive ALL had a lower probability of remaining in first continuous remission than children with CDK4-negative ALL *(213)*, but no prognostic relevance was found for CDK2.

In summary, few clinical studies on CDKs have been published, but CDK4 seems to show promise as a prognostic marker in some adenocarcinomas. However, further studies are required.

8. CELL CYCLE REGULATORS AND SENSITIVITY TO CYTOSTATIC AGENTS AND RADIATION

Since cell cycle regulators also influence sensitivity to agents that either cause arrest of the cell cycle or induce apoptosis (*see* above), one might presume an intrinsic dependency between these. Sensitivity of cells towards cytostatic agents or radiation until now has been studied mainly with respect to p53 status. Loss of p53 function in tumor cells indeed confers increased resistance towards chemotherapy or radiation *(268,381–383)*. Now the connection between E2F and p53 via p19[ARF] has been revealed, and both of them induce either p21 or apoptosis, a co-stimulatory effect is most likely to occur when cells with a normal p53 and Rb are being treated with growth factors together with cytostatic agents, as has indeed been reported for taxol and radiation *(92,384)*. One might predict that deregulation of the pRb pathway would render tumor cells with intact p19[ARF]-p53 more sensitive to these agents, whereas mutation of p19[ARF] alone would eliminate any co-stimulative effect of growth factors via E2F. Inventories of this kind have hardly been made, but might well turn out to be essential for assessment of a more effective drug therapy.

9. CONCLUSION

The previous extensive overview of the current literature on the clinical value of cell cycle regulators makes clear that there are many promising results. However, even for those markers close to clinical diagnostic or prognostic application, there are important drawbacks to the published studies. First, most studies are immunohistochemical in nature. Although there are distinct advantages to this technique, such as the fact that it is morphological in nature and can deal with intra-tumor heterogeneity, is easy, and is relatively cheap, there are certainly drawbacks. Antibodies may not be fully sensitive and specific, and between labs there are many differences in tissue pretreatment, antibodies used, and staining protocols. Besides, it may be better to directly detect genetic alterations than immunohistochemical accumulation such as in the case of p53 and cyclin D_1. Second, almost all studies were retrospective and relatively small, and therefore bigger prospective studies on the most promising variables are urgently needed. Third, little attention has been paid to reproducibility of the assays. Usually, some estimation of percentage positive cells or rough 2- or 4-tiered grouping has been applied instead of reliable countings using, e.g., stereological principles (138). Therefore, there are many methodological differences between the various studies, and consequently no uniform clinical thresholds have been established. Fourth, the very clearly present problem of intra-tumor heterogeneity has largely been neglected. This can basically be overcome by sound sampling strategies (138), but this will require substantial attention in future studies. Fifth, most studies have addressed a single marker or only a few markers. In view of the extremely complicated cell cycle machinery with its many interactions and feedbacks, such studies can hardly be extected to yield clinically relevant information. Future studies should leave this approach behind and try to arrive at expression profiling of tumors (using immunohistochemistry or microarray analysis) incorporating all known cell cycle regulators, using multivariate data analysis to figure out which combination of changes determines proliferation. In view of these drawbacks, the answer to the question of which cell cycle regulator can at the moment be clinically used must simply be negative.

For now, it therefore seems more appropriate to focus on the functional end result of the complicated cell cycle machinery: cell division or not. Counting mitoses, as the morphologically recognizable end stage of the successfully completed cell cycle, or assessment of Ki67 or cyclin A labeling index (both being good markers for cells dedicated to proliferation) are quite appropriate for this (108). Mitoses counting especially is already applied in many clinical situations as its methological issues have been well-studied (385–389). One must realize, however, that although these markers are extremely useful in risk evaluation, they do not reveal the mechanism behind the failure of control over proliferation and apoptosis.

ACKNOWLEDGMENTS

The authors' research is supported by grants from the Netherlands Cancer Foundation. We thank Yvonne Duiker for tremendous help with literature searches and assistance with preparing the manuscript. Search strategy for abstracts consisted of PubMed searches using key words "prognosis-cell cycle feature" (e.g., prognosis-cyclin D_1) as per 1/10/2000, considering expression studies published in English where it was clear from the abstract whether low or high feature values were favorable or unfavorable. Although we have attemped to be complete, the abundance of literature will no doubt have caused us to miss some important papers. We would appreciate being notified of such omissions.

REFERENCES

1. Hanahan D, Weinberg RA. The hallmarks of cancer. *Cell* 2000;100:57–70.
2. Pardee AB. G1 events and regulation of cell proliferation. *Science* 1989;246:603–608.
3. Jackman MR, Pines JN. Cyclins and the G2/M transition. *Cancer Surv* 1997;29:47–73.
4. Morgan DO. Cyclin-dependent kinases: engines, clocks, and microprocessors. *Ann Rev Cell Dev Biol* 1997;13:261–291.
5. Sherr CJ. D-type cyclins. *TIBS* 1995;20:187–190.
6. Altucci L, Addeo R, Cicatiello L, Dauvois S, Parker MG, Truss M, et al. 17beta-Estradiol induces cyclin D1 gene transcription, $p36^{D1}$-$p34^{cdk4}$ complex activation and p105Rb phosphorylation during mitogenic stimulation of G(1)-arrested human breast cancer cells. *Oncogene* 1996;12:2315–2324.
7. Brown JR, Nigh E, Lee RJ, Ye H, Thompson MA, Saudou F, et al. Fos family members induce cell cycle entry by activating cyclin D1. *Mol Cell Biol* 1998;18:5609–5619.
8. Herber B, Truss M, Beato M, Muller R. Inducible regulatory elements in the human cyclin D1 promoter. *Oncogene* 1994;9:2105–2107.
9. Hunter T. Oncoprotein networks. *Cell* 1997;88:333–346.
10. Lukas J, Bartkova J, Bartek J. Convergence of mitogenic signalling cascades from diverse classes of receptors at the cyclin D-cyclin-dependent kinase-pRb-controlled G1 checkpoint. *Mol Cell Biol* 1996;16:6917–6925.
11. Roussel MF. Key effectors of signal transduction and G1 progression. *Adv Cancer Res* 1998;74:1–24.
12. Watanabe G, Albanese C, Lee RJ, Reutens A, Vairo G, Henglein B, Pestell RG. Inhibition of cyclin D1 kinase activity is associated with E2F-mediated inhibition of cyclin D1 promoter activity through E2F and Sp1. *Mol Cell Biol* 1998;18:3212–3222.
13. Assoian RK. Anchorage-dependent cell cycle progression. *J Cell Biol* 1997;136:1–4.
14. Bottazzi ME, Assoian RK. The extracellular matrix and mitogenic growth factors control G1 phase cyclins and cyclin-dependent kinase inhibitors. *Trends Cell Biol* 1997;7:348–352.
15. Schlaepfer DD, Hanks SK, Hunter T, van der Geer P. Integrin-mediated signal transduction linked to Ras pathway by GRB2 binding to focal adhesion kinase. *Nature* 1994;372:786–791.
16. St.Croix B, Sheehan CE, Rak JW, Florenes VA, Slingerland JM, Kerbel RS. E-Cadherin-dependent growth suppression is mediated by the cyclin-dependent kinase inhibitor $p27^{KIP1}$. *J Cell Biol* 1998;142:557–571.
17. Arber N, Doki Y, Han EK, Sgambato A, Zhou P, Kim NH, et al. Antisense to cyclin D1 inhibits the growth and tumorigenicity of human colon cancer cells. *Cancer Res* 1997;57:1569–1574.
18. Lukas J, Bartkov J, Rohde M, Strauss M, Bartek J. Cyclin D1 is dispensable for G1 control in retinoblastoma gene-deficient cells independently of cdk4 activity. *Mol Cell Biol* 1995;15:2600–2611.
19. Quelle DE, Ashmun RA, Shurtleff SA, Kato JY, Bar-Sagi D, Roussel MF, Sherr CJ. Overexpression of mouse D-type cyclins accelerates G1 phase in rodent fibroblasts. *Genes Dev* 1993;7:1559–1571.
20. Weinberg RA. The retinoblastoma protein and cell cycle control. *Cell* 1995;81:323–330.
21. Beijersbergen RL, Carlee L, Kerkhoven RM, Bernards R. Regulation of the retinoblastoma protein-related p107 by G1 cyclin complexes. *Genes Dev* 1995;9:1340–1353.
22. Herrer RE, Sah VP, Williams BO, Makel TP, Weinberg RA, Jacks T. Altered cell cycle kinetics, gene expression, and G1 restriction point regulation in Rb-deficient fibroblasts. *Mol Cell Biol* 1996;16:2402–2407.

23. Muller H, Lukas J, Schneider A, Warthoe P, Bartek J, Eilers M, Strauss M. Cyclin D1 expression is regulated by the retinoblastoma protein. *Proc Natl Acad Sci USA* 1994;91:2945–2949.

24. Ohtani K, DeGregori J, Nevins JR. Regulation of the cyclin E gene by transcription factor E2F1. *Proc Natl Acad Sci USA* 1995;92:12146–12150.

25. Schulze A, Zerfass K, Spitkovsky D, Middendorp S, Berges J, Helin K, et al. Cell cycle regulation of the cyclin A gene promoter is mediated by a variant E2F site. *Proc Natl Acad Sci USA* 1995;92:11264–11268.

26. Kitagaw M, Higashi H, Jung HK, Suzuki-Takahashi I, Iked M, Tamai K, et al. The consensus motif for phosphorylation by cyclin D1-Cdk4 is different from that for phosphorylation by cyclin A/E-Cdk2. *EMBO J* 1996;15:7060–7069.

27. Ohtsubo M, Theodoras AM, Schumacher J, Roberts JM, Pagano M. Human cyclin E, a nuclear protein essential for the G1-to-S phase transition. *Mol Cell Biol* 1995;15:2612–2624.

28. Resnitzky D, Reed SI. Different roles for cyclin D1 and E in regulation of the G1-to-S transition. *Mol Cell Biol* 1995;15:3463–3469.

29. Bernards R. E2F: a nodal point in cell cycle regulation. *Biochim Biophys Acta* 1997;1333:M33–M40.

30. Hurford RK Jr, Cobrinik D, Lee MH, Dyson N. pRB and p107/p130 are required for the regulated expression of different sets of E2F responsive genes. *Genes Dev* 1997;11:1447–1463.

31. Moberg K, Starz MA, Lees JA. E2F-4 switches from p130 to p107 and pRB in response to cell cycle reentry. *Mol Cell Biol* 1996;16:1436–1449.

32. Connell-Crowley L, Elledge SJ, Harper JW. G1 cyclin-dependent kinases are sufficient to initiate DNA synthesis in quiescent human fibroblasts. *Curr Biol* 1998;8:65–68.

33. Johnson DG, Schwarz JK, Cress WD, Nevins JR. Expression of transcription factor E2F1 induces quiescent cells to enter S phase. *Nature* 1993;365:349–352.

34. Yan Z, DeGregori J, Shohet R, Leone G, Stillman B, Nevins JR, Williams RS. Cdc6 is regulated by E2F and is essential for DNA replication in mammalian cells. *Proc Natl Acad Sci USA* 1998;95:3603–3608.

35. Romanowski P, Madine MA. Mechanisms restricting DNA replication to once per cell cycle: the role of Cdc6p and ORC. *Trends Cell Biol* 1997;7:9–10.

36. Guadagno TM, Newport JW. Cdk2 kinase is required for entry into mitosis as a positive regulator of Cdc2-cyclin B kinase activity. *Cell* 1996;84:73–82.

37. Krek W, Xu G, Livingston DM. Cyclin A-kinase regulation of E2F-1 DNA binding function underlies suppression of an S phase checkpoint. *Cell* 1995;83:1149–1158.

38. Hunter T, Pines J. Cyclins and cancer II: Cyclin D and CDK inhibitors come of age. *Cell* 1994;79:573–582.

39. Diehl JA, Sherr CJ. A dominant-negative cyclin D1 mutant prevents nuclear import of cyclin-dependent kinase 4 (CDK4) and its phosphorylation by CDK-activating kinase. *Mol Cell Biol* 1997;17:7362–7374.

40. Hoyt MA. Eliminating all obstacles: regulated proteolysis in the eukaryotic cell cycle. *Cell* 1997;91:149–151.

41. Won KA, Reed SI. Activation of cyclin E/CDK2 is coupled to site-specific autophosphorylation and ubiquitin-dependent degradation of cyclin. *EMBO J* 1996;15:4182–4193.

42. Elledge SJ, Winston J, Harper JW. A question of balance: the role of cyclin-kinase inhibitors in development and tumorigenesis. *Trends Cell Biol* 1996;6:388–392.

43. Harper JW. Cyclin dependent kinase inhibitors. *Cancer Surv* 1997;29:91–107.

44. Sherr CJ, Roberts JM. Inhibitors of mammalian G1 cyclin-dependent kinases. *Genes Dev* 1995;9:1149–1163.

45. Coleman KG, Wautlet BS, Morrissey D, Mulheron J, Sedman SA, Brinkley P, et al. Identification of CDK4 sequences involved in cyclin D1 and p16 binding. *J Biol Chem* 1997;272:18869–18874.

46. Sherr CJ. G1 phase progression: cycling on cue. *Cell* 1994;79:551–555.
47. Sherr CJ. Cancer cell cycles. *Science* 1996;274:1672–1677.
48. Blain SW, Montalvo E, Massague J. Differential interaction of the cyclin-dependent kinase (Cdk) inhibitor p27^{Kip1} with cyclin A-Cdk2 and cyclin D2-Cdk4. *J Biol Chem* 1997; 272:25863–25872.
49. Harper JW, Elledge SJ, Keyomarsi K, Dynlacht B, Tsai LH, Zhang P, et al. Inhibition of cyclin-dependent kinases by p21. *Mol Biol Cell* 1995;6:387–400.
50. LaBaer J, Garrett MD, Stevenson LF, Slingerland JM, Sandhu C, Chou HS, et al. New functional activities for the p21 family of CDK inhibitors. *Genes Dev* 1997;11:847–862.
51. Sandhu C, Garbe J, Bhattacharya N, Daksis J, Pan CH, Yaswen P, et al. Transforming growth factor beta stabilizes p15^{INK4B} protein, increases p15^{INK4B}-cdk4 complexes, and inhibits cyclin D1-cdk4 association in human mammary epithelial cells. *Mol Cell Biol* 1997;17:2458–2467.
52. Planas-Silva MD, Weinberg RA. Estrogen-dependent cyclin E-cdk2 activation through p21 redistribution. *Mol Cell Biol* 1997;17:4059–4069.
53. Prall OWJ, Sarcevic B, Musgrove EA, Watts CKW, Sutherland RL. Estrogen-induced activation of Cdk4 and Cdk2 during G1-S phase progression is accompanied by increased cyclin D1 expression and decreased cyclin-dependent kinase inhibitor association with cyclin E-Cdk2. *J Biol Chem* 1997;272:10882–10894.
54. Hashemolhosseini S, Nagamine Y, Morley SJ, Desrivieres S, Mercep L, Ferrari S. Rapamycin inhibition of the G1 to S transition is mediated by effects on cyclin D1 mRNA and protein stability. *J Biol Chem* 1998;273:14424–14429.
55. Dulic V, Stein GH, Farahi Far D, Reed SI. Nuclear accumulation of p21^{Cip1} at the onset of mitosis: a role at the G2/M-phase transition. *Mol Cell Biol* 1998;18:546–557.
56. Niculescu AB, Chen X, Smeets M, Hengst L, Prives C, Reed SI. Effects of p21(Cip1/Waf1) at both the G1/S and the G2/M cell cycle transitions: pRb is a critical determinant in blocking DNA replication and in preventing endoreduplication. *Mol Cell Biol* 1998;18:629–643.
57. Levine AJ. p53, the cellular gatekeeper for growth and division. *Cell* 1997;88:323–331.
58. O'Connor PM. Mammalian G1 and G2 phase checkpoints. *Cancer Surv* 1997;29:151–182.
59. Zwijssen RM, Klompmakers R, Wientjes EB, Kristel PM, van den Burg B, Michalides RJ. Cyclin D1 triggers autonomous growth of breast cancer cells by governing cell cycle exit. *Mol Cell Biol* 1996;16:2554–2560.
60. Michalides R. Cell cycle regulators: mechanisms and their role in aetiology, prognosis, and treatment of cancer. *J Clin Pathol* 1999;52:555–568.
61. Hall M, Peters G. Genetic alterations of cyclins, cyclin-dependent kinases, and Cdk inhibitors in human cancer. *Adv Cancer Res* 1996;68:67–108.
62. Hosokawa Y, Suzuki R, Joh T, Maeda Y, Nakamura S, Kodera Y, Arnold A, Seto M. A small deletion in the 3'-untranslated region of the cyclin D1/PRAD1/bcl-1 oncogene in a patient with chronic lymphocytic leukemia. *Int J Cancer* 1998;76:791–796.
63. Betticher DC, Thatcher N, Altermatt HJ, Hoban P, Ryder WD, Heighway J. Alternate splicing produces a novel cyclin D1 transcript. *Oncogene* 1995;11:1005–1011.
64. Sawa H, Ohshima TA, Ukita H, Murakami H, Chiba Y, Kamada H, et al. Alternatively spliced forms of cyclin D1 modulate entry into the cell cycle in an inverse manner. *Oncogene* 1998;16:1701–1712.
65. He J, Allen JR, Collins VP, Allalunis-Turner MJ, Godbout R, Day RS, James CD. CDK4 amplification is an alternative mechanism to p16 gene homozygous deletion in glioma cell lines. *Cancer Res* 1994;54:5804–5807.
66. Schmidt EE, Ichimura K, Reifenberger G, Collins VP. CDKN2 (p16/MTS1) gene deletion or CDK4 amplification occurs in the majority of glioblastomas. *Cancer Res* 1994;54: 6321–6324.
67. Tsao H, Benoit E, Sober AJ, Thiele C, Haluska FG. Novel mutations in the p16/CDKN2A binding region of the cyclin-dependent kinase-4 gene. *Cancer Res* 1998;58:109–113.

68. Bartek J, Bartkova J, Lukas J. The retinoblastoma protein pathway and the restriction point. *Curr Opin Cell Biol* 1996;8:805–814.

69. Snijders PJF, van Duin M, Walboomers JMM, Steenbergen RDM, Risse EKJ, Helmerhorst TJM, et al. Telomerase activity exclusively in cervical carcinomas and a subset of cervical intraepithelial neoplasia grade III lesions: strong association with elevated messenger RNA levels of its catalytic subunit and high-risk human papillomavirus DNA. *Cancer Res* 1998;58:3812–3818.

70. Tang R, Cheng A-J, Wang J-Y, Wang TC. Close correlation between telomerase expression and adenomatous polyp progression in multistep colorectal carcinogenesis. *Cancer Res* 1998;58:4052–4054.

71. Alevizopoulos K, Vlach J, Hennecke S, Amati B. Cyclin E and c-Myc promote cell proliferation in the presence of p16^{INK4a} and of hypophosphorylated retinoblastoma family proteins. *EMBO J* 1997;16:5322–5333.

72. Sofer-Levi Y, Resnitzky D. Apoptosis induced by ectopic expression of cyclin D1 but not cyclin E. *Oncogene* 1996;13:2431–2437.

73. Hinds PW, Dowdy SF, Eaton EN, Arnold A, Weinberg RA. Function of a human cyclin gene as an oncogene. *Proc Natl Acad Sci USA* 1994;91:709–713.

74. Mueller A, Odze R, Jenkins TD, Shahsesfaei A, Nakagawa H, Inomoto T, Rustgi AK. A transgenic mouse model with cyclin D1 overexpression results in cell cycle, epidermal growth factor receptor and p53 abnormalities. *Cancer Res* 1997;57:5542–5549.

75. Lovec H, Grzeschiczek A, Kowalski MB, Moroy T. Cyclin D1/bcl-1 cooperates with myc genes in the generation of B-cell lymphoma in transgenic mice. *EMBO J* 1994;13:3487–3495.

76. Robles AI, Larcher F, Whalin RB, Murillas R, Richie E, Gimenez-Conti IB, et al. Expression of cyclin D1 in epithelial tissues of transgenic mice results in epidermal hyperproliferation and severe thymic hyperplasia. *Proc Natl Acad Sci USA* 1996;93:7634–7638.

77. Wang TC, Cardiff RD, Zukerberg L, Lees E, Arnold A, Schmidt EV. Mammary hyperplasia and carcinoma in MMTV-cyclin D1 transgenic mice. *Nature* 1994;369:669–671.

78. Bortner DM, Rosenberg MP. Induction of mammary gland hyperplasia and carcinomas in transgenic mice expressing human cyclin E. *Mol Cell Biol* 1997;17:453–459.

79. Sicinski P, Donaher JL, Parker SB, Li T, Fazeli A, Gardner H, et al. Cyclin D1 provides a link between development and oncogenesis in the retina and breast. *Cell* 1995;82:621–630.

80. Fantl V, Stamp G, Andrews A, Rosewell I, Dickson C. Mice lacking cyclin D1 are small and show defects in eye and mammary gland development. *Genes Dev* 1995;9:2364–2372.

81. Zwijsen RM, Wientjens E, Klompmaker R, Van der Sman J, Bernards R, Michalides RJ. CDK-independent activation of estrogen receptor by cyclin D1. *Cell* 1997;88:405–415.

82. Neuman E, Ladha MH, Lin N, Upton TM, Miller SJ, DiRenzo J, et al. Cyclin D1 stimulation of estrogen receptor transcriptional activity independent of cdk4. *Mol Cell Biol* 1997;17:5338–5347.

83. Sicinski P, Donaher JL, Geng Y, Parker SB, Gardner H, Park MY, et al. Cyclin D2 is an FSH-responsive gene involved in gonadal cell proliferation and oncogenesis. *Nature* 1996;384:470–474.

84. Jacks T, Fazeli A, Schmitt EM, Bronson RT, Goodell MA, Weinberg RA. Effects of an Rb mutation in the mouse. *Nature* 1992;359:295–300.

85. Zhou P, Jiang W, Weghorst CM, Weinstein IB. Overexpression of Cyclin D1 enhances gene amplification. *Cancer Res* 1996;56:36–39.

86. Sherr CJ, Roberts JM. CDK inhibitors: positive and negative regulators of G1-phase progression. *Genes Dev* 1999;13:1501–1502.

87. De Jong JS, Van Diest PJ, Michalides RJAM, Baak JPA. Concerted expression of the genes coding for p21 and cyclin D1 is associated with growth inhibition and differentiation in various carcinomas. *Mol Pathol* 1999;52:78–83.

88. De Boer CJ, van Krieken JH, Schuuring E, Kluin PM. Bcl-1/cyclin D1 in malignant lymphoma. *Ann Oncol* 1997;8:109–117.
89. Dillon DA, Howe CL, Bosari S, Costa J. The molecular biology of breast cancer: accelerating clinical applications. *Crit Rev Oncog* 1998;9:125–140.
90. Mowat MRA. p53 in tumor progression: life, death, and everything. *Adv Cancer Res* 1998;74:25–48.
91. Weber JD, Taylor LJ, Roussel MF, et al. Nucleolar Arf sequesters Mdm2 and activates p53. *Nat Cell Biol* 1999;1:20–26.
92. Coco Martin JM, Balkenende A, Verschoor T, Lallemand F, Michalides R. Cyclin D1 overexpression enhances radiation-induced apoptosis and radiosensitivity in a breast tumor cell line. *Cancer Res* 1999;59:1134–1140.
93. Yoo SS, Carter D, Turner BC, Sasaki CT, Son YH, Wilson LD, et al. Prognostic significance of cyclin D1 protein levels in early-stage larynx cancer treated with primary radiation. *Int J Cancer* 2000;90:22–28.
94. McGill G, Fisher DE. p53 and cancer therapy: a double-edged sword. *J Clin Inv* 1999;104:223–224.
95. Banerjee D, Schnieders B, Fu JZ, Adhikari D, Zhao SC, Bertino JR. Role of E2F-1 in chemosensitivity. *Cancer Res* 1998;58:4292–4296.
96. Fearon ER. Human cancer syndromes: clues to the origin and nature of cancer. *Science* 1997;278:1043–1050.
97. Califano J, van der Riet P, Westra W, Nawroz H, Clayman G, Piantadosi S, et al. Genetic progression model for head and neck cancer: implications for field cancerization. *Cancer Res* 1996;56:2488–2492.
98. Michalides R. Deregulation of cyclin D1 in cancer, in *The Biology of Tumors* (Mihich E, Croce C, eds.), Plenum Press, New York, 1998, pp. 127–145.
99. Buerger H, Otterbach F, Simon R, Poremba C, Diallo R, Decker T, et al. Comparative genomic hybridization of ductal carcinoma in situ of the breast-evidence of multiple genetic pathways. *J Pathol* 1999a;187:396–402.
100. Buerger H, Otterbach F, Simon R, Schafer KL, Poremba C, Diallo R, et al. Different genetic pathways in the evolution of invasive breast cancer are associated with distinct morphological subtypes. *J Pathol* 1999b;189:521–526.
101. Buerger H, Simon R, Schafer KL, Diallo R, Littmann R, Poremba C, et al. Genetic relation of lobular carcinoma in situ, ductal carcinoma in situ, and associated invasive carcinoma of the breast. *Mol Pathol* 2000;53:118–121.
102. Dosaka-Akita H, Hu SX, Fujino M, Harada M, Kinoshita I, Xu HJ, et al. Altered retinoblastoma protein expression in nonsmall cell lung cancer: its synergistic effects with altered ras and p53 protein status on prognosis. *Cancer* 1997;79:1329–1337.
103. Yoo GH, Xu HJ, Brennan JA, Westra W, Hruban RH, Koch W, et al. Infrequent inactivation of the retinoblastoma gene despite frequent loss of chromosome 13q in head and neck squamous cell carcinoma. *Cancer Res* 1994;54:4603–4606.
104. Olshan AF, Weissler MC, Pei H, Conway K, Anderson S, Fried DB, Yarbrough WG. Alterations of the p16 gene in head and neck cancer: frequency and association with p53, PRAD-1 and HPV. *Oncogene* 1997;14:811–818.
105. Aaltomaa S, Eskelinen M, Lipponen P. Expression of cyclin A and D proteins in prostate cancer and their relation to clinopathological variables and patient survival. *Prostate* 1999;38:175–182.
106. Ito Y, Takeda T, Sakon M, Monden M, Tsujimoto M, Matsuura N. Expression and prognostic role of cyclin-dependent kinase 1 (cdc2) in hepatocellular carcinoma. *Oncology* 2000;59:68–74.
107. Wolowiec D, Berger F, Ffrench P, Bryon PA, Ffrench M. CDK1 and cyclin A expression is linked to cell proliferation and associated with prognosis in non-Hodgkin's lymphomas. *Leuk Lymphoma* 1999;35:147–157.

108. Van Diest PJ, Brugal G, Baak JPA. Proliferation markers in tumours: interpretation and clinical value. *J Clin Pathol* 1998;51:716–724.

109. Noguchi T, Dobashi Y, Minehara H, Itoman M, Kameya T. Involvement of cyclins in cell proliferation and their clinical implications in soft tissue smooth muscle tumors. *Am J Pathol* 2000;156:2135–2147.

110. Handa K, Yamakawa M, Takeda H, Kimura S, Takahashi T. Expression of cell cycle markers in colorectal carcinoma: superiority of cyclin A as an indicator of poor prognosis. *Int J Cancer* 1999;84:225–233.

111. Aaltomaa S, Lipponen P, Eskelinen M, Ala-Opas M, Kosma VM. Prognostic value and expression of p21(waf1/cip1) protein in prostate cancer. *Prostate* 1999;39:8–15.

112. Kallakury BV, Sheehan CE, Rhee SJ, Fisher HA, Kaufman RP Jr, Rifkin MD, Ross JS. The prognostic significance of proliferation-associated nucleolar protein p120 expression in prostate adenocarcinoma: a comparison with cyclins A and B1, Ki-67, proliferating cell nuclear antigen, and p34cdc2. *Cancer* 1999;85:1569–1576.

113. Brien TP, Depowski PL, Sheehan CE, Ross JS, McKenna BJ. Prognostic factors in gastric cancer. *Mod Pathol* 1998;11:870–877.

114. Furihata M, Ishikawa T, Inoue A, Yoshikawa C, Sonobe H, Ohtsuki Y, et al. Determination of the prognostic significance of unscheduled cyclin A overexpression in patients with esophageal squamous cell carcinoma. *Clin Cancer Res* 1996;2:1781–1785.

115. Yasunaga M, Tabira Y, Kondo K, Okuma T, Kitamura N. The prognostic significance of cell cycle markers in esophageal cancer after neoadjuvant chemotherapy. *Dis Esophagus* 1999;12:120–127.

116. Dobashi Y, Shoji M, Jiang SX, Kobayashi M, Kawakubo Y, Kameya T. Active cyclin A-CDK2 complex, a possible critical factor for cell proliferation in human primary lung carcinomas. *Am J Pathol* 1998;153:963–972.

117. Volm M, Koomagi R. Relevance of proliferative and pro-apoptotic factors in non-small-cell lung cancer for patient survival. *Br J Cancer* 2000;82:1747–1754.

118. Volm M, Koomagi R, Rittgen W. Clinical implications of cyclins, cyclin-dependent kinases, RB and E2F1 in squamous-cell lung carcinoma. *Int J Cancer* 1998;79:294–299.

119. Volm M, Rittgen W, Drings P. Prognostic value of ERBB-1, VEGF, cyclin A, FOS, JUN and MYC in patients with squamous cell lung carcinomas. *Br J Cancer* 1998;77:663–669. Published erratum *Br J Cancer* 1998;77:1198.

120. Furihata M, Ohtsuki Y, Sonobe H, Shuin T, Yamamoto A, Terao N, Kuwahara M. Cyclin A overexpression in carcinoma of the renal pelvis and ureter including dysplasia: immunohistochemical findings in relation to prognosis. *Clin Cancer Res* 1997;3:1399–1404.

121. Molendini L, Benassi MS, Magagnoli G, Merli M, Sollazzo MR, Ragazzini P, et al. Prognostic significance of cyclin expression in human osteosarcoma. *Int J Oncol* 1998;12:1007–1011.

122. Huuhtanen RL, Blomqvist CP, Bohling TO, Wiklund TA, Tukiainen EJ, Virolainen M, et al. Expression of cyclin A in soft tissue sarcomas correlates with tumor aggressiveness. *Cancer Res* 1999;59:2885–2890.

123. Huuhtanen RL, Wiklund TA, Blomqvist CP, Bohling TO, Virolainen MJ, Tribukait B, Andersson LC. A high proliferation rate measured by cyclin A predicts a favourable chemotherapy response in soft tissue sarcoma patients. *Br J Cancer* 1999;81:1017–1021.

124. Kim SH, Lewis JJ, Brennan MF, Woodruff JM, Dudas M, Cordon-Cardo C. Overexpression of cyclin D1 is associated with poor prognosis in extremity soft-tissue sarcomas. *Clin Cancer Res* 1998;4:2377–2382.

125. Megha T, Lazzi S, Ferrari F, Vatti R, Howard CM, Cevenini G, et al. Expression of the G2-M checkpoint regulators cyclin B1 and P34CDC2 in breast cancer: a correlation with cellular kinetics. *Anticancer Res* 1999;19:163–169.

126. Murakami H, Furihata M, Ohtsuki Y, Ogoshi S. Determination of the prognostic significance of cyclin B1 overexpression in patients with esophageal squamous cell carcinoma. *Virchows Arch* 1999;434:153–158.

127. Suhardja AS, Kovacs KT, Rutka JT. Molecular pathogenesis of pituitary adenomas: a review. *Acta Neurochir (Wien)* 1999;141:729–736.
128. Kudoh S, Kumaravel TS, Kuramavel B, Eguchi M, Asaoku H, Dohy H, et al. Protein expression of cell cycle regulator, p27Kip1, correlates with histopathological grade of non-Hodgkin's lymphoma. *Jpn J Cancer Res* 1999;90:1262–1269.
129. Yatabe Y, Nakamura S, Seto M, Kuroda H, Kagami Y, Suzuki R, et al. Clinicopathologic study of PRAD1/cyclin D1 overexpressing lymphoma with special reference to mantle cell lymphoma. A distinct molecular pathologic entity. *Am J Surg Pathol* 1996;20:1110–1122.
130. Swerdlow SH, Yang WI, Zukerberg LR, Harris NL, Arnold A, Williams ME. Expression of cyclin D1 protein in centrocytic/mantle cell lymphomas with and without rearrangement of the BCL1/cyclin D1 gene. *Hum Pathol* 1995;26:999–1004.
131. Yatabe Y, Suzuki R, Tobinai K, Matsuno Y, Ichinohasama R, Okamoto M, et al. Significance of cyclin D1 overexpression for the diagnosis of mantle cell lymphoma: a clinicopathologic comparison of cyclin D1-positive MCL and cyclin D1-negative MCL-like B-cell lymphoma. *Blood* 2000;95:2253–2261.
132. Gillett CE, Lee AH, Millis RR, Barnes DM. Cyclin D1 and associated proteins in mammary ductal carcinoma in situ and atypical ductal hyperplasia. *J Pathol* 1998;184:396–400.
133. Mommers ECM, Van Diest PJ, Leonhart AM, Meijer CJLM, Baak JPA. Expression of proliferation and apoptosis related proteins in usual ductal hyperplasia of the breast. *Hum Pathol* 1998;29:1539–1545.
134. Weinstat-Saslow D, Merino MJ, Manrow RE, Lawrence JA, Bluth RF, Wittenbel KD, et al. Overexpression of cyclin D mRNA distinguishes invasive and in situ breast carcinomas from non-malignant lesions. *Nat Med* 1995;1:1257–1260.
135. Simpson JF, Quan DE, O'Malley F, Odom-Maryon T, Clarke PE. Amplification of CCND1 and expression of its protein product, cyclin D1, in ductal carcinoma in situ of the breast. *Am J Pathol* 1997;151:161–168.
136. Oyama T, Kashiwabara K, Yoshimoto K, Arnold A, Koerner FC. Frequent overexpression of the cyclin D1 oncogene in invasive lobular carcinoma of the breast. *Cancer Res* 1998;58:2876–2880.
137. Michalides R, Hageman PH, van Tinteren H, Houben L, Wientjens E, Klompmaker R, Peterse J. A clinico-pathological study on overexpression of cyclin D1 and of p53 in a series of 248 patients with operable breast cancer. *Br J Cancer* 1996;73:728–734.
138. Van Diest PJ, Van Dam P, Henzen-Logmans SC, Berns E, Van der Burg MEL, Green J, Vergote I. A scoring system for immunohistochemical staining: consensus report of the task force for basic research of the EORTC-GCCG. *J Clin Pathol* 1997a;50:801–804.
139. Seshadri R, Lee CS, Hui R, McCaul K, Horsfall DJ, Sutherland RL. Cyclin D1 amplification is not associated with reduced overall survival in primary breast cancer but may predict early relapse in patients with features of good prognosis. *Clin Canc Res* 1996;2:1177–1184.
140. Courjal F, Louason G, Speiser P, Katsaros D, Zeillinger R, Theillet C. Cyclin gene amplification and overexpression in breast and ovarian cancers: evidence for the selection of cyclin D1 in breast and cyclin E in ovarian tumors. *Int J Cancer* 1996;69:247–253.
141. Cuny M, Kramar A, Courjal F, Johannsdottir V, Iacopetta B, Fontaine H, et al. Relating genotype and phenotype in breast cancer: an analysis of the prognostic significance of amplification at eight different genes or loci and of p53 mutations. *Cancer Res* 2000;60:1077–1083.
142. Tsuda H, Hirohashi S, Shimosato Y, Hirota T, Tsugane S, Yamamoto H, et al. Correlation between long-term survival in breast cancer patients and amplification of two putative oncogene-coamplification units: hst-1/int-2 and c-erbB-2/ear-1. *Cancer Res* 1989;49:3104–3108.
143. Schuuring E, Verhoeven E, Tinteren H van, Peterse JL, Nunnink B, Thunnissen FBJM, et al. Amplification of genes within the chromosome 11q13 region is indicative of poor prognosis in patients with operable breast cancer. *Cancer Res* 1992;52:5229–5234.

144. An HX, Beckmann MW, Reifenberger G, Bender HG, Niederacher D. Gene amplification and overexpression of CDK4 in sporadic breast carcinomas is associated with high tumor cell proliferation. *Am J Pathol* 1999;154:113–118.
145. Nielsen NH, Emdin SO, Cajander J, Landberg G. Deregulation of cyclin E D1 in breast cancer is associated with inactivation of the retinoblastoma protein. *Oncogene* 1997;14:295–304.
146. Reed W, Fllrenes VA, Holm R, Hannisdal E, Nesland JM. Elevated levels of p27, p21 and cyclin D1 correlate with positive oestrogen and progesterone receptor status in node-negative breast carcinoma patients. *Virchows Arch* 1999;435:116–124.
147. Kenny FS, Hui R, Musgrove EA, Gee JM, Blamey RW, Nicholson RI, et al. Overexpression of cyclin D1 messenger RNA predicts for poor prognosis in estrogen receptor-positive breast cancer. *Clin Cancer Res* 1999;5:2069–2076.
148. Utsumi T, Yoshimura N, Maruta M, Takeuchi S, Ando J, Mizoguchi Y, Harada N. Correlation of cyclin D1 MRNA levels with clinico-pathological parameters and clinical outcome in human breast carcinomas. *Int J Cancer* 2000;89:39–43.
149. Hui R, Cornish AL, McClelland RA, Robertson JF, Blamey RW, Musgrove EA, et al. Cyclin D1 and estrogen receptor messenger RNA levels are positively correlated in primary breast cancer. *Clin Canc Res* 1996;2:923–928.
150. Pelosio P, Barbareschi M, Bonoldi E, Marchetti A, Verderio P, Caffo O, et al. Clinical significance of cyclin D1 expression in patients with node-positive breast carcinoma treated with adjuvant therapy. *Ann Oncol* 1996;7:695–703.
151. Doki Y, Imoto M, Han EK, Sgambato A, Weinstein IB. Increased expression of the p27[KIP1] protein in human esophageal cancer cell lines that over-express cyclin D1. *Carcinogenesis* 1997;18:1139–1148.
152. Nadal A, Jares P, Cazorla M, Fernandez PL, Sanjuan X, Hernandez L, et al. p21[WAF1/Cip1] expression is associated with cell differentiation but not with p53 mutations in squamous cell carcinomas of the larynx. *J Pathol* 1997;183:156–163.
153. McIntosh GG, Anderson JJ, Milton I, Steward M, Parr AH, Thomas MD, et al. Determination of the prognostic value of cyclin D1 overexpression in breast cancer. *Oncogene* 1995;11:885–891.
154. Maeda K, Chung YS, Kang SM, Ogawa M, Onoda N, Nakata B, et al. Overexpression of cyclin D1 and p53 associated with disease recurrence in colorectal adenocarcinoma. *Int J Cancer* 1997;74:310–315.
155. Sutter T, Doi S, Carnevale KA, Arber N, Weinstein IB. Expression of cyclin D1 and E in human colon adenocarcinomas. *J Med* 1997;28:285–309.
156. Bartkova J, Lukas J, Strauss M, Bartek J. The PRAD-1/cyclin D1 oncogene product accumulates aberrantly in a subset of colorectal carcinomas. *Int J Cancer* 1994;58:568–573.
157. Zhang T, Nanney LB, Luongo C, Lamps L, Heppner KJ, DuBois RN, Beauchamp RD. Concurrent overexpression of cyclin D1 and cyclin-dependent kinase 4 (Cdk4) in intestinal adenomas from multiple intestinal neoplasia (Min) mice and human familial adenomatous polyposis patients. *Cancer Res* 1997;57:169–175.
158. Palmqvist R, Stenling R, Oberg A, Landberg G. Expression of cyclin D1 and retinoblastoma protein in colorectal cancer. *Eur J Cancer* 1998;34:1575–1581.
159. Gansauge S, Gansauge F, Ramadani M, Stobbe H, Rau B, Harada N, Beger HG. Overexpression of cyclin D1 in human pancreatic carcinoma is associated with poor prognosis. *Cancer Res* 1997;57:1634–1637.
160. Gansauge F, Gansauge S, Schmidt E, Muller J, Beger HG. Prognostic significance of molecular alterations in human pancreatic carcinoma: an immunohistological study. *Langenbecks Arch Surg* 1998;383:152–155.
161. Naka T, Kobayashi M, Ashida K, Toyota N, Kaneko T, Kaibara N. Aberrant p16[INK4] expression related to clinical stage and prognosis in patients with pancreatic cancer. *Int J Oncol* 1998;12:1111–1116.

162. Kallakury BV, Sheehan CE, Ambros RA, Fisher HA, Kaufman RP, Ross JS. The prognostic significance of p34^{cdc2} and cyclin D1 protein expression in prostate adenocarcinoma. *Cancer* 1997;80:753–763.

163. Hui AM, Cui X, Makuuchi M, Li X, Shi YZ, Takayama T. Decreased p27(Kip1) expression and cyclin D1 overexpression, alone and in combination, influence recurrence and survival of patients with resectable extrahepatic bile duct carcinoma. *Hepatology* 1999;30:1167–1173.

164. Ito Y, Matsuura N, Sakon M, Miyoshi E, Noda K, Takeda T, et al. Expression and prognostic roles of the G1-S modulators in hepatocellular carcinoma: p27 independently predicts the recurrence. *Hepatology* 1999;30:90–99.

165. Peng SY, Chou SP, Hsu HC. Association of downregulation of cyclin D1 and of overexpression of cyclin E with p53 mutation, high tumor grade and poor prognosis in hepatocellular carcinoma. *J Hepatol* 1998;29:281–289.

166. Blok P, Craanen ME, Van Diest PJ, Dekker WJ, Tytgat GN. Lack of cyclin D1 overexpression in gastric carcinogenesis. *Histopathol* 2000;36:151–155.

167. Jang SJ, Park YW, Park MH, Lee JD, Lee YY, Jung TJ, et al. Expression of cell-cycle regulators, cyclin E and p21$^{WAF1/CIP1}$, potential prognostic markers for gastric cancer. *Eur J Surg Oncol* 1999;25:157–163.

168. Muller W, Noguchi T, Wirtz HC, Hommel G, Gabbert HE. Expression of cell-cycle regulatory proteins cyclin D1, cyclin E, and their inhibitor p21$^{WAF1/CIP1}$ in gastric cancer. *J Pathol* 1999;189:186–193.

169. Takano Y, Kato Y, van Diest PJ, Masuda M, Mitomi H, Okayasu I. Cyclin D2 overexpression and lack of p27 correlate positively and cyclin E inversely with a poor prognosis in gastric cancer cases. *Am J Pathol* 2000;156:585–594.

170. Takano Y, Kato Y, Masuda M, Ohshima Y, Okayasu I. Cyclin D2, but not cyclin D1, overexpression closely correlates with gastric cancer progression and prognosis. *J Pathol* 1999;189:194–200.

171. Hedberg Y, Davoodi E, Roos G, Ljungberg B, Landberg G. Cyclin-D1 expression in human renal-cell carcinoma. *Int J Cancer* 1999;84:268–272.

172. Bringuier PP, Tamimi Y, Schuuring E, Schaliken J. Expression of cyclin D1 and EMS1 in bladder tumours; relationship with chromosome 11q13 amplification. *Oncogene* 1996; 12:1747–1753.

173. Niehans GA, Kratzke RA, Froberg MK, Aeppli DM, Nguyen PL, Geradts J. G1 checkpoint protein and p53 abnormalities occur in most invasive transitional cell carcinomas of the urinary bladder. *Br J Cancer* 1999;80:1175–1184.

174. Shin KY, Kong G, Kim WS, Lee TY, Woo YN, Lee JD. Overexpression of cyclin D1 correlates with early recurrence in superficial bladder cancers. *Br J Cancer* 1997;75:1788–1792.

175. Wagner U, Suess K, Luginbuhl T, Schmid U, Ackermann D, Zellweger T, et al. Cyclin D1 overexpression lacks prognostic significance in superficial urinary bladder cancer. *J Pathol* 1999;188:44–50.

176. Diebold J, Mosinger K, Peiro G, Pannekamp U, Kaltz C, Baretton GB, Meier W, Lohrs U. 20q13 and cyclin D1 in ovarian carcinomas. Analysis by fluorescence in situ hybridization. *J Pathol* 2000;190:564–571.

177. Akervall JA, Michalides RJ, Mineta H, Balm A, Borg A, Dictor MR, et al. Amplification of cyclin D1 in squamous cell carcinoma of the head and neck and the prognostic value of chromosomal abnormalities and cyclin D1 overexpression. *Cancer* 1997;79(2):380–389.

178. Nogueira CP, Dolan RW, Gooey J, Byahatti S, Vaughan CW, Fuleihan NS, et al. Inactivation of p53 and amplification of cyclin D1 correlate with clinical outcome in head and neck cancer. *Laryngoscope* 1998;108:345–350.

179. Kyomoto R, Kumazawa H, Toda Y, Sakaida N, Okamura A, Iwanaga M, et al. Cyclin-D1-gene amplification is a more potent prognostic factor than its protein over-expression in human head-and-neck squamous-cell carcinoma. *Int J Cancer* 1997;74:576–581.

180. Michalides RJ, Van Veelen N, Hart A, Loftus B, Wientjens E, Balm A. Overexpression of cyclin D1 correlates with recurrence in a group of forty-seven operable squamous cell carcinomas of the head and neck. *Cancer Res* 1995;55:975–978.

181. Michalides R, van Veelen N, Kristel P, Hart A, Loftus B, Hilgers F, Balm A. Overexpression of cyclin D1 indicates a poor prognosis in squamous cell carcinoma of the head and neck. *Arch Oto Head Neck Surg* 1997;123:497–502.

182. Pignataro L, Pruneri G, Carboni N, Capaccio P, Cesana BM, Neri A, Buffa R. Clinical relevance of cyclin D1 protein overexpression in laryngeal squamous cell carcinoma. *J Clin Oncol* 1998;16:3069–3077.

183. Pruneri G, Pignataro L, Carboni N, Buffa R, Di Finizio D, Cesana BM, Neri A. Clinical relevance of expression of the CIP/KIP cell-cycle inhibitors p21 and p27 in laryngeal cancer. *J Clin Oncol* 1999;17:3150–3159.

184. Bellacosa A, Almadori G, Cavallo S, Cadoni G, Galli J, Ferrandina G, et al. Cyclin D1 gene amplification in human laryngeal squamous cell carcinomas: prognostic significance and clinical implications. *Clin Cancer Res* 1996;2:175–180.

185. Anayama T, Furihata M, Ishikawa T, Ohtsuki Y, Ogoshi S. Positive correlation between p27[Kip1] expression and progression of human esophageal squamous cell carcinoma. *Int J Cancer* 1998;79:439–443.

186. Gramlich TL, Fritsch CR, Maurer D, Eberle M, Gansler TS. Differential polymerase chain reaction assay of cyclin D1 gene amplification in esophageal carcinoma. *Diagn Mol Pathol* 1994;3:255–259.

187. Ishikawa T, Furihata M, Ohtsuki Y, Murakami H, Inoue A, Ogoshi S. Cyclin D1 overexpression related to retinoblastoma protein expression as a prognostic marker in human oesophageal squamous cell carcinoma. *Br J Cancer* 1998;77:92–97.

188. Itami A, Shimada Y, Watanabe G, Imamura M. Prognostic value of p27(Kip1) and CyclinD1 expression in esophageal cancer. *Oncology* 1999;57:311–317.

189. Kuwahara M, Hirai T, Yoshida K, Yamashita Y, Hihara J, Inoue H, Toge T. p53, p21(Waf1/Cip1) and cyclin D1 protein expression and prognosis in esophageal cancer. *Dis Esophagus* 1999;12:116–119.

190. Masuda M, Hirakawa N, Nakashima T, Kuratomi Y, Komiyama S. Cyclin D1 overexpression in primary hypopharyngeal carcinomas. *Cancer* 1996;78:390–395.

191. Matsumoto M, Furihata M, Ishikawa T, Ohtsuki Y, Ogoshi S. Comparison of deregulated expression of cyclin D1 and cyclin E with that of cyclin-dependent kinase 4 (CDK4) and CDK2 in human oesophageal squamous cell carcinoma. *Br J Cancer* 1999;80:256–261.

192. Naitoh H, Shibata J, Kawaguchi A, Kodama M, Hattori T. Overexpression and localization of cyclin D1 mRNA and antigen in esophageal cancer. *Am J Pathol* 1995;146:1161–1169.

193. Nakagawa H, Zukerberg L, Togawa K, Meltzer SJ, Nishihara T, Rustgi AK. Human cyclin D1 oncogene and esophageal squamous cell carcinoma. *Cancer* 1995;76:541–549.

194. Sarbia M, Stahl M, Fink U, Heep H, Dutkowski P, Willers R, et al. Prognostic significance of cyclin D1 in esophageal squamous cell carcinoma patients treated with surgery alone or combined therapy modalities. *Int J Cancer* 1999;84:86–91.

195. Shimada Y, Imamura M, Watanabe G, Uchida S, Harada H, Makino T, Kano M. Prognostic factors of oesophageal squamous cell carcinoma from the perspective of molecular biology. *Br J Cancer* 1999;80:1281–1288.

196. Shinozaki H, Ozawa S, Ando N, Tsuruta H, Terada M, Ueda M, Kitajima M. Cyclin D1 amplification as a new predictive classification for squamous cell carcinoma of the esophagus, adding gene information. *Clin Cancer Res* 1996;2:1155–1161.

197. Takeuchi H, Ozawa S, Ando N, Shih CH, Koyanagi K, Ueda M, Kitajima M. Altered p16/MTS1/CDKN2 and cyclin D1/PRAD-1 gene expression is associated with the prognosis of squamous cell carcinoma of the esophagus. *Clin Cancer Res* 1997;3:2229–2236.

198. Samejima R, Kitajima Y, Yunotani S, Miyazaki K. Cyclin D1 is a possible predictor of sensitivity to chemoradiotherapy for esophageal squamous cell carcinoma. *Anticancer Res* 1999;19:5515–5521.

199. Hirai T, Kuwahara M, Yoshida K, Osaki A, Toge T. The prognostic significance of p53, p21 (Waf1/Cip1), and cyclin D1 protein expression in esophageal cancer patients. *Anticancer Res* 1999;19:4587–4591.

200. Ikeda G, Isaji S, Chandra B, Watanabe M, Kawarada Y. Prognostic significance of biologic factors in squamous cell carcinoma of the esophagus. *Cancer* 1999;86:1396–1405.

201. Mineta H, Miura K, Suzuki I, Takebayashi S, Misawa K, Ueda Y, Ichimura K. p27 expression correlates with prognosis in patients with hypopharyngeal cancer. *Anticancer Res* 1999; 19:4407–4412.

202. Nishimura G, Tsukuda M, Zhou LX, Furukawa S, Baba Y. Cyclin D1 expression as a prognostic factor in advanced hypopharyngeal carcinoma. *J Laryngol Otol* 1998;112:552–555.

203. Kuo MY, Lin CY, Hahn LJ, Cheng SJ, Chiang CP. Expression of cyclin D1 is correlated with poor prognosis in patients with areca quid chewing-related oral squamous cell carcinomas in Taiwan. *J Oral Pathol Med* 1999;28:165–169.

204. Wong RJ, Keel SB, Glynn RJ, Varvares MA. Histological pattern of mandibular invasion by oral squamous cell carcinoma. *Laryngoscope* 2000;110:65–72.

205. Caputi M, Groeger AM, Esposito V, Dean C, De Luca A, Pacilio C, et al. Prognostic role of cyclin D1 in lung cancer. Relationship to proliferating cell nuclear antigen. *Am J Respir Cell Mol Biol* 1999;20:746–750.

206. Keum JS, Kong G, Yang SC, Shin DH, Park SS, Lee JH, Lee JD. Cyclin D1 overexpression is an indicator of poor prognosis in resectable non-small cell lung cancer. *Br J Cancer* 1999;81:127–132.

207. Betticher DC, Heighway J, Hasleton PS, Altermatt HJ, Ryder WD, Cerny T, Thatcher N. Prognostic significance of CCND1 (cyclin D1) overexpression in primary resected non-small-cell lung cancer. *Br J Cancer* 1996;73:294–300.

208. Nishio M, Koshikawa T, Yatabe Y, Kuroishi T, Suyama M, Nagatake M, et al. Prognostic significance of cyclin D1 and retinoblastoma expression in combination with p53 abnormalities in primary, resected non-small cell lung cancers. *Clin Cancer Res* 1997;3:1051–1058.

209. Brambilla E, Moro D, Gazzeri S, Brambilla C. Alterations of expression of Rb, p16(INK4A) and cyclin D1 in non-small cell lung carcinoma and their clinical significance. *J Pathol* 1999;188:351–360.

210. Kwa HB, Michalides RJ, Dijkman JH, Mooi WJ. The prognostic value of NCAM, p53 and cyclin D1 in resected non-small cell lung cancer. *Lung Cancer* 1996;14:207–217.

211. Yang WI, Chung KY, Shin DH, Kim YB. Cyclin D1 protein expression in lung cancer. *Yonsei Med J* 1996;37:142–150.

212. Sallinen SL, Sallinen PK, Kononen JT, Syrjakoski KM, Nupponen NN, Rantala IS, et al. Cyclin D1 expression in astrocytomas is associated with cell proliferation activity and patient prognosis. *J Pathol* 1999;188:289–293.

213. Volm M, Koomagi R, Stammler G, Rittgen W, Zintl F, Sauerbrey A. Prognostic implications of cyclins (D1, E, A), cyclin-dependent kinases (CDK2, CDK4) and tumor-suppressor genes (pRB, p16^{INK4A}) in childhood acute lymphoblastic leukemia. *Int J Cancer* 1997;74:508–512.

214. Houldsworth J, Reuter V, Bosl GJ, Chaganti RS. Aberrant expression of cyclin D2 is an early event in human male germ cell tumorigenesis. *Cell Growth Differ* 1997;8:293–299.

215. Sauerbrey A, Hafer R, Zintl F, Volm M. Analysis of cyclin D1 in de novo and relapsed childhood acute lymphoblastic leukemia. *Anticancer Res* 1999;19:645–649.

216. Antonescu CR, Leung DH, Dudas M, Ladanyi M, Brennan M, Woodruff JM, Cordon-Cardo C. Alterations of cell cycle regulators in localized synovial sarcoma: A multifactorial study with prognostic implications. *Am J Pathol* 2000;156:977–983.

217. Scott KA Walker RA. Lack of cyclin E immunoreactivity in non-malignant breast and association with proliferation in breast cancer. *Br J Cancer* 1997;76:1288–1292.
218. Keyomarsi K, O'Leary N, Molnar G, Lees E, Fingert HJ, Pardee AB. Cyclin E, a potential prognostic marker for breast cancer. *Cancer Res* 1994;54:380–385.
219. Catzavelos C, Bhattacharya N, Ung YC, Wilson JA, Roncari L, Sandhu C, et al. Decreased levels of the cell-cycle inhibitor p27[Kip1] protein: prognostic implications in primary breast cancer. *Nature Med* 1997;3:227–230.
220. Tan P, Cady B, Wanner M, Worland P, Cukor B, Magi-Galluzzi C, et al. The cell cycle inhibitor p27 is an independent prognostic marker in small (T1a,b) invasive breast carcinomas. *Cancer Res* 1997;57:1259–1263.
221. Fredersdorf S, Burns J, Milne AM, Packham G, Fallis L, Gillett CE, et al. High level expression of p27(kip1) and cyclin D1 in some human breast cancer cells: inverse correlation between the expression of p27(kip1) and degree of malignancy in human breast and colorectal cancers. *Proc Natl Acad Sci USA* 1997;94:6380–6385.
222. Porter PL, Malone KE, Heagerty PJ, Alexander GM, Gatti LA, Firpo EJ, et al. Expression of cell-cycle regulators p27[Kip1] and cyclin E, alone and in combination, correlate with survival in young breast cancer patients. *Nat Med* 1997;3:222–225.
223. Nielsen NH, Arnerlov C, Emdin SO, Landberg G. Cyclin E overexpression, a negative prognostic factor in breast cancer with strong correlation to oestrogen receptor status. *Br J Cancer* 1996;74:874–880.
224. Nielsen NH, Arnerlov C, Cajander S, Landberg G. Cyclin E expression and proliferation in breast cancer. *Anal Cell Pathol* 1998;17:177–188.
225. Yasui W, Kudo Y, Demba S, Yokozaki H, Tahara E. Reduced expression of cyclin-dependent kinase inhibitor p27Kip1 is associated with advanced stage and invasiveness of gastric carcinomas. *Jpn J Cancer Res* 1997;88:625–629.
226. Sakaguchi T, Watanabe A, Sawada H, Yamada Y, Yamashita J, Matsuda M, et al. Prognostic value of cyclin E and p53 expression in gastric carcinoma. *Cancer* 1998;82:1238–1243.
227. Fukuse T, Hirata T, Naiki H, Hitomi S, Wada H. Prognostic significance of cyclin E overexpression in resected non-small cell lung cancer. *Cancer Res* 2000;60:242–244.
228. Mishina T, Dosaka-Akita H, Hommura F, Nishi M, Kojima T, Ogura S, et al. Cyclin E expression, a potential prognostic marker for non-small cell lung cancers. *Clin Cancer Res* 2000;6:11–16.
229. Furihata M, Ohtsuki Y, Sonobe H, Shuin T, Yamamoto A, Terao N, Kuwahara M. Prognostic significance of cyclin E and p53 protein overexpression in carcinoma of the renal pelvis and ureter. *Br J Cancer* 1998;77:783–788.
230. Erlanson M, Portin C, Linderholm B, Lindh J, Roos G, Landberg G. Expression of cyclin E and the cyclin-dependent kinase inhibitor p27 in malignant lymphomas-prognostic implications. *Blood* 1998;92:770–777.
231. Yokozawa T, Towatari M, Iida H, Takeyama K, Tanimoto M, Kiyoi H, et al. Prognostic significance of the cell cycle inhibitor p27[Kip1] in acute myeloid leukemia. *Leukemia* 2000;14:28–33.
232. Dellas A, Schultheiss E, Leivas MR, Moch H, Torhorst J. Association of p27[Kip1], cyclin E and c-myc expression with progression and prognosis in HPV-positive cervical neoplasms. *Anticancer Res* 1998;18:3991–3998.
233. Eguchi N, Fujii K, Tsuchida A, Yamamoto S, Sasaki T, Kajiyama G. Cyclin E overexpression in human gallbladder carcinomas. *Oncol Rep* 1999;6:93–96.
234. Lu X, Toki T, Konishi I, Nikaido T, Fujii S. Expression of p21[WAF1/CIP1] in adenocarcinoma of the uterine cervix: a possible immunohistochemical marker of a favorable prognosis. *Cancer* 1998;82:2409–2417.
235. Shimizu M, Nikaido T, Toki T, Shiozawa T, Fujii S. Clear cell carcinoma has an expression pattern of cell cycle regulatory molecules that is unique among ovarian adenocarcinomas. *Cancer* 1999;85:669–677.

236. Chang WY, Birch L, Woodham C, Gold LI, Prins GS. Neonatal estrogen exposure alters the transforming growth factor-beta signaling system in the developing rat prostate and blocks the transient p21(cip1/waf1) expression associated with epithelial differentiation. *Endocrinology* 1999;140:2801–2813.

237. Natsugoe S, Nakashima S, Matsumoto M, Xiangming C, Okumura H, Kijima F, et al. Expression of p21WAF1/Cip1 in the p53-dependent pathway is related to prognosis in patients with advanced esophageal carcinoma. *Clin Cancer Res* 1999;5:2445–2449.

238. Nita ME, Nagawa H, Tominaga O, Tsuno N, Hatano K, Kitayama J, et al. p21$^{Waf1/Cip1}$ expression is a prognostic marker in curatively resected esophageal squamous cell carcinoma, but not p27^{Kip1}, p53, or Rb. *Ann Surg Oncol* 1999;6:481–488.

239. Lam KY, Law S, Tin L, Tung PH, Wong J. The clinicopathological significance of p21 and p53 expression in esophageal squamous cell carcinoma: an analysis of 153 patients. *Am J Gastroenterol* 1999;94:2060–2068.

240. Osaki T, Kimura T, Tatemoto Y, Dapeng L, Yoneda K, Yamamoto T. Diffuse mode of tumor cell invasion and expression of mutant p53 protein but not of p21 protein are correlated with treatment failure in oral carcinomas and their metastatic foci. *Oncology* 2000;59:36–43.

241. Hirvikoski P, Kellokoski JK, Kumpulainen EJ, Virtaniemi JA, Johansson RT, Kosma VM. Downregulation of p21/WAF1 is related to advanced and dedifferentiated laryngeal squamous cell carcinoma. *J Clin Pathol* 1999;52:440–444.

242. Qiu H, Sirivongs P, Rothenberger M, Rothenberger DA, Garcia-Aguilar J. Molecular prognostic factors in rectal cancer treated by radiation and surgery. *Dis Colon Rectum* 2000;43:451–459.

243. Zirbes TK, Baldus SE, Moenig SP, Nolden S, Kunze D, Shafizadeh ST, et al. Prognostic impact of p21/waf1/cip1 in colorectal cancer. *Int J Cancer* 2000;89:14–18.

244. Ropponen KM, Kellokoski JK, Lipponen PK, Pietilainen T, Eskelinen MJ, Alhava EM, Kosma VM. p21/WAF1 expression in human colorectal carcinoma: association with p53, transcription factor AP-2 and prognosis. *Br J Cancer* 1999;81:133–140.

245. Barbareschi M, Pelosio P, Caffo O, Buttita F, Pellegrini S, Barbazza R, et al. Cyclin-D1 gene amplification and expression in breast carcinoma: relation with clinicopathologic characteristics and with retinoblastoma gene product, p53 and p21^{WAF1} immunohistochemical expression. *Int J Cancer (Pred Oncol)* 1997;74;171–174.

246. Mathoulin-Portier MP, Viens P, Cowen D, Bertucci F, Houvenaeghel G, Geneix J, et al. Prognostic value of simultaneous expression of p21 and mdm2 in breast carcinomas treated by adjuvant chemotherapy with antracyclin. *Oncol Rep* 2000;7:675–680.

247. Anttila MA, Kosma VM, Hongxiu J, Puolakka J, Juhola M, Saarikoski S, Syrjanen K. p21/WAF1 expression as related to p53, cell proliferation and prognosis in epithelial ovarian cancer. *Br J Cancer* 1999;79:1870–1878.

248. Costa MJ, Hansen CL, Walls JE, Scudder SA. Immunohistochemical markers of cell cycle control applied to ovarian and primary peritoneal surface epithelial neoplasms: p21(WAF1/CIP1) predicts survival and good response to platinin-based chemotherapy. *Hum Pathol* 1999;30:640–647.

249. Schmider A, Gee C, Friedmann W, Lukas JJ, Press MF, Lichtenegger W, Reles A. p21 (WAF1/CIP1) protein expression is associated with prolonged survival but not with p53 expression in epithelial ovarian carcinoma. *Gynecol Oncol* 2000;77:237–242.

250. Werness BA, Freedman AN, Piver MS, Romero-Gutierrez M, Petrow E. Prognostic significance of p53 and p21(waf1/cip1) immunoreactivity in epithelial cancers of the ovary. *Gynecol Oncol* 1999;75:413–418.

251. Baekelandt M, Holm R, Trope CG, Nesland JM, Kristensen GB. Lack of independent prognostic significance of p21 and p27 expression in advanced ovarian cancer: an immunohistochemical study. *Clin Cancer Res* 1999;5:2848–2853.

252. Kaye PV, Radebold K, Isaacs S, Dent DM. Expression of p53 and p21waf1/cip1 in gastric carcinoma: lack of inter-relationship or correlation with prognosis. *Eur J Surg Oncol* 2000;26:39–43.

253. Ikeguchi M, Saito H, Kondo A, Tsujitani S, Maeta M, Kaibara N. Mutated p53 protein expression and proliferative activity in advanced gastric cancer. *Hepatogastroenterology* 1999;46:2648–2653.

254. Baretton GB, Klenk U, Diebold J, Schmeller N, Lohrs U. Proliferation- and apoptosis-associated factors in advanced prostatic carcinomas before and after androgen deprivation therapy: prognostic significance of p21/WAF1/CIP1 expression. *Br J Cancer* 1999;80:546–555.

255. Nio Y, Dong M, Uegaki K, Hirahara N, Minari Y, Sasaki S, et al. Comparative significance of p53 and WAF/1-p21 expression on the efficacy of adjuvant chemotherapy for resectable invasive ductal carcinoma of the pancreas. *Pancreas* 1999;18:117–126.

256. Vonlanthen S, Heighway J, Kappeler A, Altermatt HJ, Borner MM, Betticher DC. p21 is associated with cyclin D1, p16^{INK4a} and pRb expression in resectable non-small cell lung cancer. *Int J Oncol* 2000;16:951–957.

257. Aikawa H, Sato M, Fujimura S, Takahashi H, Endo C, Sakurada A, et al. MDM2 expression is associated with progress of disease and WAF1 expression in resected lung cancer. *Int J Mol Med* 2000;5:631–633.

258. Karjalainen JM, Eskelinen MJ, Kellokoski JK, Reinikainen M, Alhava EM, Kosma VM. p21(WAF1/CIP1) expression in stage I cutaneous malignant melanoma: its relationship with p53, cell proliferation and survival. *Br J Cancer* 1999;79:895–902.

259. Smolewski P, Niewiadomska H, Krykowski E, Robak T. Expression of p21 and MDM-2 proteins on tumor cells in responding and non-responding patients with Hodgkin's disease. *Neoplasma* 1999;46:212–218.

260. Zhang A, Ohshima K, Sato K, Kanda M, Suzumiya J, Shimazaki K, et al. Prognostic clinicopathologic factors, including immunologic expression in diffuse large B-cell lymphomas. *Pathol Int* 1999;49:1043–1052.

261. Chow NH, Tzai TS, Cheng HL, Liu HS, Chan SH, Tong YC. The clinical value of p21$^{WAFI/CIP1}$ expression in superficial bladder cancer. *Anticancer Res* 2000;20:1173–1176.

262. Korkolopoulou P, Christodoulou P, Konstantinidou AE, Thomas-Tsagli E, Kapralos P, Davaris P. Cell cycle regulators in bladder cancer: a multivariate survival study with emphasis on p27^{Kip1}. *Hum Pathol* 2000;31:751–760.

263. Kirla R, Salminen E, Huhtala S, Nuutinen J, Talve L, Haapasalo H, Kalim H. Prognostic value of the expression of tumor suppressor genes p53, p21, p16 and prb, and Ki-67 labelling in high grade astrocytomas treated with radiotherapy. *J Neurooncol* 2000;46:71–80.

264. Han EK, Begemann M, Sgambato A, Soh JW, Doki Y, Xing WQ, Liu W, Weinstein IB. Increased expression of cyclin D1 in a murine mammary epithelial cell line induces p27^{kip1}, inhibits growth and enhances apoptosis. *Cell Growth Differ* 1996;7:699–710.

265. Catzavelos C, Tsao MS, DeBoer G, Bhattacharya N, Shepherd FA, Slingerland JM. Reduced expression of the cell cycle inhibitor p27Kip1 in non-small cell lung carcinoma: a prognostic factor independent of Ras. *Cancer Res* 1999;59:684–688.

266. Gillett CE, Smith P, Peters G, Lu X, Barnes DM. Cyclin-dependent kinase inhibitor p27Kip1 expression and interaction with other cell cycle-associated proteins in mammary carcinoma. *J Pathol* 1999;187:200–206.

267. Tsuchiya A, Zhang GJ, Kanno M. Prognostic impact of cyclin-dependent kinase inhibitor p27^{kip1} in node-positive breast cancer. *J Surg Oncol* 1999;70:230–234.

268. Wu SG, el-Deiry WS. p53 and chemosensitivity. *Nat Med* 1996;2:255–256.

269. Barbareschi M, van Tinteren H, Mauri FA, Veronese S, Peterse H, Maisonneuve P, et al. p27(kip1) expression in breast carcinomas: an immunohistochemical study on 512 patients with long-term follow-up. *Int J Cancer* 2000;89:236–241.

270. Loda M, Cukor B, Tam SW, Lavin P, Firentino M, Draetta GF, Jessup JM, Pagano M. Increased proteasome-dependent degradation of the cyclin-dependent kinase inhibitor p27 in aggressive colorectal carcinomas. *Nat Med* 1997;3:231–234.

271. Palmqvist R, Stenling R, Oberg A, Landberg G. Prognostic significance of p27(Kip1) expression in colorectal cancer: a clinico-pathological characterization. *J Pathol* 1999;188:18–23.

272. Thomas GV, Szigeti K, Murphy M, Draetta G, Pagano M, Loda M. Down-regulation of p27 is associated with development of colorectal adenocarcinoma metastases. *Am J Pathol* 1998;153:681–687.

273. Tenjo T, Toyoda M, Okuda J, Watanabe I, Yamamoto T, Tanaka K, et al. Prognostic significance of p27(kip1) protein expression and spontaneous apoptosis in patients with colorectal adenocarcinomas. *Oncology* 2000;58:45–51.

274. Yao J, Eu KW, Seow-Choen F, Cheah PY. Down-regulation of p27 is a significant predictor of poor overall survival and may facilitate metastasis in colorectal carcinomas. *Int J Cancer* 2000;89:213–216.

275. Mori M, Mimori K, Shiraishi T, Tanaka S, Ueo H, Sugimachi K, Akiyoshi T. p27 expression and gastric carcinoma. *Nature Med* 1997;3:593.

276. Ohtani M, Isozaki H, Fujii K, Nomura E, Niki M, Mabuchi H, et al. Impact of the expression of cyclin-dependent kinase inhibitor p27Kip1 and apoptosis in tumor cells on the overall survival of patients with non-early stage gastric carcinoma. *Cancer* 1999;85:1711–1718.

277. Kwon OJ, Kang HS, Suh JS, Chang MS, Jang JJ, Chung JK. The loss of p27 protein has an independent prognostic significance in gastric cancer. *Anticancer Res* 1999;19:4215–4220.

278. Cote RJ, Shi YF, Groshen S, Feng A-C, Cordon-Cardo C, Skinner DG, Lieskovsky G. Association of p27Kip1 levels with recurrence and survival in patients with stage C prostate carcinoma. *J Nat Canc Inst* 1998;90:916–920.

279. De Marzo AM, Meeker AK, Epstein JI, Coffy DS. Prostate stem cell compartments: expression of the cell cycle inhibitor p27^{Kip1} in normal, hyperplastic, and neoplastic cells. *Am J Pathol* 1998;153:911–919.

280. Tsihlias J, Kapsta LR, DeBoer G, Morava-Protzer I, Zbieranowski I, Bhattacharya N, et al. Loss of cyclin-dependent kinase inhibitor p27^{Kip1} is a novel prognostic factor in localized human prostate adenocarcinoma. *Cancer Res* 1998;58:542–548.

281. Yang RM, Naitoh J, Murphy M, Wang HJ, Phillipson J, deKernion JB, et al. Low p27 expression predicts poor disease-free survival in patients with prostate cancer. *J Urol* 1998;159:941–945.

282. Erdamar S, Yang G, Harper JW, Lu X, Kattan MW, Thompson TC, Wheeler TM. Levels of expression of p27^{KIP1} protein in human prostate and prostate cancer: an immunohistochemical analysis. *Mod Pathol* 1999;12:751–755.

283. Masciullo V, Sgambato A, Pacilio C, Pucci B, Ferrandina G, Palazzo J, et al. Frequent loss of expression of the cyclin-dependent kinase inhibitor p27 in epithelial ovarian cancer. *Cancer Res* 1999;59:3790–3794.

284. Singh SP, Lipman J, Goldman H, Ellis FH Jr, Aizenman L, Cangi MG, et al. Loss or altered subcellular localization of p27 in Barrett's associated adenocarcinoma. *Cancer Res* 1998;58:1730–1735.

285. Hui AM, Li X, Shi YZ, Torzilli G, Takayama T, Makuuchi M. p27(Kip1) expression in normal epithelia, precancerous lesions, and carcinomas of the gallbladder: association with cancer progression and prognosis. *Hepatology* 2000;31:1068–1072.

286. Shamma A, Doki Y, Tsujinaka T, Shiozaki H, Inoue M, Yano M, et al. Loss of p27(KIP1) expression predicts poor prognosis in patients with esophageal squamous cell carcinoma. *Oncology* 2000;58:152–158.

287. Fan GK, Fujieda S, Sunaga H, Tsuzuki H, Ito N, Saito H. Expression of protein p27 is associated with progression and prognosis in laryngeal cancer. *Laryngoscope* 1999;109:815–820.

288. Venkatesan TK, Kuropkat C, Caldarelli DD, Panje WR, Hutchinson JC Jr, Chen S, Coon JS. Prognostic significance of p27 expression in carcinoma of the oral cavity and oropharynx. *Laryngoscope* 1999;109:1329–1333.

289. Oka K, Suzuki Y, Nakano T. Expression of p27 and p53 in cervical squamous cell carcinoma patients treated with radiotherapy alone. *Cancer* 2000;88:2766–2773.

290. Esposito V, Baldi A, De Luca A, Groger AM, Loda M, Giordano GG, et al. Prognostic role of the cyclin-dependent kinase inhibitor p27 in non-small cell lung cancer. *Cancer Res* 1997;57:3381–3385.

291. Ishihara S, Minato K, Hoshino H, Saito R, Hara F, Nakajima T, Mori M. The cyclin-dependent kinase inhibitor p27 as a prognostic factor in advanced non-small cell lung cancer: its immunohistochemical evaluation using biopsy specimens. *Lung Cancer* 1999;26:187–194.

292. Taga S, Osaki T, Ohgami A, Imoto H, Yoshimatsu T, Yoshino I, et al. Prognostic value of the immunohistochemical detection of p16^{INK4} expression in nonsmall cell lung carcinoma. *Cancer* 1997;80:389–395.

293. Okamoto A, Hussain SP, Hagiwara K, Spillare EA, Rusin MR, Demetrick DJ, et al. Mutations in the p16$^{INK4/MTS1/CDKN2}$, p15$^{INK4B/MTS2}$, and p18 genes in primary and metastatic lung cancer. *Cancer Res* 1995;55:1448–1451.

294. Yatabe Y, Masuda A, Koshikawa T, Nakamura S, Kuroishi T, Osada H, et al. p27^{KIP1} in human lung cancers: differential changes in small cell and non-small cell carcinomas. *Cancer Res* 1998;58:1042–1047.

295. Gazzeri S, Gouyer V. Inactivation of RB gene and pRB function in lung cancer, in *Lung Tumors: Fundamental Biology and Clinical Management*, Brambilla C, Brambilla E, eds. Marcel Dekker, New York, 1998.

296. Sanchez-Beato M, Saez AI, Martinez JC, Mateo MS, Sanchez LS, Villuendas R, et al. Cyclin-dependent kinase inhibitor p27^{kip1} in lymphoid tissue: p27^{kip1} expression is inversely proportional to the proliferative index. *Am J Pathol* 1997;151:151–160.

297. Fuse T, Tanikawa M, Nakanishi M, Ikeda K, Tada T, Inagaki H, et al. p27^{Kip1} expression by contact inhibition as a prognostic index of human glioma. *J Neurochem* 2000;74:1393–1399.

298. Cavalla P, Piva R, Bortolotto S, Grosso R, Cancelli I, Chio A, Schiffer D. p27/kip1 expression in oligodendrogliomas and its possible prognostic role. *Acta Neuropathol (Berl)* 1999; 98:629–634.

299. Taniguchi T, Chikatsu N, Takahashi S, Fujita A, Uchimaru K, Asano S, et al. Expression of p16^{INK4A} and p14^{ARF} in hematological malignancies. *Leukemia* 1999;13:1760–1769.

300. Hussussian CJ, Struewing JP, Goldstein AM, Higgins PA, Ally DS, Sheahan MD, et al. Germline p16 mutations in familial melanoma. *Nat Genet* 1994;8:15–21.

301. Straume O, Sviland L, Akslen LA. Loss of nuclear p16 protein expression correlates with increased tumor cell proliferation (Ki-67) and poor prognosis in patients with vertical growth phase melanoma. *Clin Cancer Res* 2000;6:1845–1853.

302. Chana JS, Grover R, Wilson GD, Hudson DA, Forders M, Sanders R, Grobbelaar AO. An analysis of p16 tumour suppressor gene expression in acral lentiginous melanoma. *Br J Plast Surg* 2000;53:46–50.

303. Straume O, Akslen LA. Alterations and prognostic significance of p16 and p53 protein expression in subgroups of cutaneous melanoma. *Int J Cancer* 1997;74:535–539.

303a. Klaes R, Friedrich T, Spitkovsky D, et al. Overexpression of p16 (INK4A) as a specific marker for dysplastic and neoplastic epithelial cells of the cervix uteri. *Int J Cancer* 2001;92:276–284.

304. Salvesen HB, Das S, Akslen LA. Loss of nuclear p16 protein expression is not associated with promoter methylation but defines a subgroup of aggressive endometrial carcinomas with poor prognosis. *Clin Cancer Res* 2000;6:153–159.

305. Dong Y, Walsh MD, McGuckin MA, Cummings MC, Gabrielli BG, Wright GR, et al. Reduced expression of retinoblastoma gene product (pRB) and high expression of p53 are associated with poor prognosis in ovarian cancer. *Int J Cancer* 1997;74:407–415.

306. Barbieri F, Cagnoli M, Ragni N, Pedulla F, Foglia G, Alama A. Expression of cyclin D1 correlates with malignancy in human ovarian tumours. *Br J Cancer* 1997;75:1263–1268.

307. Hu YX, Watanabe H, Ohtsubo K, Yamaguchi Y, Ha A, Okai T, Sawabu N. Frequent loss of p16 expression and its correlation with clinicopathological parameters in pancreatic carcinoma. *Clin Cancer Res* 1997;3:1473–1477.
308. Volm M, Koomagi R, Mattern J. Prognostic value of p16^{INK4A} expression in lung adenocarcinoma. *Anticancer Res* 1998;18:2309–2312.
309. Xu L, Sgroi D, Sterner CJ, Beauchamp RL, Pinney DM, Keel S, et al. Mutational analysis of CDKN2 (MTS1/p16^{ink4}) in human breast carcinomas. *Cancer Res* 1994;54:5262–5264.
310. Dublin EA, Patel NK, Gillett CE, Smith P, Peters G, Barnes DM. Retinoblastoma and p16 proteins in mammary carcinoma: their relationship to cyclin D1 and histopathological parameters. *Int J Cancer* 1998;79:71–75.
311. Tsujie M, Yamamoto H, Tomita N, Sugita Y, Ohue M, Sakita I, et al. Expression of tumor suppressor gene p16(INK4) products in primary gastric cancer. *Oncology* 2000;58:126–136.
312. Huang CI, Taki T, Higashiyama M, Kohno N, Miyake M. p16 protein expression is associated with a poor prognosis in squamous cell carcinoma of the lung. *Br J Cancer* 2000; 82:374–380.
313. Kawabuchi B, Moriyama S, Hironaka M, Fujii T, Koike M, Moriyama H, et al. p16 inactivation in small-sized lung adenocarcinoma: its association with poor prognosis. *Int J Cancer* 1999;84:49–53.
314. Kratzke RA, Greatens TM, Rubins JB, Maddaus MA, Niewoehner DE, Niehans GA, Geradts J. Rb and p16INK4a expression in resected non-small cell lung tumors. *Cancer Res* 1996;56:3415–3420.
315. Groeger AM, Caputi M, Esposito V, De Luca A, Bagella L, Pacilio C, et al. Independent prognostic role of p16 expression in lung cancer. *J Thorac Cardiovasc Surg* 1999;118:529–535.
316. Hommura F, Dosaka-Akita H, Kinoshita I, Mishina T, Hiroumi H, Ogura S, et al. Predictive value of expression of p16^{INK4A}, retinoblastoma and p53 proteins for the prognosis of non-small-cell lung cancers. *Br J Cancer* 1999;81:696–701.
317. Gorgoulis VG, Zacharatos P, Kotsinas A, Liloglou T, Kyroudi A, Veslemes M, et al. Alterations of the p16-pRb pathway and the chromosome locus 9p21-22 in non-small-cell lung carcinomas: relationship with p53 and MDM2 protein expression. *Am J Pathol* 1998; 153:1749–1765.
318. Mekki Y, Catallo R, Bertrand Y, Manel AM, Ffrench P, Baghdassarian N, et al. Enhanced expression of p16ink4a is associated with a poor prognosis in childhood acute lymphoblastic leukemia. *Leukemia* 1999;13:181–189.
319. Kees UR, Burton PR, Lu C, Baker DL. Homozygous deletion of the p16/MTS1 gene in pediatric acute lymphoblastic leukemia is associated with unfavorable clinical outcome. *Blood* 1997;89:4161–4166.
320. Diccianni MB, Batova A, Yu J, Vu T, Pullen J, Amylon M, Pollock BH, Yu AL. Shortened survival after relapse in T-cell acute lymphoblastic leukemia patients with p16/p15 deletions. *Leuk Res* 1997;21:549–558.
321. Yamada Y, Hatta Y, Murata K, Sugawara K, Ikeda S, Mine M, et al. Deletions of p15 and/or p16 genes as a poor-prognosis factor in adult T-cell leukemia. *J Clin Oncol* 1997;15: 1778–1785.
322. Garcia-Sanz R, Gonzalez M, Vargas M, Chillon MC, Balanzategui A, Barbon M, et al. Deletions and rearrangements of cyclin-dependent kinase 4 inhibitor gene p16 are associated with poor prognosis in B cell non-Hodgkin's lymphomas. *Leukemia* 1997;11:1915–1920.
323. Gronbaek K, de Nully Brown P, Moller MB, Nedergaard T, Ralfkiaer E, Moller P, et al. Concurrent disruption of p16^{INK4a} and the ARF-p53 pathway predicts poor prognosis in aggressive non-Hodgkin's lymphoma. *Leukemia* 2000 Oct;14(10):1727–1735.
324. Guenova M, Rassidakis GZ, Gorgoulis VG, Angelopoulou MK, Siakantaris MR, Kanavaros P, et al. p16^{INK4A} is regularly expressed in Hodgkin's disease: comparison with retinoblas-

toma, p53 and MDM2 protein status, and the presence of Epstein-Barr virus. *Mod Pathol* 1999;12:1062–1071.

325. Takita J, Hayashi Y, Nakajima T, Adachi J, Tanaka T, Yamaguchi N, et al. The p16 (CDKN2A) gene is involved in the growth of neuroblastoma cells and its expression is associated with prognosis of neuroblastoma patients. *Oncogene* 1998;17:3137–3143.

326. Bortolotto S, Chiado-Piat L, Cavalla P, Bosone I, Chio A, Mauro A, Schiffer D. CDKN2A/p16 inactivation in the prognosis of oligodendrogliomas. *Int J Cancer* 2000;88:554–557.

327. Puduvalli VK, Kyritsis AP, Hess KR, Bondy ML, Fuller GN, Kouraklis GP, et al. Patterns of expression of Rb and p16 in astrocytic gliomas, and correlation with survival. *Int J Oncol* 2000;17:963–969.

328. Orlow I, Drobnjak M, Zhang ZF, Lewis J, Woodruff JM, Brennan MF, Cordon-Cardo C. Alterations of INK4A and INK4B genes in adult soft tissue sarcomas: effect on survival. *J Natl Cancer Inst* 1999;91:73–79.

329. Miettinen H, Kononen J, Sallinen P, Alho H, Helen P, Helin H, et al. CDKN2/p16 predicts survival in oligodendrogliomas: comparison with astrocytomas. *J Neurooncol* 1999; 41:205–211.

330. Orlow I, LaRue H, Osman I, Lacombe L, Moore L, Rabbani F, et al. Deletions of the INK4A gene in superficial bladder tumors. Association with recurrence. *Am J Pathol* 1999;155: 105–113.

331. Faderl S, Kantarjian HM, Manshouri T, Chan CY, Pierce S, Hays KJ, et al. The prognostic significance of p16INK4a/p14ARF and p15INK4b deletions in adult acute lymphoblastic leukemia. *Clin Cancer Res* 1999;5:1855–1861.

332. Wong IH, Ng MH, Huang DP, Lee JC. Aberrant p15 promoter methylation in adult and childhood acute leukemias of nearly all morphologic subtypes: potential prognostic implications. *Blood* 2000;95:1942–1949.

333. Zhou M, Gu L, Yeager AM, Findley HW. Incidence and clinical significance of CDKN2/MTS1/P16^{ink4A} and MTS2/P15^{ink4B} gene deletions in childhood acute lymphoblastic leukemia. *Pediatr Hematol Oncol* 1997;14:141–150.

334. Quesnel B, Guillerm G, Vereecque R, Wattel E, Preudhomme C, Bauters F, et al. Methylation of the p15(INK4b) gene in myelodysplastic syndromes is frequent and acquired during disease progression. *Blood* 1998;91:2985–2990.

335. Berns EM, de Klein A, van Putten WL, van Staveren IL, Bootsma A, Klijn JG, Foekens JA. Association between RB-1 gene alterations and factors of favourable prognosis in human breast cancer, without effect on survival. *Int J Cancer* 1995;64:140–145.

336. Pietilainen T, Lipponen P, Aaltomaa S, Eskelinen M, Kosma VM, Syrjanen K. Expression of retinoblastoma gene protein (Rb) in breast cancer as related to established prognostic factors and survival. *Eur J Cancer* 1995;31A:329–333.

337. Sawan A, Randall B, Angus B, Wright C, Henry JA, Ostrowski J, et al. Retinoblastoma and p53 gene expression related to relapse and survival in human breast cancer: an immunohistochemical study. *J Pathol* 1992;168(1):23–28.

338. Poller DN, Baxter KJ, Shepherd NA. p53 and Rb1 protein expression: are they prognostically useful in colorectal cancer? *Br J Cancer* 1997;75:87–93.

339. Naka T, Toyota N, Kaneko T, Kaibara N. Protein expression of p53, p21WAF1, and Rb as prognostic indicators in patients with surgically treated hepatocellular carcinoma. *Anticancer Res* 1998;18:555–564.

340. Vargas MP, Vargas HI, Kleiner DE, Merino MJ. Adrenocortical neoplasms: role of prognostic markers MIB-1, P53, and RB. *Am J Surg Pathol* 1997;21:556–562.

341. Dokiya F, Ueno K, Ma S, Eizuru Y, Furuta S, Ohyama M. Retinoblastoma protein expression and prognosis in laryngeal cancer. *Acta Otolaryngol* 1998;118:759–762.

342. Girod SC, Pfeiffer P, Ries J, Pape HD. Proliferative activity and loss of function of tumour suppressor genes as 'biomarkers' in diagnosis and prognosis of benign and preneoplastic oral lesions and oral squamous cell carcinoma. *Br J Oral Maxillofac Surg* 1998;36:252–260.

343. Guerry M, Vabre L, Talbot M, Mamelle G, Leridant AM, Hill C, et al. Prognostic value of histological and biological markers in pharyngeal squamous cell carcinoma: a case-control study. *Br J Cancer* 1998;77:1932–1936.

344. Hashimoto N, Tachibana M, Dhar DK, Yoshimura H, Nagasue N. Expression of p53 and RB proteins in squamous cell carcinoma of the esophagus: their relationship with clinicopathologic characteristics. *Ann Surg Oncol* 1999;6:489–494.

345. Ikeguchi M, Oka S, Gomyo Y, Tsujitani S, Maeta M, Kaibara N. Clinical significance of retinoblastoma protein (pRB) expression in esophageal squamous cell carcinoma. *J Surg Oncol* 2000;73:104–108.

346. Zur Hausen A, Sarbia M, Heep H, Willers R, Gabbert HE. Retinoblastoma-protein (prb) expression and prognosis in squamous-cell carcinomas of the esophagus. *Int J Cancer* 1999;22;84:618–622.

347. Cordon-Cardo C, Wartinger D, Petrylak D, Dalbagni G, Fair WR, Fuks Z, Reuter VE. Altered expression of the retinoblastoma gene product: prognostic indicator in bladder cancer. *J Natl Cancer Inst* 1992;84:1251–1256.

348. Cote RJ, Dunn MD, Chatterjee SJ, Stein JP, Shi SR, Tran QC, et al. Elevated and absent pRb expression is associated with bladder cancer progression and has cooperative effects with p53. *Cancer Res* 1998;58:1090–1094.

349. Grossman HB, Liebert M, Antelo M, Dinney CP, Hu SX, Palmer JL, Benedict WF. p53 and RB expression predict progression in T1 bladder cancer. *Clin Cancer Res* 1998;4:829–834.

350. Jahnson S, Risberg B, Karlsson MG, Westman G, Bergstrom R, Pedersen J. p53 and Rb immunostaining in locally advanced bladder cancer: relation to prognostic variables and predictive value for the local response to radical radiotherapy. *Eur Urol* 1995;28:135–142.

351. Lipponen PK, Liukkonen TJ. Reduced expression of retinoblastoma (Rb) gene protein is related to cell proliferation and prognosis in transitional-cell bladder cancer. *J Cancer Res Clin Oncol* 1995;121:44–50.

352. Logothetis CJ, Xu HJ, Ro JY, Hu SX, Sahin A, Ordonez N, Benedict WF. Altered expression of retinoblastoma protein and known prognostic variables in locally advanced bladder cancer. *J Natl Cancer Inst* 1992;84:1256–1261.

353. Pollack A, Czerniak B, Zagars GK, Hu SX, Wu CS, Dinney CP, et al. Retinoblastoma protein expression and radiation response in muscle-invasive bladder cancer. *Int J Radiat Oncol Biol Phys* 1997;39:687–695.

354. Tetu B, Fradet Y, Allard P, Veilleux C, Roberge N, Bernard P. Prevalence and clinical significance of HER/2neu, p53 and Rb expression in primary superficial bladder cancer. *J Urol* 1996;155:1784–1788.

355. Xu HJ, Quinlan DC, Davidson AG, Hu SX, Summers CL, Li J, Benedict WF. Altered retinoblastoma protein expression and prognosis in early-stage non-small-cell lung carcinoma. *J Natl Cancer Inst* 1994;86:695–699.

356. Xu HJ, Cagle PT, Hu SX, Li J, Benedict WF. Altered retinoblastoma and p53 protein status in non-small cell carcinoma of the lung: potential synergistic effects on prognosis. *Clin Cancer Res* 1996;2:1169–1176.

357. Volm M, Stammler G. Retinoblastoma (Rb) protein expression and resistance in squamous cell lung carcinomas. *Anticancer Res* 1996;16:891–894.

358. Wurl P, Meye A, Berger D, Lautenschlager C, Bache M, Holzhausen HJ, et al. Significance of retinoblastoma and mdm2 gene expression as prognostic markers for soft-tissue sarcoma. *Langenbecks Arch Surg* 1998;383:99–103.

359. Cance WG, Brennan MF, Dudas ME, Huang CM, Cordon-Cardo C. Altered expression of the retinoblastoma gene product in human sarcomas. *N Engl J Med* 1990;323:1457–1462.

360. Benassi MS, Molendini L, Gamberi G, Sollazzo MR, Ragazzini P, Merli M, et al. Altered G1 phase regulation in osteosarcoma. *Int J Cancer* 1997;74:518–522.
361. Kornblau SM, Xu HJ, Zhang W, Hu SX, Beran M, Smith TL, et al. Levels of retinoblastoma protein expression in newly diagnosed acute myelogenous leukemia. *Blood* 1994; 84:256–261.
362. Kornblau SM, Andreeff M, Hu SX, Xu HJ, Patel S, Theriault A, et al. Low and maximally phosphorylated levels of the retinoblastoma protein confer poor prognosis in newly diagnosed acute myelogenous leukemia: a prospective study. *Clin Cancer Res* 1998; 4:1955–1963.
363. Morente MM, Piris MA, Abraira V, Acevedo A, Aguilera B, Bellas C, Fraga M, et al. Adverse clinical outcome in Hodgkin's disease is associated with loss of retinoblastoma protein expression, high Ki67 proliferation index, and absence of Epstein-Barr virus-latent membrane protein 1 expression. *Blood* 1997;90:2429–2436.
364. Sanchez E, Chacon I, Plaza MM, Munoz E, Cruz MA, Martinez B, et al. Clinical outcome in diffuse large B-cell lymphoma is dependent on the relationship between different cell-cycle regulator proteins. *J Clin Oncol* 1998;16:1931–1939.
365. Sauerbrey A, Stammler G, Zintl F, Volm M. Expression and prognostic value of the retinoblastoma tumour suppressor gene (RB-1) in childhood acute lymphoblastic leukaemia. *Br J Haematol* 1996;94:99–104.
366. Tsai T, Davalath S, Rankin C, Radich JP, Head D, Appelbaum FR, Boldt DH. Tumor suppressor gene alteration in adult acute lymphoblastic leukemia (ALL). Analysis of retinoblastoma (Rb) and p53 gene expression in lymphoblasts of patients with de novo, relapsed, or refractory ALL treated in Southwest Oncology Group studies. *Leukemia* 1996;10:1901–1910.
367. Massaro-Giordano M, Baldi G, De Luca A, Baldi A, Giordano A. Differential expression of the retinoblastoma gene family members in choroidal melanoma: prognostic significance. *Clin Cancer Res* 1999;5:1455–1458.
368. Leoncini L, Bellan C, Cossu A, Claudio PP, Lazzi S, Cinti C, et al. Retinoblastoma-related p107 and pRb2/p130 proteins in malignant lymphomas: distinct mechanisms of cell growth control. *Clin Cancer Res* 1999 Dec;5(12):4065–4072.
369. Susini T, Baldi F, Howard CM, Baldi A, Taddei G, Massi D, et al. Expression of the retinoblastoma-related gene Rb2/p130 correlates with clinical outcome in endometrial cancer. *J Clin Oncol* 1998;16:1085–1093.
370. Zheng W, Cao P, Zheng M, Kramer EE, Godwin TA. p53 overexpression and bcl-2 persistence in endometrial carcinoma: comparison of papillary serous and endometrioid subtypes. *Gynecol Oncol* 1996;61:167–174.
371. Ramael M, Lemmens G, Eerdekens C, Buysse C, Deblier I, Jacobs W, van Marck E. Immunoreactivity for p53 protein in malignant mesothelioma and non-neoplastic mesothelium. *J Pathol.* 1992;168:371–375.
372. Polkowski W, Baak JP, van Lanschot JJ, Meijer GA, Schuurmans LT, Ten Kate FJ, et al. Clinical decision making in Barrett's oesophagus can be supported by computerized immunoquantitation and morphometry of features associated with proliferation and differentiation. *J Pathol* 1998;184:161–168.
373. Van Sandick JW, Baak JP, van Lanschot JJ, Polkowski W, ten Kate FJ, Obertop H, Offerhaus GJ. Computerized quantitative pathology for the grading of dysplasia in surveillance biopsies of Barrett's oesophagus. *J Pathol* 2000;190:177–183.
374. Thor AD, Moore DH II, Edgerton SM, Kawasaki ES, Reihsaus E, Lynch HT, et al. Accumulation of p53 tumor suppressor gene protein: an independent marker of prognosis in breast cancers. *J Natl Cancer Inst* 1992;84:845–855.
375. Andersen TI, Holm R, Nesland JM, Heimdal KR, Ottestad L, Borresen AL. Prognostic significance of TP53 alterations in breast carcinoma. *Br J Cancer* 1993;68:540–548.
376. Maeda K, Chung Y, Kang S, Ogawa M, Onoda N, Nishiguchi Y, et al. Cyclin D1 overexpression and prognosis in colorectal adenocarcinoma. *Oncology* 1998;55:145–151.

377. Kobayashi S, Koide Y, Endo M, Isono K, Ochiai T. The p53 gene mutation is of prognostic value in esophageal squamous cell carcinoma patients in unified stages of curability. *Am J Surg* 1999;177:497–502.

378. Louie DC, Offit K, Jaslow R, Parsa NZ, Murty VV, Schluger A, Chaganti RS. p53 overexpression as a marker of poor prognosis in mantle cell lymphomas with t(11;14) (q13;q32). *Blood* 1995;86:2892–2899.

379. Xiong Y, Zhang H, Beach D. Subunit rearrangement of the cyclin-dependent kinase is associated with cellular transformation. *Genes Dev* 1993;7:1572–1583.

380. Sui L, Dong Y, Ohno M, Goto M, Inohara T, Sugimoto K, et al. Inverse Expression of Cdk4 and p16 in Epithelial Ovarian Tumors. *Gynecol Oncol* 2000;79:230–237.

381. Aas T, Borresen AL, Geisler S, Smith-Sorensen B, Johnsen H, Varhaug JE, et al. Specific P53 mutations are associated with de novo resistance to doxorubicin in breast cancer patients. *Nat Med* 1996;2:811–814.

382. Righetti SC, Della Torre G, Pilotti S, Menard S, Ottone F, Colnaghi MI, et al. A comparative study of p53 gene mutations, protein accumulation, and response to cisplatin-based chemotherapy in advanced ovarian carcinoma. *Cancer Res* 1996;56:689–693.

383. Rusch V, Klimstra D, Venkatraman E, Oliver J, Martini N, Gralla R, et al. Aberrant p53 expression predicts clinical resistance to cisplatin-based chemotherapy in locally advanced non-small cell lung cancer. *Cancer Res* 1995;55:5038–5042.

384. Blagosklonny MV, el-Deiry WS. Acute overexpression of wt p53 facilitates anticancer drug-induced death of cancer and normal cells. *Int J Cancer* 1998;75:933–940.

385. Bergers E, Jannink I, Van Diest PJ, Baak JPA. Influence of fixation delay on mitotic activity and flow cytometric %S-phase. *Hum Pathol* 1997;28:95–100.

386. Van Diest PJ, Baak JPA, Matze-Cok P, Wisse-Brekelmans ECM, Galen CM van, Kurver PHJ, et al. Reproducibility of mitosis counting in 2469 breast cancer specimens: results from the Multicenter Morphometric Mammary Carcinoma Project. *Hum Pathol* 1992; 23:603–607.

387. Jannink I, Van Diest PJ, Baak JPA. Comparison of the prognostic value of Mitotic Activity Index (MAI), random MAI (rMAI), M/V-index, and random M/V-index (rM/V-index) in breast cancer patients. *Hum Pathol* 1995;26:1086–1092.

388. Jannink I, Van Diest PJ, Baak JPA. Comparison of the prognostic value of mitotic frequency and mitotic activity index in breast cancer. *Breast* 1996;5:31–36.

389. Jannink I, Risberg B, Van Diest PJ, Baak JPA. Heterogeneity of mitoses counting in breast cancer. *Histopathology* 1996;29:421–428.

390. Michaelides R, van Tinteren H, Balkenende A, et al. Cyclin A is a prognostic indicator in early stage breast cancer with and without tamoxifen treatment. *Br J Cancer* 2002;86: 402–408.

10 Cell Cycle Regulators as Targets of Anticancer Therapy

Mikhail V. Blagosklonny, MD, PhD

CONTENTS

INTRODUCTION
CELL CYCLE AND GROWTH FACTORS
TARGETING SIGNAL TRANSDUCTION
TARGETING CDKs
REFERENCES

1. INTRODUCTION

In recent years, dramatic progress has been made in our understanding of the cell cycle regulation and signal transduction, thus facilitating the development of mechanism-based therapeutics. Compounds are becoming available that target almost every key regulator that governs the entry into S phase and mitosis: from growth factors to cyclin-dependent kinases. Given the increasing number of experimental therapeutic compounds, I will limit the discussion to those therapeutic agents that are undergoing at least Phase I clinical evaluation.

Semi-paradoxically, standard chemotherapy also targets cell cycle regulators. For example, DNA damaging drugs induce p53, which in turn trans-activates p21, an inhibitor of cyclin dependent kinase 2 (CDK 2) and cdc2. The former kinase is required for the entry into S phase and cdc2 is required for the onset of mitosis. DNA-damaging drugs also activate pathways leading to degradation and downregulation of cyclin D1 (1). In addition, DNA-damage-activated Chk1 kinase results in inhibition of cyclin B/cdc 2. Similarly, microtubule-active drugs such as paclitaxel (Taxol) or the Vinca alkaloids activate mitotic checkpoint and affect numerous cell cycle regulators. Standard chemotherapy affects these regulators indirectly and has many other cytotoxic effects, precluding precise targeting of cell cycle regulators.

From: *Cancer Drug Discovery and Development:*
Cell Cycle Inhibitors in Cancer Therapy: Current Strategies
Edited by: A. Giordano and K. J. Soprano © Humana Press Inc., Totowa, NJ

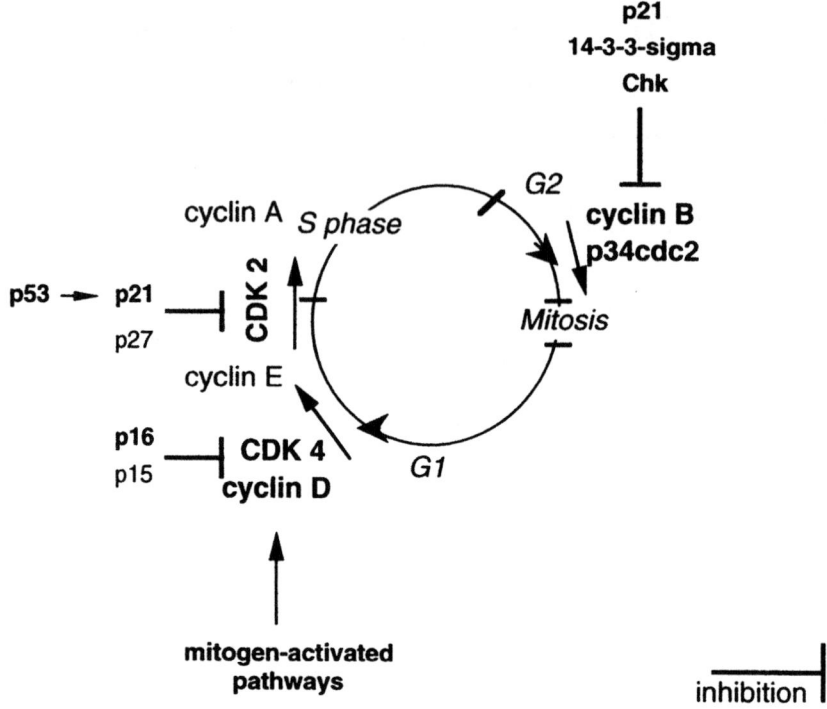

Fig. 1. Cell cycle regulators as drug targets.

2. CELL CYCLE AND GROWTH FACTORS

The cell cycle is driven by the cyclins, unstable proteins that activate cyclin-dependent kinases (CDK) *(2)*. As cells proceed through the cycle, four major cyclins are produced sequentially (D, E, A, and B), and they activate corresponding CDKs. The three D cyclins (cyclin D_1, D_2, D_3) and cyclin E drive cells into S-phase by activating kinases: CDK-2, -4, and -6. Progression through S phase requires cyclin A *(3,4)*. After completion of DNA synthesis, cells enter G_2 phase in preparation for mitosis. Cyclin B accumulates, translocates into the nucleus, and activates p34cdc2 kinase. B-type cyclins associate with p34cdc2 to trigger entry into mitosis. At the onset of mitosis, cyclin B/cdc2 phosphorylates laminin, a nuclear membrane protein, thus dissolving the nuclear envelope, and causes condensation of chromosomes.

Growth factors are necessary to initiate and maintain the transition through G_1 phase of the cell cycle toward S phase. In normal cells, withdrawal of growth factors prevents the initiation of S phase. The point at G_1 at which commitment occurs and the cell no longer requires growth factors to complete the cell cycle has been termed the restriction point *(5)*.

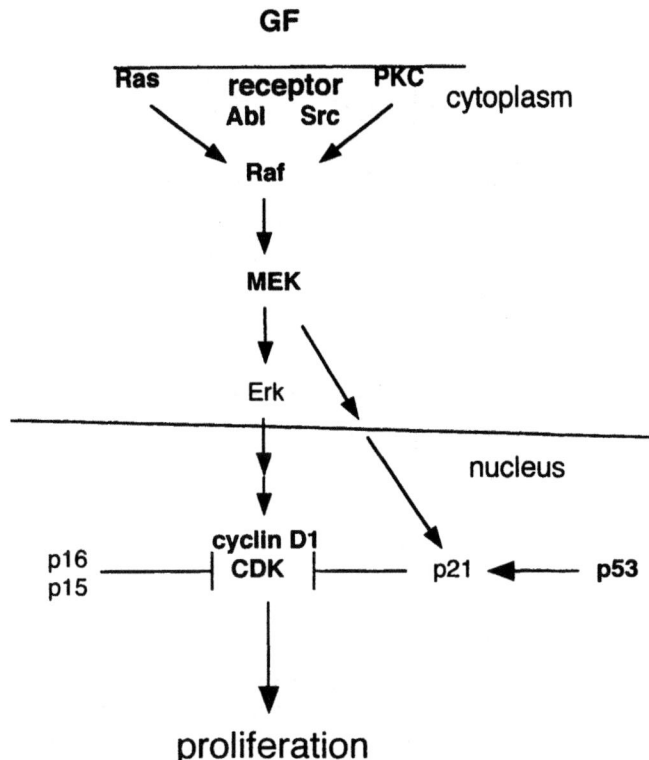

Fig. 2. From growth signaling to cell proliferation. In bold: potential therapeutic targets.

Growth factors activate their receptors and other tyrosine kinases, Ras and related proteins, mitogen activated pathways culminating in transcriptional induction of numerous genes, including cyclin D *(6–8)*. Therefore, cyclins D are growth-factor sensors (Fig. 1). In other words, growth factor-dependent progression through G_1 phase is mediated by induction of the cyclins D. Growth factors regulate cyclin D_1 by several mechanisms: 1) transcriptional induction of cyclin D_1 by growth factors that is dependent on the Ras/Raf-1/Mek/ERK pathway *(3,9–12)*. 2) Stabilization and accumulation of the cyclin D protein. In the absence of growth factor signaling, cyclin D_1 is rapidly degraded by the proteasome. The pathway that sequentially involves Ras, phosphatidylinositol-3-OH kinase (PI3K), and protein kinase B (Akt) prevented degradation of cyclin D_1 *(13,14)*. 3) Translocation of cyclin D to the nucleus and assemble with their catalytic partners, CDK-4 and CDK-6 *(15)*.

Receptors of growth factors, which extracellular domains bind growth factors, are located on the cellular membrane. Once activated by growth factors, they transduce the proliferative signal through a network of mitogen activated kinases (Fig. 2). The mitogen-activated protein kinase (MAPK) superfamily is currently

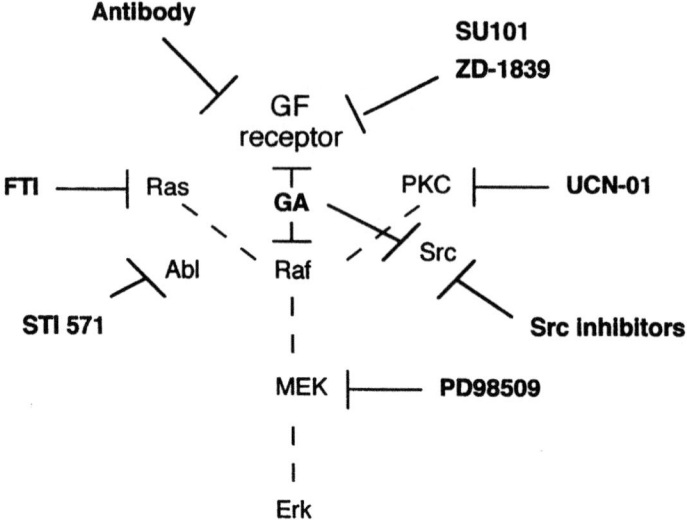

Fig. 3. Targeting growth signaling pathways. In bold: molecular therapeutics.

comprised of three pathways, including classical MAPK, also called ERK, stress activated protein kinases, known as JNK, and osmotic shock-regulated kinase, or p38 *(16)*. The classical MAPK module consists of three sequentially acting protein kinases, Raf-1, MEK, and ERK (Extracellular Ligand Regulated Kinases). Raf-1 kinase has a central role in regulating proliferation, differentiation, and apoptosis. Raf-1 is downstream of Ras, and tyrosine kinases, such as Src and Abl. Protein kinase C (PKC) activates Raf-1 by direct phosphorylation, which requires formation of Ras-Raf complexes *(17)*. The activation of mitogen-activated pathways results in accumulation of cyclin D and activation of CDK-4 and CDK-6.

Autocrine secretion of growth factors (platelet-derived growth factor [PDGF]/ sis, insulin-like growing factor [IGF], epithelial growth factor [EGF], transforming growth factor-α [TGF-α]), overexpression of their receptors, activation of the Ras protooncoprotein by mutations, and overactivation of mitogenic kinases (Src, Raf, Abl, etc.) are hallmarks of cancer *(7)*. Therefore, they are appealing targets of novel experimental therapeutics (Fig. 3).

3. TARGETING SIGNAL TRANSDUCTION

3.1. Inhibitors of Growth Factors and Their Receptors

3.1.1. SURAMIN

Suramin, a synthetic polysulfonated anionic compound, abrogates the activity of a variety of growth factors and is the first drug shown to exert its anticancer activity by blocking autocrine loops involved in malignant transformation *(18)*. Multiple potential mechanisms of action of suramin against tumors, including the ability to bind growth factors that are necessary for tumor angiogenesis, were also suggested. Outpatient treatment with suramin plus hydrocortisone is tolerated and provides moderate palliative benefit and delay in disease progression for patients with symptomatic hormone-refractory prostate cancer *(19)*. However, no objective tumor responses were observed in some other clinical trials *(20)*.

3.1.2. ANTIBODIES AGAINST GF RECEPTORS

Monoclonal antibodies (MAbs) against the extracellular domain of HER-2 and EGF receptors were developed and show effects in breast cancer patients *(21,22)*. HER-2 expression is unregulated and activated in 25–30% of human breast cancers. Overexpression of HER-2 generally correlates with the severity of the disease. Trastuzumab, a MAb, is directed against the extracellular domain of HER-2 *(23)*. This drug is indicated primary to patients whose tumor samples overexpress HER-2. Binding of MAb to HER-2 causes internalization and degradation of HER-2 is associated with upregulation of the CDK inhibitor p27. In addition, trastuzumab may induce immune cell-mediated cytotoxicity against target cells. C225, a human/mouse chimeric antibody *(22)*, and E7.6.3, a fully human antibody, have also been developed against the EGF receptor. They prevent binding EGF to its receptor, and cause tumor regression in mouse xenograft tumor assays. In preliminary trial results, complete responses were noted in head and neck cancers when C225 was combined with radiotherapy. Antibodies against either EGF receptor or HER-2 receptor appears to be especially effective in combination with doxorubicin, paclitaxel (Taxol), or docetaxel *(22,24)*. The mechanism of the synergy between anti-GF receptor antibodies and chemotherapy is unclear. In theory, we would expect rather an antagonism. Thus, if inhibition of EGF signaling causes growth arrest, such cells would be protected against cell cycle-dependent chemotherapy with paclitaxel. The most reasonable explanation is that paclitaxel and antibodies each target different subpopulations of cancer cells. Cells that are resistant to Taxol are sensitive to anti-HER-2 and vice versa. The combination of trastuzumab with doxorubicin has higher cardiotoxicity *(25)*. Cardiomyopathy caused by trastuzumab may be explained taking into account that myocardial cells express HER-3 and HER-2 receptors.

Anti-HER-2 MAb was used to deliver geldanamycin, an experimental therapeutic that depletes HER-2, by coupling geldanamycin to this MAb *(26)*. This could enhance the capacity of the antibody to downregulate HER-2 and also to avoid site effects of geldanamycin *(27)*.

3.1.3. INHIBITORS OF RECEPTOR KINASES

Several human tumors, including gliomas and breast carcinomas, strongly express receptor to PDGF *(28)*. SU101 inhibits the receptor PDGF-R/Flk-1 family of receptor tyrosine kinases *(29)*. SU101 decreased PDGF-stimulated proliferation and delayed tumor growth in mice. It is important to emphasize that SU101 possesses one additional mechanism of action in vivo. The major metabolite of SU101 is an inhibitor of dihydro-orotate dehydrogenase, thus blocking *de novo* pyrimidine synthesis. This mechanism of action, similar to antimetabolites may also contribute to the antiproliferative activity of SU101. In a Phase I study, SU101 was administered as a 24-h infusion weekly *(30)*. A maximum-tolerated dose was not reached because the large fluid volume required for administration of the drug prevented escalation to dose-limiting toxicity. An objective response was observed in a patient with malignant glioma, a tumor type characterized by high levels of PDGFβ-receptor. SU-101 is currently in Phase II development for treating glioblastomas.

The EGF receptor is also the target for the development of inhibitors of the intracellular tyrosine kinase domain *(31)*. In addition to growth arrest, inhibitors of EGF tyrosine kinase can induce apoptosis *(32,33)*. Competitive inhibitors of ATP binding to the receptor (ZD-1839 and CP-358,774) are currently in clinical trials *(31)*. According their mechanism of action, the dermatological toxicity was observed. Also irreversible inhibitors of the EGF receptor kinase have been developed (PD-168,393).

3.1.4. INHIBITORS OF RAS

Mutations in the Ras oncogene occur very frequently in a number of human cancers. Mutated forms of Kirsten-ras (K-Ras) and N-Ras are found in solid tumors (lung, colon, pancreas, and brain) and leukemias, whereas mutant Harvey-ras (H-Ras) alleles are found in only a small subset of bladder, head, and neck tumors *(6)*. Ras proteins carry an essential lipid moiety—a farnesyl group—at their C-termini. Inhibition of Ras farnesylation blocks Ras localization to the plasma membrane. Farnesyltransferase, an enzyme that catalyzes the first step in the posttranslational modification of Ras and a number of other polypeptides therefore can be an important target for the development of anticancer agents.

Potent farnesyltransferase inhibitors (FTI) were developed. These compounds prevented Ras localization on the cellular membrane, and therefore affect tumor growth. They have demonstrated significant antitumor activity against experimental models of human cancer. Treatment of five different human pancreatic cancer cell lines with FTI such as L-744,832 resulted in accumulation of cells G_2/M with high levels of cyclin B1/cdc2 kinase activity *(34)*. This indicates that cell cycle arrest is downstream from the DNA damage-inducible G_2/M cell cycle checkpoint. In addition, sensitive cell lines undergo apoptosis *(34)*, cell death mediated by caspases *(35,36)*. The effects of FTIs were associated with changes in posttranslational processing of H-Ras an N-Ras, but not K-Ras *(34)*. It should be noted that K-Ras is the Ras gene most frequently mutated in human cancers thus limiting usefulness of FTIs. Treatment of K-Ras transgenic mice with

L-744,832 caused inhibition of tumor growth in the absence of systemic toxicity *(37)*. Although FTase activity was inhibited in tumors from the treated mice, unprocessed K-Ras was not detected. Even though the FTI L-744,832 can inhibit tumor growth in this model, K-Ras may not be the sole mediator of the biological effects of the FTI *(37)*.

We can reach several conclusions: 1) The similar effects of structurally distinct FTIs indicates that anti-tumor activity by inhibiting FT (as intended); and 2) FTIs were originally expected to induce growth arrest rather than cell death. However, FTIs induce apoptosis in cancer cells *(34,38,39)*. FTIs are not Ras-specific inhibitors because the transferase reaction is essential not only to the function of Ras, but also to the function of at least several dozens other farnesyl proteins *(40)*.

Several different FTIs are currently undergoing evaluation administered either orally or intravenously *(41)*. The doses achieved in the clinic with L-778,123 and SCH 66336 were sufficient to inhibit protein farnesylation in white blood cells and cells of the buccal mucosa. Dose-limiting toxicities involving bone marrow and the gastrointestinal tract, indicating that FTIs inhibit proliferation and/or survival of normal proliferating cells. Following treatment with SCH66336, partial response was observed in a patient with previously treated metastatic non-small cell lung cancer (NSCLC), who remained in the study for 14 mo *(42)*. A highly potent and selective novel class of nonthiol-containing peptidomimetics inhibits human tumor growth in whole animals. Their combinations with cytotoxic agents is more beneficial than monotherapy *(43)*.

Importantly that FTI may exert anti-Ras activities in the absence of mutations in Ras gene. Although 25% of human cancers harbor oncogenic Ras mutations, such mutations are not found in astrocytomas. The activation of receptor tyrosine kinases in malignant human astrocytoma cells results in functional upregulation of the Ras signaling pathway and increased levels of activated Ras *(38)*. The FTI L-744,832 demonstrates both cytostatic and cytotoxic effects on astrocytoma cells, and cells expressing a truncated EGF receptor common in high-grade astrocytomas demonstrate increased sensitivity to the agent *(38)*. Finally, angiogenesis in astrocytomas has been shown to be dependent on secretion of vacular endothelial growth factor (VEGF) by tumor cells. L-744,832 potently inhibits the secretion of VEGF under hypoxic conditions. These combinations of mechanisms suggest that these tumors, despite the absence of oncogenic Ras mutations, will be amenable to growth inhibition by FTIs, through a combination of anti-proliferative, pro-apoptotic, and anti-angiogenic effects *(38)*.

3.1.5. INHIBITORS OF MEK

In the mitogen-activated pathway, MEK phosphorylates and activates ERKs (Fig. 1). Constitutive activation of ERKs has been observed in 50 tumor cell lines (36%) in tissue-specific manner: cell lines derived from pancreas, colon, lung, ovary, and kidney showed a high degree of ERK activation, while those derived from brain, esophagus, stomach, liver, and of hematopoietic origin showed low degree of ERK activation *(44)*. ERKs were constitutively activated in primary human tumors derived from kidney, colon, and lung tissues, but not from liver tissue. The activation of ERKs was completely associated with the activation of MEK, indicating that this activation is a result of the upstream signaling *(44)*.

Inhibitors of MEK suppress tumor cell growth in mouse models *(45)*. MEK inhibitors such as PD098059 are designed to exert cytostatic or preferably cytotoxic activity. This inhibition was demonstrated in normal fibroblasts and cells transformed by oncogenes whose activity strictly depends on MEK *(46)*. Although the MAPK pathway is essential for normal proliferation, PD 098509 does not arrest growth of some cancer cell lines such as A431 cancer cells *(47)*. Given that tumor cells can cycle in the absence of normal mitogen stimuli, limited inhibi-tion of MEK can be considered for the selective arrest of normal cells for the protection of normal cells against cell cycle-dependent chemotherapy *(48)*.

3.1.6. INHIBITORS OF BCR-ABL

The median survival in after the onset of blast crisis chronic myelogenous leukemia (CML) is about 3–5 mo *(49)*. CML is characterized by a reciprocal 9:22 chromosomal translocation, known as the Philadelphia chromosome (Ph), which fuses the truncated Bcr gene to the truncated c-Abl kinase *(50)*. A fusion gene, Bcr-Abl, encodes a chimeric protein, p210BCR-ABL. This fusion protein is a constitutively active protein tyrosine kinase that induces growth factor independence and leukemogenesis *(51)*. The Ph chromosome translocation may give rise to different BCR/ABL fusion proteins including p190, which is associated with lymphoblastic leukemia *(52)*. The expression of the BCR-ABL chimeric gene prevents apoptosis in response to a variety of anticancer agents including high-dose Ara C, etoposide, paclitaxel, actinomycin D, staurosporine, and proteasome inhibitors. In contrast, Abl kinase inhibitors cause selective apoptosis in Bcr-Abl expressing cells. Also Abl kinase inhibitors have been shown to increase the sensitivity of Bcr-Abl expressing cells to chemotherapeutic agents *(53–65)*. STI 571, an inhibitor of the Abl kinase, has demonstrated high efficacy in the treatment of Ph (+) CML *(65)*.

3.1.7. INHIBITORS OF HSP90

A number of protein kinases, including Raf-1, p60v-src, and p185ErbB-2, Akt, CDK-4, p210Bcr-Abl depends upon the chaperone protein heat-shock protein 90 (Hsp90) for proper function and stability *(66–68)*. The benzoquinone ansamycin geldanamycin (GA) and the macrocyclic antifungal antibiotic radicol bind to Hsp90 and specifically inhibit this chaperone's function, resulting in degradation of HSP90-associated proteins *(69)*. These unrelated compounds both bind to the N-terminal ATP/ADP-binding domain of Hsp90, and inhibit the inherent ATPase activity of Hsp90, which is essential for its function in vivo *(67,70,71)*. Also, Hsp90 participates in the achievement of the mutated conformation of mutant p53 that can be pharmacologically antagonized by drugs targeting Hsp90 *(72)*. Inhibition of Hsp90 leads to the depletion of mutant p53 but not wild-type p53 in breast, prostate, and leukemia cell lines *(73)*. Exposure to GA caused degradation of mutant p53 *(73)*. GA restored p53 polyubiquitination and degradation of mutant p53 by the proteasome *(74,75)*. A novel radicicol oxime derivative, radicicol 6-oxime (KF25706) competed with GA for binding to Hsp90 and showed potent antiproliferative activities against various human tumor cell lines and inhibited v-Src- and K-Ras-activated signaling *(68)*. In addition, Hsp90 family chaperone-associated proteins, ErbB-2, Raf-1, CDK-4, and mutant p53, were depleted by GA analogs and KF25706 at a doses comparable to that required for antiproliferative activity *(68,76)*. Depletion of the Bcr-Abl protein at doses of GA as low as 30 n*M* selectively induce apoptosis in Bcr-Abl positive cells and sensitized these cells to standard chemotherapy (Blagosklonny et al., submitted). Growth inhibitory effects of GA and its analogs including 17-allylamino,17-demethoxygeldanamycin (17AA-geldanamycin) depends on depletion of these proteins *(76,77)*. 17AA-geldanamycin is the first inhibitor of Hsp90 that enters a Phase I clinical trial in cancer.

4. TARGETING CDKS

4.1. Overview

The retinoblastoma protein (Rb) is a central regulatory protein in the G_1-to-S transition *(78)*. Inactivation of Rb through hyperphosphorylation by CDKs complexes such as cyclin D/CDK 4 and cyclin E/CDK 2 causes the release of the E2F transcription factor, which in turn controls the transcription of genes required for the G_1-to-S transition *(79,80)*. Conversely, hypo-phosphorylated forms of Rb bind to the E2F family of transcription factors preventing their action and, complexed to E2F, act as active transcriptional repressors preventing cell cycle progression *(81)*. Inappropriately activated E2F-1 triggers apoptosis in several tissues of Rb-deficient mice *(82)*. Oligopeptides that prevent interaction of cyclin A/cdk2 and E2F killed certain transformed but not normal cells *(83,84)*.

Inhibitors of CDKs can be subdivided into two groups: direct and indirect inhibitors. Direct inhibitors bind to CDK and inhibit their kinase activity. Indirect inhibitors induce endogenous proteins, inhibitors of CDK, such as p16, p21, p27, p57, or downregulate cyclins, usually cyclin D. Importantly that even direct inhibitors are partly inhibit CDKs by indirect mechanism. Thus, "direct" kinase inhibitors flavopiridol and UCN-01 also upregulate p21, p27, and downregulate cyclin D.

4.2. Direct Inhibitors

4.2.1. FLAVOPIRIDOL

Flavopiridol (L86-8275) is a semisynthetic flavonoid that binds to the ATP-binding pocket of the kinase and blocks both CDK-1, CDK-2, and CDK-4 *(85,86)*. Inhibition of CDK-4 is partially indirect because flavopiridol causes transcriptional repression of cyclin D1, preceding the inhibition of CD-4 activity *(87)*. High concentrations of flavopiridol (300–500 n*M*) induce apoptosis in most cancer cells regardless of tissue origin, including breast *(88)*, non-small cell lung *(89)*, esophageal cancer cells *(90)*, prostate cancer cells *(91)*, and leukemia cells *(92,93)*. Flavopiridol can induce apoptosis, with caspase-8 playing a key role. In human lung carcinoma cells, which lack procaspase-8, flavopiridol treatment leads to mitochondrial depolarization in the absence of cytochrome c release, followed by the activation of caspase-3 and cell death *(94)*.

Flavopiridol is currently undergoing clinical evaluation *(95)*. In the Phase I clinical trial, one patient with refractory renal cancer achieved a partial response, and plasma concentrations of 300–500 n*M* flavopiridol, which inhibit CDK activity in vitro, were safely achieved *(96)*. As a single agent, however, flavopiridol was ineffective in metastatic renal cancer in a recent Phase II trial *(97)*. Phase I and II clinical trials of flavopiridol have largely employed a 3-d continuous infusion of the drug every 14 d. In patients, flavopiridol does not cause significant hematologic toxicity, but it has also only occasionally produced cytotoxic tumor responses. In the case of lung cancer, although the nanomolar concentrations achieved in vivo are frequently at levels adequate for cell cycle arrest, they are below the levels required for apoptosis. New bolus dosing schedules are being explored with the hope of achieving higher steady-state levels.

The mitotic kinase p34cdc2 is very sensitive to flavopiridol *(98)*. Therefore, one would predict that flavopiridol will inhibit entry into mitosis and/or accelerate exit from mitosis, thus antagonizing the effects of taxanes. In fact, it has been reported that the pretreatment cells with flavopiridol prevented mitotic arrest and cytotoxicity caused by paclitaxel *(99)*, whereas administration of flavopiridol simultaneously or after paclitaxel increased the cytotoxicity of paclitaxel *(99)*.

Flavopiridol inhibits transcription *(100)*. Flavopiridol binds to duplex DNA and most closely resembles cytotoxic antineoplastic intercalators. Not surprisingly, the transcriptional inhibitor flavopiridol induces p53 *(100)*. Similarly, that may explain downregulation of cyclin D by flavopiridol.

Several new inhibitors have been generated from a small molecule library of substituted purines. This approach led to the discovery of purvalanol B, which is more potent than flavopiridol and which shows a high degree of selectivity for CDKs *(101)*. In addition to substituted purines and pyrimidines, other novel classes of cdk inhibitors have been reported, including those equipotent for

CDK-4, CDK-2, and cdc2, and those that demonstrate over 100-fold selectivity for CDK-4 *(102)*. Several of these compounds display high selectivity to CDKs.

4.2.2. UCN-01

UCN-01 (7-hydroxystaurosporine) UCN-01 was initially developed as a potent inhibitor of protein kinase C (PKC). At low doses (25 nM), UCN-01 is a relatively selective inhibitor of PKCa *(103–105)*. However, PKC is not likely to play a direct role in the growth arrest by UCN-01 *(106)*. UCN-01 also modulates other kinases, including CDKs and Chk1 kinase *(107–110)*. Inhibition of Chk1 results in indirect activation of cdc2 kinase *(110,111)*. UCN-01 causes p53-independent induction of p21 and p27, and it can cause reduction of CDK-4 expression levels with subsequent redistribution of p27 from CDK-4 to CDK-2 *(112,113)*. Staurosporine blocks cell progression through G_1 between the cyclin D and cyclin E restriction points, indicating CDKs as a potential target *(114)*. In human cells, G_1 arrest is most pronounced in cells expressing wild-type Rb. In non-small lung cancer cell lines, the sensitivity to UCN-01 correlated with their Rb status *(113)*. Regardless of Rb status, breast cancer cell lines could not be arrested by low doses of UCN-01 that arrested normal breast cells *(115)*. However, Rb status determined G_1 vs non-G_1 cell cycle arrest by high doses of UCN-01 *(115)*. Rb might be necessary but not sufficient for G_1 growth arrest by low doses of UCN-01. This dependence on Rb suggests that inhibition of CDK-4 may partially be the basis for its cytostatic activity.

UCN-01 is presently being evaluated in clinical trials *(116)*. UCN-01 at low doses selectively inhibits endothelial proliferation and angiogenic hypoxic response *(117)*. Inhibition of proliferation of endothelial cells by low doses of UCN-01 (10–30 nM) may be explained by inhibition of PKCa *(117)*. VEGF activates PKC-dependent, but Ras-independent, Raf-MEK-MAP kinase pathway for proliferation of endothelial cells *(118)*.

Following DNA damage, UCN-01 can abrogate the G_2 checkpoint, leading to mitotic catastrophe *(109,111,119)*. Thus, UCN-01 prevented G_2 arrest in cells lacking p53. It has been demonstrated that UCN-01 inhibits Chk1, and this inhibition occurs at low doses of UCN-01 *(110,120)*. Furthermore, this abrogation increases the toxicity of cytotoxic doses of DNA damaging drugs *(95,109,111)*. Certain cell lines demonstrated synergistic interactions with combinations of UCN-01 (20–150 nM) and thiotepa, mitomycin C, cisplatin, melphalan, topotecan, gemcitabine, fludarabine, or 5-FU *(121)*. UCN-01 combinations with paclitaxel and vincristine, or topoisomerase II inhibitors, adriamycin and etoposide, resulted in additive toxicity. Cells with mutant p53 were significantly more susceptible to the supra-additive effects of DNA-damaging agents and UCN-01 combinations, than cells expressing wt p53 *(121)*.

4.3. Indirect Inhibitors

4.3.1. ACTIVATORS OF PKC

PKC-mediated activation of the Raf-1/MAPK pathway may simultaneously induce cyclin D_1 and p21 *(122)*. Dramatic induction of p21 determines growth arrest caused by the PKC activator phorbol ester (PMA) PMA in a cell-type dependent manner. Leukemia blasts lacking p53 are especially sensitive to PMA-induced p21 *(123–125)*. Also, PMA induces growth arrest in SKBr3 breast cancer and LNCaP cancer cells *(126–130)*. Clinical applications of PMA were recently studied in leukemia. It was well-known for more than 20 years that PMA inhibits growth and induces differentiation of leukemia cells in vitro *(131,132)*. Even so, PMA has been reluctantly considered for clinical use due to its potential side effects, including a possible tumor-promoter activity. Recently, a remarkable potency of PMA in the treatment of refractory leukemia and its low toxicity for the patients has been demonstrated *(133,134)*.

4.3.2. DNA DAMAGING AGENTS

These numerous drugs are cornerstone of standard chemotherapy. DNA damage induce p53 and p21, which inhibits CDK-2 and cdc-2. DNA damage also downregulates cyclin D_1 and activates Chk1 in p53-independent mechanism. Wt p53 is induced by radiation (gamma-radiation, UV-light) and DNA damaging agents including clinically useful doxorubicin, daunomycin, etoposide, topotecan, actinomycin D, mitomycin C, bleomycin, cisplatin, carboplatin, cyclophosphamide, melphalan, chlorambucil, busulfan, ifosfamide, and the nitrosoureas. DNA strand breaks appear to be the most important lesion triggering elevation of p53 protein levels *(135,136)*. Antimetabolites such as 5-fluorouracil (5-FU), cytosine arabinoside (AraC), methotrexate, also cause p53 and p21 accumulation and p53-dependent arrest *(61,137–139)*.

4.3.3. PROTEASOME INHIBITORS

Proteasomal inhibitors block degradation of p53 and inhibitors of CDKs (p21, p27, p57) which are normally degraded by the proteasome *(140–145)*. Inhibitors of the proteasome cause rapid cell death *(61,143,145–147)*. The association between p53, p21, and p27 accumulation and apoptosis has led to the suggestion that apoptosis may depend on this accumulation *(143–145)*. However, wt p53, p21, and p27 appears to play no role in proteasome inhibitor-induced apoptosis, even though both wt p53 accumulation and apoptosis are caused by inhibition of the proteasome. Wt p53 is neither sufficient nor essential for apoptosis that is caused by proteasome inhibitors *(61)*. Thus, the accumulation of proteasome-degraded proteins such as p53, p21, and p27 is a marker of efficient inhibition of the proteasome, and therefore is tightly associated with apoptosis caused by proteasome inhibitors. Induction of wt p53 and apoptosis represent two independent markers of proteasome inhibition, although p53, p21, p27 may mediate growth arrest *(61,142)*. PS-341 is the most selective proteasomal inhibitor that is effective in nanomolar concentrations *(148,149)*. In animals, PS-341 inhibits the proteasome that results in reduced tumor growth. PS-341 is currently undergoing clinical trials *(148,149)*.

4.3.4. INHIBITORS OF HISTONE DEACETYLASE

Histone acetylation provides an enzymatic mechanism to regulate transcription by affecting the interaction between DNA and histones. Histone deacetylases (HDAC) is a class of enzymes consisting of at least two subfamilies with at least 7 members *(150)*. Several histone deacetylase (HDAC) inhibitors were studied as differentiating agents since 1978 *(151)*. For example, HDAC inhibitors synergize with retinoic acid to stimulate leukemia cell differentiation *(152–154)*. Different HDAC inhibitors including butyrate, trichostatin A (TSA), oxamflatin, and FR901228 upregulate p21 *(155–157)*.

FR901228, (NSC 630176, depsipeptide) a novel histone deacetylase inhibitor *(158)* is currently undergoing clinical trials (Sandor et al., submitted). The compound is cytotoxic at nanomolar concentrations in several in vitro and in vivo models *(159,160)*. Importantly, FR901228 caused G_1 arrest and cytotoxicity at nanomolar concentrations, thus showing at least 100,000-fold higher activity than butyrate. FR901228 downregulated cyclin D_1 and unregulated CDK inhibitor p21WAF1/CIP1, resulting in inhibition of CDK activity and Rb dephosphorylation and G_1 arrest *(161)*. Cells lacking p21 did not undergo G_1 arrest, continued DNA synthesis, and were arrested in G_2/M phase of the cell cycle *(161)*. The HDAC inhibitor oxamflatin increased expression of cyclin E and p21 and decreased expression of cyclin D_1 *(162)*. It has been reported that growth arrest by butyrate was mediated by p21 in HCT116 cells *(163)*. However, p21 induction was dispensable for G_1 arrest caused by butyrate in mouse fibroblasts *(157)*. In the later study, butyrate treatment decreased cyclin E.

When cyclin D_1 is downregulated and p21 is unregulated, CDKs are inhibited, resulting in Rb dephosphorylation. Dephosphorylated Rb complexed with E2F actively blocks cyclin E expression, thus preventing the next step of cell cycle progression *(81)*. The complex of dephosphorylated Rb and E2F associates with a histone deacetylase to effect transcriptional repression *(81,164–166)*. FR901228, by inhibiting histone deacetylase, may prevent cyclin E downregulation. FR901228 treatment resulted in a unique combination: increased p21 and cyclin E accompany decreased cyclin D_1 *(161)*. Following FR901228 treatment, increased p21 counterbalanced increased cyclin E in HCT116 cells, and G_1 arrest, which is initially triggered by downregulation of cyclin D_1, thus depends on p21 expression *(161)*. In contrast, p21 induction was dispensable for G_1 arrest by butyrate in MEF cells in which butyrate downregulated cyclin E *(157)*. Thus, the opposing effects on the levels of cyclin E may determine the requirement for p21 induction. Neither G_2/M arrest nor cytotoxicity of depsipeptide depends on p21 *(161)*.

4.3.5. Inhibitors of Methylation

Tumor suppressors such as p16 and p27 that are often silenced in cancer by DNA methylation *(167)*. The methylation of DNA is an epigenetic modification that can play an important role in the control of gene expression in mammalian cells *(168)*. The enzyme DNA methyltransferase modifies base that is found mostly at CpG sites in the genome.The potent and specific inhibitor of DNA methylation, 5-aza-2'-deoxycytidine (5-asa-CdR) has been demonstrated to reactivate the expression most of tumor-suppressor genes in human tumor cell lines *(168)*. 5-asa-CdR can slow the growth of tumor cells by reactivating growth-regulatory genes such as p16 silenced by *de novo* methylation *(169)*.

Densely methylated DNA associates with transcriptionally repressive chromatin characterized by the presence of deacetylated histones. Hypermethylated genes p15 and p16 cannot be transcriptionally reactivated with TSA (a HDAC inhibitor) alone in tumor cells in which TSA alone can upregulate the expression of nonmethylated genes. Following minimal demethylation and slight gene reactivation in the presence of low-dose 5-aza-2'deoxycytidine (5Aza-dC), however, TSA treatment results in robust re-expression of each gene. Thus, although DNA methylation and histone deacetylation appear to act as synergistic layers for the silencing of genes in cancer, dense CpG island methylation is dominant for the stable maintenance of a silent state at these loci *(170)*.

REFERENCES

1. Agami R, Bernards R. Distinct initiation and maintenance mechanisms cooperate to induce G1 cell cycle arrest in response to DNA damage. *Cell* 2000;102:55–66.
2. Koepp DM, Harper JW, Elledge SJ. How the cyclin became a cyclin: regulated proteolysis in the cell cycle. *Cell* 1999;97:431–434.
3. Sherr CJ. The Pezcoller lecture: cancer cell cycle revisited. *Cancer Res* 2000;60:3689–3695.
4. Sherr CJ, Roberts JM. CDK inhibitors: positive and negative regulators of G1-phase progression. *Genes Dev* 1999;13:1501–1512.
5. Pardee AB. A restriction point for control of normal animal cell proliferation. *Proc Natl Acad Sci USA* 1974;71:1286–1290.
6. Hunter T. Oncoprotein networks. *Cell* 1997;88:333–346.
7. Hanahan D, Weinberg RA. The hallmarks of cancer. *Cell* 2000;100:57–70.
8. Sherr CJ. Cancer cell cycles. *Science* 1999;274:1672–1677.
9. Filmus J, Robles AI, Shi W, Wong MJ, Colombo LL, Conti CJ. Induction of cyclin D1 overexpression by activated ras. *Oncogene* 1994;9:3627–3633.
10. Aktas H, Cai H, Cooper GM. Ras links growth factor signaling to the cell cycle machinery via regulation of cyclin D1 and the Cdk inhibitor p27KIP1. *Mol Cell Biol* 1997;17:3850–3857.
11. Winston JT, Coats SR, Wang YZ, Pledger WJ. Regulation of the cell cycle machinery by oncogenic ras. *Oncogene* 1996;12:127–134.
12. Surmacz E, Reiss K, Sell C, Baserga R. Cyclin D1 messenger RNA is inducible by platelet-derived growth factor in cultured fibroblasts. *Cancer Res* 1992;52:4522–4525.
13. Diehl JA, Zindy F, Sherr CJ. Inhibition of cyclin D1 phosphorylation on threonine-286 prevents its rapid degradation via the ubiquitin-proteasome pathway. *Genes Dev* 1997; 11:957–972.

14. Diehl JA, Cheng M, Roussel MF, Sherr CJ. Glycogen synthase kinase-3beta regulates cyclin D1 proteolysis and subcellular localization. *Genes Dev* 1998;12:3499–3511.
15. Cheng M, Sexl V, Sherr CJ, Roussel MF. Assembly of cyclin D-dependent kinase and titration of p27Kip1 regulated by mitogen-activated protein kinase kinase (MEK1). *Proc Natl Acad Sci USA* 1998;95:1091–1096.
16. Marshall CJ. Specificity of receptor tyrosine kinase signaling: transient versus sustained extracellular signal-regulated kinase activation. *Cell* 1995;80:179–185.
17. Marais R, Light Y, Mason C, Paterson H, Olson MF, Marshall CJ. Requirement of Ras GTP-Raf complexes for activation of Raf-1 by protein kinase C. *Science* 1998;280:109–112.
18. LaRocca RV, Cooper MR, Uhrich M, Danesi R, Walther MM, Linehan WM, Myers CE. Use of suramin in treatment of prostatic carcinoma refractory to conventional hormonal manipulation. *Urol Clin North Am* 1991;18:123–129.
19. Small EJ, Meyer M, Marshall ME, Reyno LM, Meyers FJ, Natale RB, et al. Suramin therapy for patients with symptomatic hormone refractory prostate cancer: results of a randomized phase III trial comparing suramin plus hydrocortisone to placebo plus hydrocortisone. *J Clin Oncol* 2000;18:1440–1450.
20. Gradishar WJ, Soff G, Liu J, Cisneros A, French S, Rademaker A, et al. A pilot trial of suramin in metastatic breast cancer to assess antiangiogenic activity in individual patients. *Oncology* 2000;58:324–333.
21. Baselga J, Tripathy D, Mendelsohn J, Baugman S, Benz CC, Dantis L, et al. Phase II study of weekly intravenous trastuzumab (Herceptin) in patients with HER2/neu-overexpressing metastatic breast cancer. *Semin Oncol* 1999;26:78–83.
22. Fan Z, Mendelsohn J. Therapeutic application of anti-growth factor receptors antibodies. *Curr Opin Oncol* 1998;10:67–73.
23. Goldenberg MM. Trastuzumab, a recommbinant DNA-derived humanized monoclonal antibody, a novel agent for the treatment of metastatic breast cancer. *Clin Ther* 1999; 21:309–318.
24. Burris HA. Docetaxel (Taxotere) in HER-2-positive patients and in combination with trastuzumab (Herceptin). *Semin Oncol* 2000;27 (2 Suppl 3):19–23.
25. Ewer MS, Gibbs HR, Swafford J, Benjamin RS. Cardiotoxicity in patients receiving trastuzumab (Herceptin): primary toxicity, synergistic or sequential stress, or surveillance artifact? *Semin Oncol* 1999;26:96–101.
26. Mandler R, Wu C, Sausville EA, Roettinger AJ, Newman DJ, Ho DK, et al. Immunoconjugates of geldanamycin and anti-HER2 monoclonal antibodies: antiproliferative activity on human breast carcinoma cell lines. *J Natl Cancer Inst* 2000;92:1573–1581.
27. Mendelsohn J. Use of an antibody to target geldanamycin. *J Natl Cancer Inst* 2000;92: 1549–1551.
28. Hermanson M, Funa K, Hartman M, Claesson-Welsh L, Heldin CH, Westermark B, Nister M. Platelet-derived growth factor and its receptors in human glioma tissue: expression of messenger RNA and protein suggests the presence of autocrine and paracrine loops. *Cancer Res* 1992;52:3213–3219.
29. Gibbs JB. Mechanism-based target identification and drug discovery in cancer. *Science* 2000;287:1969–1973.
30. Eckhardt SG, Rizzo J, Sweeney KR, Cropp G, Baker SD, Kraynak MA, et al. Phase I and pharmacologic study of the tyrosine kinase inhibitor SU101 in patients with advanced solid tumors. *J Clin Oncol* 1999;17:1095–1104.
31. Fry DW. Inhibition of the epidermal growth factor receptor family of tyrosine kinases as an approach to cancer chemotherapy: progression from reversible to irreversible inhibitors. *Pharmacol Ther* 1999;82:207–218.
32. Moyer JD, et al. Induction of apoptosis and cell cycle arrest by CP-358,774, an inhibitor of epidermal growth factor receptor tyrosine kinase. *Cancer Res* 1997;57:4838–4848.

33. Ciardiello F, Caputo R, Bianco R, Damiano V, Pomatico G, De Placido S, et al. Antitumor effect and potentiation of cytotoxic drugs activity in human cancer cells by ZD-1839 (Iressa), an epidermal growth factor receptor-selective tyrosine kinase inhibitor. *Clin Cancer Res* 2000;6:2053–2063.

34. Song SY, Meszoely IM, Coffey RJ, Pietenpol JA, Leach SD. K-Ras-independent effects of the farnesyl transferase inhibitor L-744,832 on cyclin B1/Cdc2 kinase activity, G2/M cell cycle progression and apoptosis in human pancreatic ductal adenocarcinoma cells. *Neoplasia* 2000;2:261–272.

35. Blagosklonny MV. Cell death beyond apoptosis. *Leukemia* 2000;14:1502–1508.

36. Fadeel B, Orrenius S, Zhivotovsky B. The most unkindest cut of all: on the multiple roles of mammalian caspases. *Leukemia* 2000;14:1514–1525.

37. Omer CA, Chen Z, Diehl RE, Conner MW, Chen HY, Trumbauer ME, et al. Mouse mammary tumor virus-Ki-rasB transgenic mice develop mammary carcinomas that can be growth-inhibited by a farnesyl:protein transferase inhibitor. *Cancer Res* 2000;60:2680–2688.

38. Feldkamp MM, Lau N, Guha A. Growth inhibition of astrocytoma cells by farnesyl trans-ferase inhibitors is mediated by a combination of anti-proliferative, pro-apoptotic and anti angiogenic effects. *Oncogene* 1999;18:7514–7526.

39. Suzuki N, Urano J, Tamanoi F. Farnesyltransferase inhibitors induce cytochrome c release and caspase 3 activation preferentially in transformed cells. *Proc Natl Acad Sci USA* 1998;95:15356–15361.

40. Oliff A. Farnesyltranssferase inhibitors: targeting the molecular basis of cancer. *Biochim Biophys Acta* 1999;1423:C19–C30.

41. Ferrante K, Winograd B, Canetta R. Promising new developments in cancer chemotherapy. *Cancer Chemother Pharmacol* 1999;43:61–68.

42. Adjei AA, Erlichman C, Davis JN, Cutler DL, Sloan JA, Marks RS, et al. A Phase I trial of the farnesyl transferase inhibitor SCH66336: evidence for biological and clinical activity. *Cancer Res* 2000;60:1871–1877.

43. Sun J, Blaskovich MA, Knowles D, Qian Y, Ohkanda J, Bailey RD, et al. Antitumor efficacy of a novel class of non-thiol-containing peptidomimetic inhibitors of farnesyltransferase and geranylgeranyltransferase I: combination therapy with the cytotoxic agents cisplatin, Taxol, and gemcitabine. *Cancer Res* 1999;59:4919–4926.

44. Hoshino R, Chatani Y, Yamori T, Tsuruo T, Oka H, Yoshida O, et al. Constitutive activation of the 41-/43-kDa mitogen-activated protein kinase signaling pathway in human tumors. *Oncogene* 1999;18:813–822.

45. Sebolt-Leopold JS, Dudley DT, Herrera R, Van Becelaere K, Wiland A, Gowan RC, et al. Blockade of the MAP kinase pathway suppresses growth of colon tumors in vivo. *Nat Med* 1999;5:810–816.

46. Dudley DT, Pang SJ, Decker AJ, Bridges AJ, Saltiel AR. A synthetic inhibitor of the mitogen-activated protein kinase cascade. *Proc Natl Acad Sci USA* 1995;92:7686–7689.

47. Busse D, Doughty RS, Ramsey TT, Russell WE, Price JO, Flanagan WM, et al. Reversible G1 arrest induced by inhibition of the epidermal growth factor receptor tyrosine kinase requires up-regulation of p27KIP1 independent of MAPK activity. *J Biol Chem* 2000; 275:6987–6995.

48. Blagosklonny MV, Bishop PC, Robey R, Fojo T, Bates S. Loss of cell cycle control allows for selective microtubule drug-induced Bcl-2 phosphorylation and cytotoxicity in highly autonomous cancer cells. *Cancer Res* 2000;60:3425–3428.

49. Sokal E, Baccarani M, Russo B, et al. Staging and prognosis in chronic myelogenous leuke-mia. *Semin Hematol* 1988;25:19–61.

50. Shtivelman EB, Lifshitz B, Gale RP, Canaani E. Fused transcript of abl and bcr genes in chronic myelogennnnous leukemia. *Nature* 1985;315:550–554.

51. Huettner CS, Zhang P, Van Etten RA, Tenen DG. Reversibility of acute B-cell leukaemia induced by BCR-ABL1. *Nature Genet* 2000;24:57–60.

52. Winter SS, Greene JM, McConnell TS, Willman CL. Pre-B acute lymphoblastic leukemia with b3a2 (p210) and e1a2 (p190) BCR-ABL fusion transcripts relapsing as chronic myelogenous leukemia with a less differentiated b3a2 (p210) clone. *Leukemia* 1999;13: 2007–2011.

53. Bedi A, Barber JP, Bedi GC, el-Deiry WS, Sidransky D, Vala MS, et al. BCR-ABL-mediated inhibition of apoptosis with delay of G2/M transition after DNA damage: a mechanism of resistance to multiple anticancer agents. *Blood* 1995;86:1148–1158.

54. Druker BJ, Tamura S, Buchdunger E, Ohno S, Gegal GM, Fanning S, et al. Effects of a selective inhibitor of the Abl tyrosine kinase on the growth of Bcr-Abl positive cells. *Nature Med* 1996;2:561–566.

55. Amarante-Mendes GP, McGahon AJ, Nishioka WK, Afar DE, Witte ON, Green DR. Bcl 2-independent Bcr-Abl-mediated resistance to apoptosis: protection is correlated with upregulation of Bcl-xL. *Oncogene* 1998;16:1383–1390.

56. Amarante-Mendes GP, Naekyung Kim C, Liu L, Huang Y, Perkins CL, Green DR, Bhalla K. Bcr-Abl exerts its antiapoptotic effect against diverse apoptotic stimuli through blockage of mitochondrial release of cytochrome C and activation of caspase-3. *Blood* 1998;91:1700–1705.

57. Dan S, Naito M, Tsuruo T. Selective induction of apoptosis in Philadelphia chromosome positive chronic myelogenous leukemia cells by an inhibitor of BCR - ABL tyrosine kinase, CGP 57148. *Cell Death Differ* 1998;5:710–715.

58. Dubrez L, Eymin B, Sordet O, Droin N, Turhan AG, Solary E. BCR-ABL delays apoptosis upstream of procaspase-3 activation. *Blood* 1998;91:2415–2422.

59. Horita M, Andreu EJ, Benito A, Arbona C, Sanz C, Benet I, et al. Blockade of the Bcr-Abl kinase activity induces apoptosis of chronic myelogenous leukemia cells by suppressing signal transducer and activator of transcription 5-dependent expression of Bcl xL. *J Exp Med* 2000;191:977–984.

60. Perkins C, Kim CN, Fang G, Bhalla KN. Arsenic induces apoptosis of multidrug-resistant human myeloid leukemia cells that express Bcr-Abl or overexpress MDR, MRP, Bcl-2, or Bcl-xL. *Blood* 2000;95:1014–1022.

61. An WG, Hwang SG, Trepel JB, Blagosklonny MV. Protease inhibitor-induced apoptosis: accumulation wt p53, p21WAF1/CIP1, and induction of apoptosis are independent markers of proteasome inhibition. *Leukemia* 2000;14:1276–1283.

62. Weisberg E, Griffin JD. Mechanism of resistance to the ABL tyrosine kinase inhibitor STI571 in BCR/ABL-transformed hematopoietic cell lines. *Blood* 2000;95:3498–3505.

63. Svingen PA, Tefferi A, Kottke TJ, Kaur G, Narayanan VL, Sausville EA, Kaufmann SH. Effect of the bcr/abl kinase inhibitors AG957 and NSC 680410 on chronic myelogenous leukemia cells in vitro. *Clin Cancer Res* 2000;6:237–249.

64. Dorsey JF, Jove R, Kraker AJ, Wu J. The pyrido[2,3-d]pyrimidine derivative PD180970 inhibits p210Bcr-Abl tyrosine kinase and induces apoptosis of K562 leukemic cells. *Cancer Res* 2000;60:3127–3131.

65. Druker BJ, Lydon NB. Lessons learned from the development of an abl tyrosine kinase inhibitor for chronic myelogenous leukemia. *J Clin Invest* 2000;105:3–7.

66. Whitesell L, Mimnaugh EG, De Costa B, Myers CE, Neckers LM. Inhibition of HSP90 pp60v-src heteroprotein complex formation by benzoquinone ansamycins: essential role for stress proteins in oncogenic transformation. *PNAS* 1994;91:8324–8328.

67. Neckers L, Schulte TW, Mimnaugh E. Geldanamycin as a potential anti-cancer agent: its molecular target and biochemical activity. *Invest New Drugs* 1999;17:361–373.

68. Soga S, Neckers LM, Schulte TW, Shiotsu Y, Akasaka K, Narumi H, et al. KF25706, a novel oxime derivative of radicicol, exhibits in vivo antitumor activity via selective depletion of Hsp90 binding signaling molecules. *Cancer Res* 1999;59:2931–2938.

69. Stebbins CE, Russo AA, Schnieder C, Rosen N, Hartl FU, Pavletich NP. Crystal structure of an Hsp90-geldanamycin complex: targeting of a protein chaperone by an antitumor agent. *Cell* 1997;89:239–250.

70. Grenert JP, Sullivan WP, Fadden P, Haystead TAJ, Clark J, Mimnaugh E, et al. The amino-terminal domain of heat shock protein 90 (hsp90) that binds geldanamycin is an ATP/ADP switch domain that regulates hsp90 conformation. *J Biol Chem* 1997;272:23843–23850.

71. Roe SM, Prodromou C, O'Brien R, Ladbury JE, Piper PW, Pearl LH. Structural basis for inhibition of the Hsp90 molecular chaperone by the antitumor antibiotics radicicol and geldanamycin. *J Med Chem* 1999;42:260–266.

72. Blagosklonny MV, Toretskey J, Bohen S, Neckers LM. Conformation of mutated p53 requires functional HSP90. *Proc Natl Acad Sci USA* 1996;93:8379–8383.

73. Blagosklonny MV, Toretskey J, Neckers LM. Geldanamycin selectively destabilizes and conformationally alters mutated p53. *Oncogene* 1995;11:933–939.

74. Whitesell L, Sutphin P, An WG, Schulte T, Blagosklonny MV, Neckers L. Geldanamycin-stimulated destabolization of mutated p53 is mediated by the proteasome in vivo. *Oncogene* 1997;14:2809–2816.

75. Nagata Y, Anan T, Yoshida T, Mizukami T, Taya Y, Fujiwara T, et al. The stabilization mechanism of mutant-type p53 by impaired ubiquitination: the loss of wild type p53 function and the hsp90 association. *Oncogene* 1999;18:6037–6049.

76. An WG, Schnur RC, Neckers LM, Blagosklonny MV. Depletion of ErbB2, Raf-1 and mutant p53 proteins by geldanamycin derivatives correlates with antiproliferative activity. *Cancer Chemother Pharmacol* 1997;40:60–64.

77. Schulte TW, Neckers LM. The benzoquinone ansamycin 17-allylamino-17 demethoxygeldanamycin binds to HSP90 and shares important biologic activities with geldanamycin. *Cancer Chemother Pharmacol* 1998;42:273–279.

78. Weinberg RA. The retinoblastoma protein and cell cycle control. *Cell* 1995;81:323–330.

79. DeGregori J, Leone G, Ohtani K, Miron A, Nevins J. E2F-1 accumulation bypasses a G1 arrest resulting from the inhibition of G1 cyclin-dependent kinase activity. *Genes Dev* 1995;9:2873–2887.

80. Nevins JR. Toward an understanding of the functional complexity of the E2F and retinoblastoma families. *Cell Growth Diff* 1998;9:585–593.

81. Zhang HS, Postigo AA, Dean DC. Active transcriptional repression by the Rb-E2F complex mediates G1 arrest triggered by p16INK4a, TGFbeta, and contact inhibition. *Cell* 1999;97:53–61.

82. Tsai KY, Hu Y, Macleod KF, Crowley D, Yamasaki L, Jacks T. Mutation of E2f-1 suppresses apoptosis and inappropriate S phase entry and extends survival of Rb-deficient mouse embryos. *Mol Cell* 1998;2:293–304.

83. Chen Y-NP, Sharma SK, Ramsey TM, Jiang L, Martin MS, Baker K, et al. Selective killing of transformed cells by cyclin/cyclin-dependent kinase 2 antagonists. *Proc Natl Acad. Sci USA* 1999;96:4325–4329.

84. Lees JA, Weinberg RA. Tossing monkey wrenches into the clock: new ways of treating cancer. *Proc Natl Acad Sci USA* 1999;96:4221–4223.

85. Carlson BA, Dubay MM, Sausville EA, Brizuela L, Worland PJ. Flavopiridol induces G1 arrest with inhibition of cyclin-dependent kinase (CDK) 2 and CDK 4 in human breast carcinoma cells. *Cancer Res* 1996;56:2973–2978.

86. Bible KC, Kaufmann SH. Flavopiridol: a cytotoxic flavone that induces cell death in noncycling A549 human lung carcinoma cells. *Cancer Res* 1996;56:4856–4861.

87. Carlson B, Iahusen T, Singh S, Loaiza-Perez A, Worland PJ, Pestell R, et al. Downregulation of cyclin D1 by transcriptional repression in MCF-7 human breast carcinoma cells induced by flavopiridol. *Cancer Res* 1998;59:4634–4641.

88. Li Y, Bhuiyan M, Alhasan S, Senderowitcz AM, Sarkar FH. Induction of apoptosis and inhibition of c-erbB-2 in breast cancer cells by flavopiridol. *Clin Cancer Res* 2000;6:223–229.

89. Shapiro GI, Koestner DA, Matranga CB, Rollins BJ. Flavopiridol induces cell cycle arrest and p53-independent apoptosis in non-small cell lung cancer cell lines. *Clin Cancer Res* 1999;5:2925–2938.

90. Schrump DS, Matthews W, Chen GA, Mixon A, Altorki NK. Flavopiridol mediates cell cycle arrest and apoptosis in esophageal cancer cells. *Clin Cancer Res* 1998;2885–2890.

91. Li Y, Chinni SR, Senderowicz AM, Sarkar FH. Induction of growth inhibition and apoptosis in prostate cancer cells by flavopiridol. *Int J Oncol* 2000;17:755–759.

92. Parker BW, Kaur G, Nieves-Neira W, Taimi M, Kohlhagen G, Shimizu T, et al. Early induction of apoptosis in hematopoietic cell lines after exposure to flavopiridol. *Blood* 1998;91:458–465.

93. Byrd JC, Shinn C, Waselenko JK, Fuchs EJ, Lehman TA, Nguyen FL, et al. Flavopiridol induces apoptosis in chronic lymphocytic leukemia cells via cativation of caspase-3 without evidence of bcl-2 modulation or dependence on functional p53. *Blood* 1998;92:3804–3816.

94. Achenbach T, Muller R, Slater EP. Bcl-2 independence of flavopiridol-induced apoptosis: mitochondrial depolarization in the absence of cytochrome c release. *J Biol Chem* 2000; 3289–3297.

95. Senderowicz AM, Sausville EA. Preclinical and clinical development of cyclin-dependent kinase modulators. *J Natl Cancer Inst* 2000;92:376–387.

96. Senderowicz AM, Headlee D, Stinson SF, Lush RM, Kalil N, Villalba L, et al. Phase I trial of continuous infusion flavopiridol, a novel cyclin-dependent kinase inhibitor, in patients with refractory neoplasms. *J Clin Oncol* 1998;16:2986–2999.

97. Stadler WM, Vogelzang NJ, Amato R, Sosman J, Taber D, Liebowitz D, Vokes EE. Flavopiridol, a novel cyclin-dependent kinase inhibitor, in metastatic renal cancer: a University of Chicago Phase II Consortium study. *J Clin Oncol* 2000;18:371–375.

98. Patel V, Senderowicz AM, Pinto DJ, Igishi T, Raffeld M, Quintanilla-Martinez L, et al. Flavopiridol, a novel cyclin-dependent kinase inhibitor, suppresses the growth of head and neck squamous cell carcinomas by inducing apoptosis. *J Clin Invest* 1998;102:1674–1681.

99. Motwani M, Delohery TM, Schwartz GK. Sequential dependent enhancement of caspase activation and apoptosis by flavopiridol on paclitaxel-treated human gastric and breast cancer cells. *Clin Cancer Res* 1999;5:1876–1883.

100. Bible KC, Bible RHJ, Kottke TJ, Svingen PA, Xu K, Pang YP, et al. Flavopiridol binds to duplex DNA. *Cancer Res* 2000;60:2419–2428.

101. Gray NS, Wodicka L, Thunnissen AM, Norman TC, Kwon S, Espinoza FH, et al. Exploiting chemical libraries, structure, and genomics in the search for kinase inhibitors. *Science* 1998;281:533–538.

102. Shapiro GI, Harper JW. Anticancer drug targets: cell cycle and checkpoint control. *J Clin Invest* 1999;104:1645–1653.

103. Takahashi I, Koboyashi E, Asana K, et al. UCN-01, a selective inhibitor of protein kinase C from streptomices. *J Antibiot* 1987;40:1782–1784.

104. Seynaeve CM, Kazanietz MG, Blumberg PM, Sausville EA, Worland PJ. Differential inhibition of protein kinase C isozymes by UCN-01, a staurosporine analogue. *Mol Pharmacol* 1994;45:1207–1214.

105. Mizuno K, Noda K, Ueda Y, Hanaki H, Saido TC, Ikuta T, et al. UCN-01, an anti-tumor drug, is a selective inhibitor of the conventional PKC subfamily. *FEBS Lett* 1995;359:259–261.

106. Courage C, Budworth J, Gescher A. Comparison of ability of protein kinase C inhibitors to arrest cell growth and to alter cellular protein kinase C localisation. *Br J Cancer* 1995;71:697–704.

107. Wang Q, Worland PJ, Clark JL, Carlson BA, Sausville EA. Apoptosis in 7 hydroxystaurosporine-treated T lymphoblasts correlates with activation of cyclin-dependent kinases 1 and 2. *Cell Growth Differ* 1995;6:927–936.

108. Courage C, Bradder SM, Jones T, Schultze-Mosgau MH, Gescher A. Characterisation of novel human lung carcinoma cell lines selected for resistance to anti-neoplastic analogous of staurosporine. *Int J Cancer* 1997;73:763–768.

109. Yu L, Orlandi L, Wang P, Orr MS, Senderowicz AM, Sausville EA, et al. UCN-01 abrogates G2 arrest through a Cdc2 dependent pathway that is associated with inactivation of the Wee1Hu kinase and activation of the Cdc25C phosphatase. *J Biol Chem* 1998;273: 33455–33464.

110. Graves PR, Yu L, Schwarz JK, Gales J, Sausville EA, O'Connor P, Piwnica-Worms H. The Chk1 protein kinase and the Cdc25C regulatory pathways are targets of the anticancer agent UCN-01. *J Biol Chem* 2000;275:5600–5605.

111. Wang Q, Fan S, Eastman A, Worland PR, Sausville EA, O'Connor PM. UCN-01, a potent abrogator of G2 checkpoint function in cancer cells with disrupted p53. *J Natl Cancer Inst* 1996;88:956–965.

112. Akiyama T, Yoshida T, Tsujita T, Shimizu M, Mizukami T, Okabe M, Akinaga S. G1 phase accumulation induced by UCN-01 is associated with dephosphorylation of Rb and CDK2 proteins as well as induction of CDK inhibitor p21/Cip1/WAF1/Sdi1 in p53-mutated human epidermoid carcinoma A431 cells. *Cancer Res* 1997;57:1495–1501.

113. Mack PC, Gandara DR, Bowen C, Edelman MJ, Paglieroni T, Schnier JB, et al. RB status as a determinant of response to UCN-01 in non-small cell lung carcinoma. *Clin Cancer Res* 1999;5:2596–2604.

114. Gong J, Traganos F, Darzynkiewicz Z. Staurosporine blocks cell progression through G1 between the cyclin D and cyclin E restriction points. *Cancer Res* 1994;54:3136–3139.

115. Chen X, Lowe M, Keyomarsi K. UCN-01-mediated G1 arrest in normal but not tumor breast cells is pRb-dependent and p53-independent. *Oncogene* 1999;18:5691–5702.

116. Sausville EA, Lush RD, Headlee D, Smith AC, Figg WD, Arbuck SG, et al. Clinical pharmacology of UCN-01: initial observations and comparison to preclinical models. *Cancer Chemother Pharmacol* 1998;42:S54–S59.

117. Kruger EA, Blagosklonny MV, Dixon SC, Figg WD. UCN-01, an inhibitor of protein kinase C, selectively inhibits endothelial proliferation and angiogenic hypoxic response. *Invas Metast* 1998–1999;18:209–218.

118. Takahashi T, Ueno H, Shibuya M. VEGF activates protein kinase C-dependent, but Ras independent Raf-MEK-MAP kinase pathway for DNA synthesis in primary endothelial cells. *Oncogene* 1999;18:2221–2230.

119. Jackson JR, Gilmartin A, Imburgia C, Winkler JD, Marshall LA, Roshak A. An indolocarbazole inhibitors of human checkpoint kinase (Chk1) abrogates cell cycle arrest caused by DNA damage. *Cancer Res* 2000;60:566–572.

120. Busby EC, Leistritz DF, Abraham RT, Karnitz LM, Sarkaria JN. The radiosensitizing agent 7-hydroxystaurosporine (UCN-01) inhibits the DNA damage checkpoint kinase hChk1. *Cancer Res* 2000;60:2108–2112.

121. Monks A, Harris ED, Vaigro-Wolff A, Hose CD, Connelly JW, Sausville EA. UCN-01 enhances the in vitro toxicity of clinical agents in human tumor cell lines. *Invest New Drugs* 2000;18:95–107.

122. Blagosklonny MV. A node between proliferation, apoptosis, and growth arrest. *BioEssays* 1999;21:704–709.

123. Steinman RA, Hoffman B, Iro A, Guillouf C, Liebermann DA, El-Houseini ME. Induction of p21 (WAF-1/CIP1) during differentiation. *Oncogene* 1994;9:3389–3396.

124. Zeng YX, El-Deiry WS. Regulation of p21WAF1/CIP1 expression by p53-independent pathways. *Oncogene* 1996;12:1557–1565.

125. Blagosklonny MV, Alvarez M, Fojo A, Neckers LM. Bcl-2 protein downregulation is not required for differentiation of multidrug resistant HL60 leukemia cells. *Leukemia Res* 1996;20:101–107.

126. Powell CT, Brittis NJ, Stec D, Hug H, Heston WD, Fair WR. Persistent membrane translocation of protein kinase C alpha during 12-O-tetradecanoylphorbol-13-acetate-induced apoptosis of LNCaP human prostate cancer cells. *Cell Growth Differ* 1996;7:419–428.

127. Blagosklonny MV. The mitogen-activated protein kinase pathway mediates growth arrest or E1A-dependent apoptosis in SKBr3 human breast cancer cells. *Int J Cancer* 1998;78:511–517.
128. Blagosklonny MV, Prabhu NS, El-Deiry WS. Defects in p21WAF1/CIP1, Rb, c-myc signaling in phorbol ester-resistant cancer cells. *Cancer Res* 1997;57:320–325.
129. Mitchell KO, El-Deiry WS. Overexpression of c-myc inhibits p21WAF1/CIP1 expression and induces S-phase entry in 12-O-tetradecanoylphorbol-13-acetate (TPA)-sensitive human cancer cells. *Cell Growth Differ* 1999;10:223–230.
130. Zhao X, Gschwend JE, Powell CT, Foster RG, Day KC, Day ML. Retinoblastoma protein-dependent growth signal conflict and caspase activity are required for protein kinase c signalled apoptosis of prostate epithelial cells. *J Biol Chem* 1997;272:22751–22757.
131. Huberman E, Callaham MF. Induction of terminal differentiation in human promyelocytic leukemia cells by tumor-promoting agents. *Proc Natl Acad Sci USA* 1979;76:1293–1297.
132. Rovera G, O'Brien TG, Diamond L. Induction of differentiation in human promyelocytic leukemia cells by tumor promoters. *Science* 1979;204:868–870.
133. Han ZT, Tong YK, He LM, Zhang Y, Sun JZ, Wang TY, et al. 12-O-tetradecanoylphorbol-13-acetate (TPA)-induced increase in depressed white blood cell counts in patients treated with cytotoxic cancer chemotherapeutic drugs. *Proc Natl Acad Sci USA* 1998;95:5362–5365.
134. Han ZT, Zhu XX, Yang RY, Sun JZ, Tian GF, Liu XJ, et al. Effect of intravenous infusions of 12-O-tetradecanoylphorbol-13-acetate (TPA) in patients with myelocytic leukemia: Preliminary studies on therapeutic efficacy and toxicity. *Proc Natl Acad Sci USA* 1998;95:5357–5361.
135. Kastan MB, Onyekwere O, Sidransky D, Vogelstein B, Craig RW. Participation of p53 protein in the cellular response to DNA damage. *Cancer Res* 1991;51:6304–6311.
136. Nelson WG, Kastan MB. DNA strand breaks: the DNA template alterations that trigger p53-dependent DNA damage response pathways. *Mol Cell Biol* 1994;14:1815–1823.
137. Linke SP, Clarkin KC, Di Leonardo A, Tsou A, Wahl GM. A reversible, p53-dependent G0/G1 cell cycle arrest induced by ribonucleotide depletion in the absence of detectable DNA damage. *Genes Dev* 1996;10:934–947.
138. Pritchard DM, Watson AJ, Potten CS, Jackman AL, Hickman JA. Inhibition by uridine but not thymidine of p53-dependent intestinal apoptosis initiated by 5-fluorouracil: evidence for the involvement of RNA perturbation. *Proc Natl Acad Sci USA* 1997;94:1795–1799.
139. Bunz F, Hwang PM, Torrance C, Waldman T, Zhang Y, Dillehay L, et al. Disruption of p53 in human cancer cells alters the responses to therapeutic agents. *J Clin Invest* 1999;104:263–269.
140. Pagano M, Tam SW, Theodoras AM, Beer-Romero P, Del-Sal G, Chau V, et al. Role of the ubiquitin-proteasome pathway in regulating abundance of the cyclin-dependent kinase inhibitor p27. *Science* 1995;269:682–685.
141. Maki CG, Huibregtse JM, Howley PM. In vivo ubiquitination and proteasome-mediated degradation of p53. *Cancer Res* 1996;56:2649–2654.
142. Blagosklonny MV, Wu GS, Omura S, El-Deiry WS. Proteasome-dependent regulation of p21WAF1/CIP1 expression. *Biochem Biophys Res Comm* 1996;227:564–569.
143. Shinohara K, Tomioka M, Nakano H, Tone S, Ito H, Kawashima S. Apoptosis induction resulting from proteasome inhibition. *Biochem J* 1996;317:385–388.
144. Lopes UG, Erhardt P, Yao R, Cooper GM. p53-dependent induction of apoptosis by proteasome inhibitors. *J Biol Chem* 1997;272:12893–12896.
145. Drexler HC. Activation of the cell death program by inhibition of proteasome function. *Proc Natl Acad Sci USA* 1997;94:855–860.
146. Chandra J, Niemer I, Gilbreath J, Kliche KO, Andreeff M, Freireich EJ, et al. Proteasome inhibitors induce apoptosis in glucocorticoid-resistant chronic lymphocytic leukemic lymphocytes. *Blood* 1998;92:4220–4229.
147. Fenteany G, Schreiber SL. Lactacystin, proteasome function, and cell fate. *J Biol Chem* 1998;273:8545–8548.

148. Adams J, Palombella VJ, Elliott PJ. Proteasome inhibition: a new strategy in cancer treatment. *Investig New Drugs* 2000;18:109–121.
149. Adams J, Palombella VJ, Sausville EA, Johnson J, Destree A, Lazarus DD, et al. Proteasome inhibitors: a novel class of potent and effective antitumor agents. *Cancer Res* 1999;59:2615–2622.
150. Weidle UH, Grossmann A. Inhibition of histone deacetylases: a new strategy to target epigenetic modifications for anticancer treatment. *Anticancer Res* 2000;20:1471–1485.
151. Candido EPM, Reeves R, Davie JR. Sodium butyrate inhibits histone deacetylation in cultured cells. *Cell* 1978;14:105–113.
152. Lin RJ, Nagy L, Inoue S, Shao W, Miller WH, Evans RM. Role of the histone deacetylase complex in acute promyelocytic leukemia. *Nature* 1998;391:811–814.
153. Grignani F, De Matteis S, Nervi C, Tomassoni L, Gelmetti V, Cioce M, et al. Fusion proteins of the retinoic acid receptor-alpha recruit histone deacetylase in promyelocytic leukemia. *Nature* 1998;391:815–818.
154. Kosugi H, Towatari M, Hatano S, Kitamura K, Kiyoi H, Kinoshita T, et al. Histone deacetylase inhibitors are the potent inducer/enhancer of differentiation in acute myeloid leukemia: a new approach to anti-leukemia therapy. *Leukemia* 1999;13:1316–1324.
155. Sowa Y, Orita T, Minamikawa S, Nakano K, Mizuno T, Nomura H, Sakai T. Histone deacetylase inhibitor activates the WAF1/Cip1 gene promoter through the SP1 sites. *Biocem Biophys Res Comm* 1997;241:142–150.
156. Rajgolikar G, Chan KK, Wang HC. Effects of a novel antitumor depsipeptide, FR901228, on human breast cancer cells. *Breast Cancer Res Treat* 1998;51:29–38.
157. Vaziri C, Stice L, Faller DV. Butyrate-induced G1 arrest results from p21-independent disruption of retinoblastoma protein-mediated signals. *Cell Growth Diff* 1998;9:465–474.
158. Nakajima H, Kim YB, Terano H, Yoshida M, Horinouchi S. FR901228, a potent antitumor antibiotic, is a novel histone deacetylase inhibitor. *Exp Cell Res* 1998;241:126–133.
159. Ueda H, Manda T, Matsumoto S, Mukumoto S, Nishigaki F, Kawamura I, Shimomura K. FR901228, a novel antitumor bicyclic depsipeptide produced by Chromobacterium violaceum No. 968. Antitumor activities on experimental tumors in mice. *J Antibiot* 1994;47:315–323.
160. Wang R, Brunner T, Zhang L, Shi Y. Fungal metabolite FR901228 inhibits c-Myc and Fas ligand expression. *Oncogene* 1998;17:1503–1508.
161. Sandor V, Senderowicz A, Mertins S, Sackett D, Sausville E, Blagosklonny MV, Bates SE. P21-dependent G1 arrest with downregulation of cyclin D1 and upregulation of cyclin E by the histone deacetylase inhibitor FR901228. *Br J Cancer* 2000;83:817–825.
162. Kim YB, Lee KH, Sugita K, Yoshida M, Horinouchi S. Oxamflatin is a novel antitumor compound that inhibits mammalian histone deacetylase. *Oncogene* 1999;18:2461–2470.
163. Archer SY, Meng S, Shei A, Hodin RA. p21WAF1 is required for butyrate-mediated growth inhibition of human colon cancer cells. *Proc Natl Acad Sci USA* 1998;95:6791–6796.
164. Luo RX, Postigo AA, Dean DC. Rb interacts with histone deacetylase to repress transcription. *Cell* 1998;92:463–473.
165. Brehm A, Miska EA, McCance DJ, Reid JL, Bannister AJ, Kouzarides T. Retinoblastoma protein recruits histone deacetylase to repress transcription. *Nature* 1998;391:597–601.
166. Magnaghi-Jaulin L, Groisman R, Naguibneva I, Robin P, Lorain S, Le Villain JP, et al. Retinoblastoma protein repress transcription by recruiting a histone deacetylase. *Nature* 1998;391:601–605.
167. Baylin SB, Herman JG, Graff JR, Vertino PM, Issa JP. Alterations in DNA methylation: a fundamental aspect of neoplasia. *Adv Cancer Res* 1998;72:141–196.
168. Momparler RL, Bovenzi V. DNA methylation and cancer. *J Cell Physiol* 2000;183:145–154.

169. Bender CM, Pao MM, Jones PA. Inhibition of DNA methylation by 5-aza-2' deoxycytidine suppresses the growth of human tumor cell lines. *Cancer Res* 1998;58:95–101.
170. Cameron EE, Bachman KE, Myohanen S, Herman JG, Baylin SB. Synergy of demethylation and histone deacetylase inhibition in the re-expression of genes silenced in cancer. *Nat Genet* 1999;21:103–107.

11 Mammalian CDK Inhibitors as Targets of Ubiquitinization in Cancer

Valeria Masciullo, MD, PhD,
Kenneth J. Soprano, PhD,
and Antonio Giordano, MD, PhD

CONTENTS

1. INTRODUCTION

Within the last 10 years, several studies have clearly demonstrated that disruption of cell cycle control is one of the most frequent alterations in tumor cells leading to uncontrolled cell proliferation and tumor development *(1)*. The commitment of eukaryotic cells to enter the DNA synthetic (S) phase of the cell cycle occurs at the so-called restriction point (R) late in G_1 phase and is governed by a series of proteins called cyclins, which function as positive regulatory subunits of a family of cyclin-dependent protein kinases (CDKs) *(2)*. Each cyclin binds to and activates specific CDKs thus controlling the progression of cells through the cell cycle. While CDKs are constitutively expressed with respect to cell cycle phases, cyclin levels oscillate, being regulated mainly at the transcriptional level but also by protein degradation via the ubiquitin proteasome pathway *(1)*. The

From: *Cancer Drug Discovery and Development:*
Cell Cycle Inhibitors in Cancer Therapy: Current Strategies
Edited by: A. Giordano and K. J. Soprano © Humana Press Inc., Totowa, NJ

activity of cyclin/CDK complexes is further regulated by both positive and negative phosphorylation events *(3)*, as well as their association with specific inhibitory proteins *(2)*.

2. THE CYCLIN-DEPENDENT KINASE INHIBITORS (CKIS)

The CDK inhibitors (CKI) identified in mammalian cells are classified into two major categories *(2)*: 1) the INK4 family includes p16^{INK4A} *(4)*, p15^{INK4B} *(5)*, p18^{INK4C} *(6)*, and p19^{INK4D} *(7)*, which bind to and specifically inhibit CDK4 and CDK6, thus preventing cyclin D association; 2) the CIP/Kip family includes p21^{Waf1} *(8)*, p27^{Kip1} *(9)*, and p57^{Kip2} *(10)*, which inhibit a broader range of CDKs by binding to several cyclin/CDK complexes essential for G$_1$ progression and S-phase entry.

2.1. The INK4 Family

Because of their specificity as inhibitors of CDK4 and CDK6, this group of protein was designated INK4. The activity of CDK4 in vivo is affected by cyclin D$_1$ and p16^{INK4A} that therefore regulate G$_1$-phase progression. In particular, p16^{INK4A}, by acting upstream of cyclin D-dependent kinases, is able to inhibit their phosphorylation of pRb. In fact, overexpression of p16^{INK4A} prevents proliferation in pRb-positive cells but is ineffective in pRb-negative cells, including Mouse Embryo Fibroblasts (MEFs) derived from Rb-nullizygous mice *(11)*. Overexpression of p16^{INK4A} also is able to induce G$_1$ arrest in various cancer cell lines *(12)*. However, its activity is strictly dependent on the presence of a functional pRb and in the absence of pRb function, overexpression of p16^{INK4A} or inhibition of cyclin D-dependent kinase does not affect G$_1$ progression. p16^{INK4A} is not only an inhibitor of the cyclinD/CDK4 complex but also can interfere with its assembly by replacing progressively D-type cyclins when it is overexpressed *(13)*.

p15^{INK4B} synthesis is induced in human epithelial cells by transforming growth factor-β (TGF-β) *(5)* and is expressed ubiquitously. p18^{INK4C} and p19^{INK4D} are also expressed in several proliferating cultured cells and normal mouse tissues *(6,7)* and rely on the presence of functional pRb to arrest cell cycle *(14)*. Despite sharing similar biochemical properties, INK4 family members are not redundant but appear to respond differentially to anti-proliferative signals, showing unique expression patterns dependent on cell tissue type and differentiation stage.

The tandemly linked INK4A and INK4B genes have been localized on the chromosomal region 9p21, an area frequently affected by frameshift, nonsensense, and missense mutations. Deletions and mutations involving INK4A occur in many different types of human cancer *(15,16)*. Deletions and hypermethylation of both INK4A and INK4B are significant in the development of certain types of tumors *(17,18)*.

The INK4C and INK4D loci map to chromosomes 1p32 and 19p13 and at present there is no certain evidence that the product of either gene acts as a tumor suppressor *(19)*.

2.2. The CIP/Kip Family

Induction of p21$^{Waf1/Cip1/Sdi1}$ in mammalian cells has revealed that it can act as a potent and universal inhibitor of cdk activity and is capable of inducing growth arrest, in different physiological situations. p21 is transiently induced in the course of replicative senescence, reversible and irreversible forms of damage-induced growth arrest, and terminal differentiation of postmitotic cells; its induction is regulated through p53-dependent and -independent mechanisms *(20)*. Ectopic overexpression of p21 leads to cell growth arrest in G_1 and G_2 *(21)* and is accompanied by phenotypic markers of senescence in many cells. Similarly, increases in p21 expression are associated with antiproliferative conditions, such as the TGF-β-induced inhibition of cell growth. However, recent studies have suggested that the stoichiometric ratio of p21 to the kinase subunits defines the role of p21. When the stoichiometric ratio is low, p21 facilitates kinase complex assembly and thus promotes kinase activation. At higher stoichiometric ratios, p21 serves as a kinase inhibitor and blocks cell-cycle progression *(22)*. In contrast, association of G_1 kinases with p27, another member of the Cip/Kip family of cyclin kinase inhibitors, always results in reductions in kinase activity and in the rate of proliferation, regardless of its stoichiometric ratio. Although p21 is not a transcription factor, it is conceivable that some of its functions may be mediated by indirect effects of p21 on cellular gene expression. Thus, CDK inhibition by p21 results in dephosphorylation of pRb and inhibition of E2F transcription factors that regulate many genes involved in DNA replication and cell-cycle progression *(23)*. Accordingly, p21 was shown to be involved in radiation-induced inhibition of several E2F-regulated genes. p21 interactions with proteins other than CDKs may also have a potential effect on gene expression. For example, p21 was reported to bind c-Jun amino-terminal kinases, apoptosis signal-regulating kinase 1, and Gadd45 *(24)*. Cell cycle arrest caused by enforced p21 expression do not trigger a suicide program and, on the other hand, p53-dependent apoptosis does not require p21-induced cell cycle arrest in G_1 *(25)*.

p27^{kip1} was first identified as an inhibitor of cyclin E-CDK2 complex *(26)*. Overexpression of p27 in cultured cells arrests the cell cycle. In general, p27 expression is highest in quiescent cells and declines as cells reenter the cell cycle. Many antiproliferative signals lead to p27 accumulation, including mitogen/cytokine withdrawal, cell-cell contact, and agents such as cAMP and rapamycin. The crystal structure of p27 bound to cyclin A-CDK2 revealed that p27 inserts itself deep within the CDK catalytic site, blocking ATP access. These data support a simple model in which antiproliferative stimuli upregulate p27, followed by tight CDK inhibition and cell cycle arrest. The key role of p27^{kip1} in regulating cell proliferation is reflected in the p27 knockout mouse, which exhibits gigantism (because of increased cell number), female sterility, and increased tumorigenesis (27,28). Multiple post-transcriptional mechanisms regulate p27 abundance. p27 may be degraded by the ubiquitin-proteasome system (see below) or by translational control. Increased p27 translation rates are found in arrested (G_0) vs growing cells, and the accumulation of p27 in G_0 cells may result largely from the increased association of p27 mRNA with polyribosomes (29). p27 is also regulated by phosphorylation, and phosphorylation of p27 by cyclin E-CDK2 leads to its turnover (see below). The relative contribution of proteolytic and translational control to p27 regulation in various physiologic contexts remains largely unknown. p27 expression and/or function may also be affected by dominantly acting oncogenes. Several groups have reported that c-*myc* overexpression overcomes a p27-mediated cell cycle arrest (30). Ras activity, either alone or in concert with c-*myc*, may also downregulate p27 (31). Interestingly, the adenovirus E1A protein, which functions like c-*myc* in some transformation assays, may also inactivate p27. The most recently proposed mechanism of p27 regulation is subcellular compartmentalization. p27 appears to interact with its targets in the cell nucleus, and mislocalization of p27 in the cytoplasm might inactivate p27 by sequestering it away from relevant cellular targets (32). In fact, cytoplasmic mislocalization of p27 has been reported in human tumors and cell lines (33). Genes that inhibit cell proliferation are excellent candidates for tumor-suppressor genes. Indeed, it has been demonstrated that p27 is haplo-insufficient for tumor suppression (34) and, although homozygous inactivation of the p27 gene is extremely rare (35), single allelic p27 loss has been observed in human primary tumors. The complex post-transcriptional regulation of p27 suggests that mechanisms other than direct mutation might downregulate p27 in tumor cells. This, in fact, seems to be the case and p27 expression has now been examined in many human tumors. Evidence that p27 may be involved in human tumor progression comes largely from studies that have directly measured the expression of p27 protein in clinical tumor samples by immunohistochemistry. The cumulative data from these studies indicate that low or absent p27 protein in tumor cells is an important clinical marker of disease progression in many malignancies. The number of tumor types that have been studied for expression of p27 has steadily increased and the data across types are strikingly consistent. The prognostic value of p27 protein expression will be specifically treated in another chapter.

The p57^{kip2} protein can inhibit the kinase activities of cyclin D-cdk4, D-cdk6, E-cdk2, E-cdk3, and A-cdk2 complexes in vitro and when transfected in SaOs2 osteosarcoma cell line (p53 and pRb-) induces G_1 arrest (36). Expression of p57^{kip2} is more tissue-restricted than the other Cip/Kip family members (36). It is highly expressed during mouse embryo development especially in tissues that do not actively proliferate. Its chromosomal localization is in a region, 11p15, that undergoes frequent deletions or rearrangements in many types of cancer such as Wilm's tumor *(37,38)*. According to these data, several investigations *(39,40)* support a role for p57^{kip2} as tumor-suppressor gene.

2.3. CKIs and the Retinoblastoma Family

The three members of the retinoblastoma gene family (pRb, pRb2/p130, and p107) are among the most well-characterized substrates of the cyclin/cdk complexes *(1)*. All members of the Rb family members are nuclear phosphoproteins that regulate G$_1$ progression, are implicated in various forms of differentiation, are regulated by phosphorylation, are growth-suppressive in a cell type-dependent manner, and are critical targets for inactivation by transforming oncoproteins of DNA tumor viruses *(41)*. Each of the Rb family proteins binds to and modulates the activity of the E2F family of transcription factors essential for transcription of genes needed to progress through the S phase. However, the timing of this regulation varies between Rb family members, and they each bind to distinct members of the E2F family *(42)*.

The Rb protein acts as a major gatekeeper at the restriction point, blocking further G$_1$ progression until all systems are prepared for proliferation. The transition from a hypophosphorylated form to a hyperphosphorylated form of pRb marks the end of G$_1$ phase control by pRb. Cyclin D/cdk4/6 complexes perform the main phosphorylation of pRb and they themselves are under negative regulation by CKIs. However, several studies have demonstrated either amplification of cyclin D genes, mutations in cdks inhibiting CKI binding or mutations in the CKI itself in tumor cells. Another function promoted by pRb is inhibition of DNA synthesis. p53 itself, is a well-described transcription factor which, in response to DNA damage, transactivate p21$^{waf1/cip1}$. Dependent on its stoichiometric abundance, p21 is necessary, in equimolar amounts, for the formation of active cyclin D/cdk4 complexes *(43)*. Therefore, one important pathway to arrest cells is to prevent G$_1$-S phase progression by inhibiting Rb phosphorylation at the restriction point (R). In support of the idea of a p53-p21-pRb-E2F pathway, there are several reports demonstrating that excess pRb can overcome p53-mediated apoptosis and that p53 mediated-growth arrest is converted to apoptosis by overexpression of E2F-1 *(44)*.

Major recent investigations have revealed many disturbances in tumor cells in what is now called the Rb/cyclin D$_1$/cdk4/p16 pathway *(45)*, characterized by the same end results. For example, irregular activation of E2F transcription factor is obtained by substituting events, such as overexpression of cyclin D$_1$ or cdk4, and by functional inactivation of pRb or p16. Each of these alterations can be due to different mechanisms, either affecting the gene directly, such as deletions and mutations in p16 and Rb, or chromosomal rearrangements of cyclin D$_1$ and cdk4; or affecting expression of the gene in the case of cyclin D$_1$

overexpression due to constitutive activation by signaling pathways from activated growth factor receptors. Expression of the CKI p16^{INK4D} is also under the control of E2F. This feedback mechanism ensures the turning off of cyclin D$_1$-cdk activity at the end of early G$_1$. p16 inhibits cyclin D$_1$/cdk4 activity by competitive binding to cdk4 at the same site where cdk4 binds to cyclin D$_1$. As a net result, overstimulation of E2F, such as the one following mutation of Rb, leads to enhanced expression of p16^{INK4D}, which replaces cyclin D$_1$ in the complex with cdk4. At this point cyclin D$_1$ becomes available for proteosomal degradation, which explains why tumor cells with mutations in pRb exhibit low expression of cyclin D$_1$.

Recently an investigation on the mechanism by which pRb induces senescence has demonstrated that pRb causes a post-transcriptional accumulation of the cyclin-dependent kinase inhibitor p27^{KIP1} that is accompanied by an increase in p27^{KIP1} specifically bound to cyclin E and a concomitant decrease in cyclin E-associated kinase activity. Moreover, the ability of pRb to mantain cell cycle arrest and induce senescence is reversibly abrogated by ablation of p27^{KIP1} expression, suggesting that prolonged cell cycle arrest through the persistent and specific inhibition of cdk2 activity by p27^{KIP1} is critical for pRb-induced senescence *(46)*.

In contrast, the pRb-related proteins p107 and pRb2/p130, which also decrease cyclin E-kinase activity, do not cause an accumulation of p27^{KIP1} and induce senescence poorly. pRb2/p130 and p107 family members, in contrast to pRb, are also able to stably bind to cyclin A/cdk2 or cyclin E/cdk2 complexes. Two research groups have shown that pRb2/p130 and p107 use p21 similar sequences to bind to and inhibit the activity of cyclin/cdk complexes.

Rb2/p130 in association with E2F-4 is the most abundant E2F complex found in resting or quiescent cells in G$_0$, and helps to maintain a state of transcriptional silence *(47)*. The stability of pRb2/p130 is mostly regulated by the 26S proteasome *(48)*. Recently, we found that induction of pRb2/p130 in vivo, by a tetracycline-regulated gene expression system, specifically inhibits cyclin A- and cyclin E-associated kinase activity and by doing so induces p27^{Kip1} levels, presumably by inhibiting p27^{Kip1}-targeted proteolysis by cyclin E-Cdk2 phosphorylation of p27^{Kip1}. This suggests that pRb2/p130 and p27^{Kip1} may cooperate in regulating cellular proliferation, and both may be involved in a negative feedback regulatory loop with cyclin E *(49)*. These data are consistent with another recent study *(50)* showing an increase of both p27-cyclin E and Rb2/p130-E2F4 complexes in CA-OV3 cells whose growth was arrested by retinoic acid.

Cyclins and CKI expression is regulated at multiple levels. Temporally regulated degradation of some cyclins and CKIs, such as p27^{kip1}, p21^{waf1}, p57^{kip2}, and p19^{INK4D}, is carried out by the ubiquitin-proteasome system, which therefore represents a critical mechanism by which a wide variety of mitogenic and antimitogenic signals regulates the cell cycle.

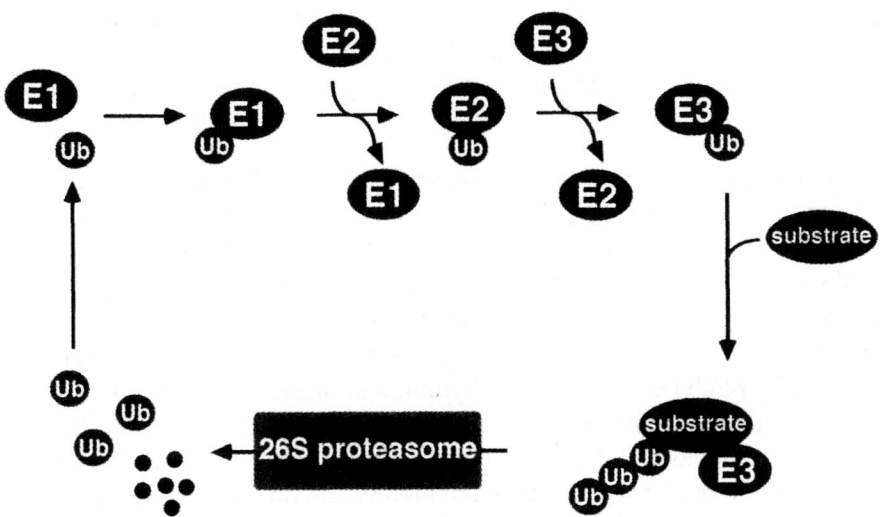

Fig. 1. The ubiquitin proteasome pathway. Degradation of a protein via the ubiquitin-proteasome pathway involves two fundamental steps: 1) generation of a polyubiquitin chain covalently conjugated to the protein substrate and 2) degradation of the tagged protein by the 26S proteasome.

3. THE UBIQUITIN PROTEASOME-MEDIATED PROTEOLYSIS

Proteolysis via the ubiquitin system is an important pathway of nonlysosomal protein degradation that controls fundamental cellular processes such as regulation of the cell cycle, differentiation, development, modulation of the immune and inflammatory response, regulation of cell surface receptors and ion channels, and DNA repair *(51–53)*. Several cellular proteins are known to be targeted by the ubiquitin system, including cyclins *(54)*; the CKIs p21 and p27 (*see* above); the tumor suppressor p53 *(55)*; the transcription factors E2F-1, E2F-4, c-myc, c-jun, c-fos, NF-κB, IκBα; and cell-surface receptors such as T-cell receptor, PDGF, EGF, and estrogen *(56)*.

An ATP-dependent proteolytic system from reticulocytes was first biochemically characterized in 1978 *(57)* with the identification of a small protein, remarkably stable to heat treatment, named APF-1, for ATP-dependent proteolysis factor 1. APF-1 was later identified as ubiquitin *(58)*, a 76-amino acid polypeptide, found to be present in several tissues and organisms, hence its name *(59)*. Proteins ligated to multi-ubiquitin chains are degraded by a 26 proteasome complex in the presence of ATP *(60)*. Specifically, conjugation of ubiquitin to the protein substrate occurs via a three-step cascade mechanism (Fig. 1):

1. Ubiquitin is activated by forming a high thioester bond with ubiquitin activating enzyme 1 (E1).

2. Activated ubiquitin is then transferred, via transacylation, to one of several ubiquitin-conjugating enzymes (Ubc or E2).
3. Finally, ubiquitin attachment to an ε-aminogroup of a reactive lysine residue in the target protein is catalyzed by the ubiquitin-protein ligase (E3).

A polyubiquitin chain is synthesized by additional transfer of ubiquitin moieties and this provides a signal for the action of the 26S proteasome complex. This complex is composed of a core, 20S catalytic subcomplex flanked by 19S regulatory subcomplexes and is able to recognize specifically ubiquitin-tagged proteins. The release of ubiquitin, a step essential for both protein degradation and ubiquitin biosynthesis (Fig. 1), is catalyzed by two classes of de-ubiquitinating enzymes: 1) the ubiquitin C-terminal hydrolases (UCHs), which are involved in the translational process of proubiquitin gene products and 2) the ubiquitin-C-terminal specific proteases (UBPs or isopeptidases). These proteases cleave between the C-terminal residue of the upstream moiety and the N-terminal residue of the following one, releasing ubiquitin from conjugates with cellular proteins or from polyubiquitin chains, thus maintaining the free pool of cellular ubiquitin.

Regarding the recognition of proteins as targets for ubiquitinization, some substrates are recognized via genetically coded primary structural motifs, while others undergo post-translational modification such as phosphorylation or associate with molecular chaperones before binding to the N-terminal binding site of E3α, the ubiquitin ligase involved in recognition via the N-terminal residue-specific ligases. The N-terminal residue of each protein stongly determines its in vivo half life in all eukaryotes and even in prokaryotes (which lack ubiquitin). This finding, also known as the N-end rule pathway (11), was the first mechanism to be discovered for substrate recognition by the ubiquitin system.

The ubiquitin proteasome pathway could be generally regulated at the level of ubiquitination or proteasome activity.

3.1. Ubiquitination

Degradation of specific substrates of the ubiquitin pathway is often regulated at the level of ubiquitination. In reality, the ubiquitination state of a protein is the result of two balancing processes: ubiquitination and deubiquitination. However, levels of ubiquitination can be regulated by several mechanisms:

1. Modification of the substrate. Post-translational phosphorylation of the substrate is required prior to ubiquitination by several proteins, such as the yeast G_1 cyclins Cln2 (62) and Cln3 (63), the yeast cyclin-dependent kinase inhibitor Sic1 (64), the mammalian G_1 cyclins D (65) and E (66), the CDK inhibitor $p27^{kip1}$ (67), and the transcriptional regulators IκBα (68) and β catenin (69). Inhibition of ubiquitination by phosphorylation has also been frequently described such as in the case of the protooncogene c-mos, whose degradation is inhibited by phosphorylation in Ser (70) or of bcl-2, which, following apoptotic

stimuli, becomes underphosphorylated and subsequently susceptible to degradation *(71)*.

2. Modulation of ubiquitination activity. Some classes of E3 enzymes may not be constitutively active but may depend on association with other factors such as viral proteins or ancillary proteins. For example, the E6-AP (E6-*associated protein*), a member of the HECT domain family of E3 enzymes, requires binding to human papillomavirus (HPV) E6 protein in order to degrade p53. Another class of E3 enzymes is involved in degradation of cyclins. The anaphase promoting complex (APC) has an ubiquitin ligase activity specific for cell cycle regulatory proteins such as cyclin B, certain anaphase inhibitors, and spindle-associated proteins, all of which are degraded at the end of mitosis. APC ability to differentially regulate degradation of various substrates is due to proteins that bind and confer to APC different substrate specificities *(72)*.

3. Deubiquitination. This process, which is essential for both the new synthesis and recycling of ubiquitin, has recently shown to play a specific regulatory role in ubiquitin-mediated proteolysis. The large number of deubiquitinating enzymes discovered suggests that some of them may have specific functions, such as in the case of DUB1 and DUB2, which affect growth regulation in mammals *(73)*. In general, deubiquitinating enzymes can either accelerate proteolysis or inhibit it, depending on which step of the pathway they are interacting with. Inhibition of proteolysis can occur by releasing ubiquitin from mistakenly tagged substrates. Alternatively, proteolysis can be accelerated by the release of free ubiquitin from biosynthetic precursors, terminal proteolytic products, or polyubiquitin chains.

3.2. Proteasome Activity

Substrate recognition by the 26S proteasome is mediated by the interaction of specific subunits of the 19s regulatory complex with the anchored polyubiquitin chain. PA28 is an additional complex that when associated with the 20S proteasome, dramatically enhances its degradation activity. PA28 expression is induced by interferon-γ (IFN-γ) and plays a specific role in the antigen degradation function of the proteasome by presenting large peptides generated by the 26S complex to the precise antigen epitopes recognized by the class I MHC complex.

4. REGULATION OF CKIS BY THE UBIQUITIN SYSTEM

Many mammalian (e.g., cyclins D, E, A, B, p27^{kip1}, p21^{waf1}, E2F, Rb, and p53) and yeast (Clns, Clbs, Sic1, and Far1) cell cycle proteins are ubiquitinated and degradated by the proteasome in vivo *(51)*. Proteolysis has been suggested as an essential mechanism in mammalian cells for the progression from G_1 through S phase, thus resulting in the onset of DNA replication. The inability of cells to enter S phase may result in cell death or improper differentiation in certain cell types.

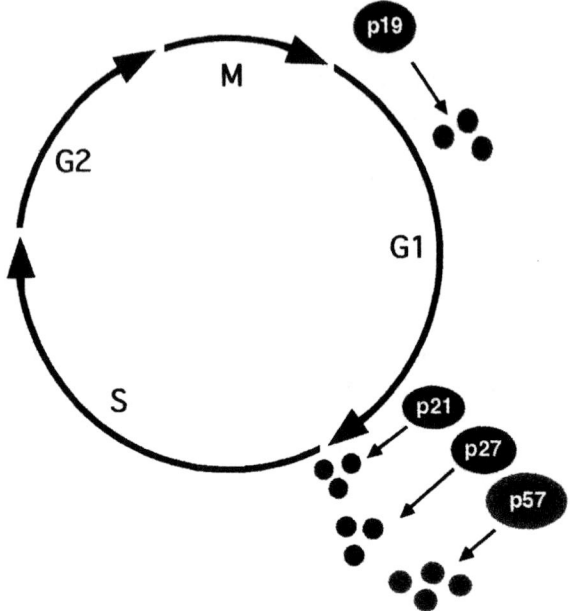

Fig. 2. Cell cycle dependent degradation of cyclin-dependent kinase inhibitors (CKIs). CKIs are indicated at the point in the mammalian cell cycle at which they appear to be degraded by ubiquitin-mediated proteolysis. Their temporally ordered degradation is critical for the proper regulation of cell cycle.

The following paragraph describes the targeted ubiquitin-mediated degradation of CKIs that negatively regulate entry into S phase (Fig. 2).

4.1. p21[wafl/cip1]

p21[wafl] belongs to the Cip/Kip family of CKIs (*see* above) and mediates cell cycle arrest in response to activation of the p53 tumor suppressor by several stimuli such as DNA damage (2). Several pieces of evidence (74–78) have indicated that p21 meets two of the basic criteria as a target of ubiquitin proteasome degradation: proteasome inhibition results in both p21 accumulation and appearance of p21-ubiquitin conjugates in vivo. The observation that proteasome-specific inhibitors such as lactacystin (LC) or MG132 were able to induce expression of p21[Wafl/Cip1] in human cancer cells regardless of their p53 status, suggested for the first time that p21 protein expression could be increased by transcriptional mechanisms as well as by inhibition of the proteasome activity (74, 75). Later, in vivo ubiquitination of p21 was demonstrated by two different approaches (76): 1) transient overexpression of ubiquitin in U2OS cells (expressing p21), followed by treatment of the cells with specific proteasome inhibitors (MG115 or lactacystin); 2) introduction of DNAs expressing both wild-type p21 and ubiquitin into SaOs2 cells (not expressing detectable levels of p21), followed by treatment with a proteasome inhibitor (MG115 or MG132). Both experiments showed the presence of ubiquitinated p21 species, demonstrating that p21 is also a target for degradation of the ubiquitin-dependent proteolytic pathway.

With regard to the mechanisms regulating p21 degradation, it appears that the proteolytic pathway of p21 is regulated by its association with CDKs and PCNA *(77)*. In fact, a p21 mutant deficient for interaction with CDKs (p21CDK-) displayed an enhanced stability and greatly reduced sensitivity to proteasome-mediated proteolysis, indicating that association with cyclin/CDK complexes may trigger p21 degradation. In contrast, a p21 mutant impaired in the interaction with PCNA (p21PCNA-) exhibited a decreased stability, suggesting that association with PCNA protects p21 from proteasome-dependent degradation. Moreover, the ability of p21 to induce growth inhibition by its CDK and PCNA binding domains is dependent on their stability, which is also determined by the ubiquitin-proteasome pathway *(78)*. Finally, p21 stability appears to be regulated by the p19^{SKP1}/p45^{SKP2}/CUL-1 (SCF) complex, which is likely to function as an E$_3$ ligase to target selectively p21 and cyclin D proteins for ubiquitin-dependent protein degradation *(79)*.

The turnover of p21 has been demonstrated to depend on its localization to the nucleus and to be essentially regulated by ubiquitination in several systems *(74–76,80–81)*. Nevertheless, it has been recently shown that direct ubiquitination of p21 is not a prerequisite for its degradation in vivo *(81)*. How p21 might be degraded independently of ubiquitin attachment is still unknown. Several hypotheses have been proposed, such as p21 interaction with binding partners that affect its turnover or, alternatively, the direct recognition and degradation by the proteasome. On the other hand, the presence of ubiquitinated p21 could be owing simply to its association with ubiquitinating enzymes such as SCF proteins complexes (SKP1 and SKP2) *(79)*. Finally, it is possible that p21 turnover is affected by proteasome inhibitors indirectly. Proteasome inhibition may indirectly stabilize p21 by affecting proteins responsible for p21 regulation.

Due to the dual role of p21 in G$_1$ and early S-phase progression, further studies are required in order to clarify the significance of p21 ubiquitination and its ability to temporally regulate the cell cycle.

4.2. p19 ^{INK4d}

One feature of p19^{INK4d}, but not of other INK4 inhibitors, is the periodic accumulation of its protein in S phase of the cell cycle *(82)*. Recently *(83)*, the periodic oscillation of p19^{INK4d} during the cell cycle was found to be regulated by the ubiquitin proteasome-dependent mechanism, allowing the p19^{INK4d} protein levels to follow the changes in its mRNA expression. Within the INK4 family, this regulation appears to be restricted only to p19^{INK4d}, whose ubiquitination is critically regulated by its physical association with CDK4 and the integrity of lysine 62 *(83)*. The ubiquitination of p19[INK4d] suggests a new mechanism of regulation of cyclin/CDK4 *(56)* complex formation, raising further questions about the mechanism leading to p19 degradation and its consequent impact on cell cycle progression.

4.3. p57 [kip2]

Of all CKIs, only p57[kip2] plays an essential role(s) for which other CKIs cannot compensate in embryonic development *(84)*. Thus far, little is known about the mechanism controlling p57[kip2] protein stability. One study has shown that p57[kip2] is degraded through the ubiquitin-proteasome pathway in osteoblastic cells stimulated to proliferation by transforming growth factor (TGF)-β1 *(85)*. More recently, it has been elucidated that TGF-β1-induced p57[kip2] proteolysis is mediated through transcription by the Smad (Smad2 or Smad3 with Smad4) pathway as shown by the accumulation of p57[kip2] following the forced expression of an inhibitory Smad called Smad7 in TGF-β1-stimulated cells *(86)*. In light of these findings and given the functional similarities between p27[kip1] and p57[kip2], an important role for the ubiquitin pathway in regulating p57[kip2] is no longer unexpected and definitely deserves further investigation.

4.4. p27 [kip1]

p27[kip1] expression is regulated primarily at the post-transcriptional level. In fact, although p27[kip1] mRNA levels are constant during the cell cycle, in proliferating cells the p27[kip1] protein undergoes rapid degradation by the ubiquitin proteasome pathway, and this proteolysis is dramatically reduced in resting cells *(87)*. Before the onset of S phase, p27 becomes a substrate of cyclin E/cdk2 complexes, resulting in phosphorylation at Thr-187 *(88)*. Phosphorylation has been shown to trigger ubiquitin-mediated degradation of p27[kip1]. In fact, p27[kip1] mutation of Thr 187 to alanine results in resistance to phosphorylation by cyclin E/cdk2 and to degradation *(89)*. Phosphorylated p27[kip1] is then polyubiquinated by an E2-E3 complex formed by Cdc34 and the SCF components p19[Skp1], Cul1, p45[Skp2] *(90–93)*, and subsequently degraded by the 26S proteasome. However, it has been shown recently that the ubiquitination process can be mediated by the ubiquitin-like protein Nedd8 and the enzymes that catalyze Nedd 8 conjugation to proteins, regardless of p27[kip1] phosphorylation status *(94)*. Phosphorylation of p27kip1 and its subsequent degradation are also instigated by Jab1, a transcriptional activator of c-Jun, which interacts with p27kip1 in the nucleus and translocate it to the cytoplasm, where it is ubiquinated and degraded *(95)*. Activated Ras is also able to induce p27[kip1] degradation through the RhoA pathway, which involves cyclinE/cdk2 *(96)* or the MAPK pathway *(97)*. By enhancing Cul1 expression, myc is also able to promote p27[kip1] ubiquitin-dependent proteolysis *(98)*, whereas p27[kip1] accumulation following retinoic-induced differentiation occurs by downregulation of the ubiquitin pathway *(99)*. Recently, a role for PTEN has been identified in downregulation of $p27^{kip1}$ ubiquitin-dependent degradation through the interaction with the ubiquitin E3 ligase SKP2 *(100)*.

Several pieces of evidence support the role of $p27^{kip1}$ degradation in controlling the G_1-S phase transition: 1) $p27^{kip1}$ overexpression arrests cells in G_1 phase in a variety of conditions *(101)* and this arrest can be overcome only by the concomitant overexpression of cyclin E; however, when a $p27^{kip1}$ mutant in Thr 187 (T187A) is ectopically overexpressed, cells arrest in G_1 and cannot be rescued by cyclin E overexpression *(89)*; 2) upon the overexpression of p45SKP2, T187A, but not $WTp27^{kip1}$, arrests cells in S phase *(93)*; 3) p45SKP2 antisense oligonucleotides prevent cell entry into S phase *(102)*.

Degradation of $p27^{Kip1}$ at the G_0-G_1 transition of the cell cycle has been shown to proceed normally in Skp2(–/–) lymphocytes, whereas $p27^{Kip1}$ proteolysis during S-G_2 phases is impaired in these Skp2-deficient cells. Both $p27^{kip1}$ and cyclin E accumulate in SKP2–/– MEFs; however, in contrast with the idea of $p27^{kip1}$ being exclusively degraded in a $p45^{Skp2}$-dependent manner, cells did not arrest in G_1 *(103)*. A recent study *(104)* has partially clarified the problem by showing that polyubiquitination of $p27^{Kip1}$ in the nucleus is dependent on Skp2 and phosphorylation of $p27^{Kip1}$ on threonine 187. However, polyubiquitination activity is also detected in the cytoplasm of Skp2(–/–) cells, even with a threonine 187 —> alanine mutant of p27(Kip1) as substrate. These results suggest that polyubiquitination activity in the cytoplasm contributes to the early phase of $p27^{Kip1}$ degradation in a Skp2-independent manner, thereby promoting cell cycle progression from G_0 to G_1.

Further studies are nevertheless necessary in order to clarify the requirement and the exclusiveness of $p27^{kip1}$ degradation in the onset of DNA replication in mammals.

5. THE UBIQUITIN SYSTEM AS A TARGET OF CANCER THERAPY

Several cell cycle regulatory proteins are degraded by the proteasome, including cyclins, CKIs, tumor-suppressor genes, oncogenes, enzymes, and other regulatory molecules.

The correct and timed production and degradation of CKIs is critical to their function and to the orderly progression of cells through the cell cycle; disruption of this perfectly synchronized mechanism leads to tumor development.

In the last few years, researchers have been trying to control tumor onset and progression by inhibiting proteasome activity. This inhibition leads to the stabilization of CKIs and, as a result, cell cycle arrest occurs and the cells undergo apoptosis. Moreover, disruption of the cell cycle involving the ubiquitin-proteasome pathway has been reported in several malignancies and frequently involves CKIs. Indeed, reduced expression of p27^{kip1} was definitely shown to correlate with enhanced and specific proteasome-dependent degradation of this protein in human primary gliomas *(105)*, lung *(106)*, and colorectal *(107)* cancer. The strong correlation between the low levels of p27kip1 and the aggressiveness of the tumor makes p27 a powerful independent prognostic parameter *(108,109)* and an interesting target of therapy.

Consequently, proteasome inhibitors have been explored for the treatment of hematologic malignancies and solid tumors *(110)*. Several natural and synthetic compounds that act as proteasome inhibitors have been reported *(111)*; however, few of them have currently progressed in clinical trials for cancer therapy.

PS-341 is the most extensively studied proteasome inhibitor *(112)* and one of the few agents to be used in clinical trials. By inhibiting the proteasome, PS-341 is able to decrease NF-κB activity and angiogenesis, to increase apoptosis and stabilize cell cycle proteins, such as p21, p53, and a variety of cyclins *(111,112)*. Moreover, PS-341 was found to decrease tumor size in a large series of cell lines such as HT-29, NCI-H23 lung, PANC-1, PC-3 prostate tumor models, and various human xenografts *(111,112)*. Moreover, PS-341 is able to overcome cellular resistance to other chemotherapeutic agents and the resistance to apoptosis exerted by bcl-2 transfection. Such results suggest a role for this drug in combination therapy with conventional chemotherapeutic agents or radiation. To date, several studies have been showing synergistic antitumor activity between PS-341 and radiation, 5-fluorouracil, doxorubicin, cisplatin, irinotecan (CPT-11), dexamethason, gemcitabine, melphalan, and paclitaxel. PS-341 has also been shown to be effective in limiting the metastatic process and angiogenesis in several experimental cancer systems. For these reasons, PS-341 has been under investigation in a Phase I clinical trial since 1998. These studies include patients with a variey of solid tumors (prostate, colorectal, renal, lung) and hematologic malignancies (multiple myeloma, non-Hodgkin's lymphoma, leukemia).

The results of this first trial have shown that PS-341 biological effects are accompanied by minimal toxic effects. Phase II single-agent trials have just been started on patients with multiple myeloma and further trials are on the way to evaluate PS-341 combination with radiation and with other agents such as gemcitabine and irinotecan.

6. CONCLUSIONS AND PERSPECTIVES

Ubiquitin-mediated protein degradation has been implicated in the pathogenesis of several diseases, including some types of cancer. However, with the broad range of ubiquitin-targeted substrates and the complexity of the enzymatic cascade involved, the future discovery of a major involvement of this pathway in the process of tumorigenesis is not unexpected.

Many problems still remain unresolved. For example, it is unclear which degradation requirements may be sufficient for entry into S phase and which mechanisms lead a process of physiological significance to become pathological. Another underexplored area is the regulation of the degradation machinery itself. Studies in yeast suggest a degradation occurring by an autocatalytic mechanism; however, phosphorylation processes also appear to be involved.

For potential clinical application, although many drugs are already under investigation in clinical trials, further studies are necessary to define the prognostic significance of these molecules and for the early identification and treatment of aggressive cancers that may develop due to dysregulation of these processes.

During the next several years, data from clinical trials will become available, and the usefulness of these novel agents targeting the ubiquitination system for the treatment of cancer and or other diseases will be clarified.

ACKNOWLEDGMENTS

The authors would like to thank M.L. Basso for her assistance in editing and Dr. A. Sgambato for critical reading of the manuscript. We also apologize in the event that any relevant publications as of 1/31/2002 were inadvertently omitted. This manuscript is supported by NIH Grants to A.G. and K.S. V.M. is supported by a fellowship from the National Cancer Institute (PHS 5 T32 CA09137).

REFERENCES

1. MacLachlan TK, Sang N, Giordano A. Cyclins, cyclin-dependent kinases and cdk inhibitors: implications in cell cycle control and cancer. *Crit Rev Eukaryot Gene Expr* 1995;5:127–156.
2. Sherr CJ, Roberts JM. Inhibitors of mammalian G1 cyclin-dependent kinases. *Genes Dev* 1995;9,1149–1163.
3. Morgan DO. Principles of CDK regulation. *Nature* 1995;374:131–134.
4. Serrano M, Hannon GJ, Beach D. A new regulatory motif in cell cycle control causing specific inhibition of cyclin D/cdk4. *Nature* 1993;366:704–707.
5. Hannon GJ, Beach D. p15INK4B is a potential effector of cell cycle arrest mediated by TGFβ. *Nature* 1994;371:257–261.
6. Hirai H, Roussel MF, Kato J, Ashmun RA, Sherr CJ. Novel INK4 proteins, p19 and p18, are specific inhibitors of cyclin D-dependent kinases CDK4 and CDK6. *Mol Cell Biol* 1995;15:2672–2681.
7. Chan FKM, Zhang J, Chen L, Shapiro DN, Winoto A. Identification of a human mouse p19, a novel cdk4/cdk6 inhibitor with homology to p16[INK4]. *Mol Cell Biol* 1995;15:2682–2688.
8. Xiong Y, Hannon H, Zhang H, Casso D, Kobayashi R, Beach D. p21 is a universal inhibitor of cyclin kinases. *Nature* 1993;366:701–704.
9. Bullrich F, MacLachlan T, Sang N, Druck T, Veronese ML, Allen SL, et al. Chromosomal mapping of members of the cdc2 family of protein kinases, cdk3, cdk6, PISSLRE, and PITALRE, and a cdk inhibitor, p27kip1, to regions involved in human cancer. *Cancer Res* 1995;55:1199–1205.
10. Lee MH, Reynisdottir I, Massague J. Cloning of p57kip2, a cylin-dependent kinase inhibitor with unique domain structure and tissue distribution. *Genes Dev* 1995;9:639–649.
11. Medema R, Herrera RE, Lam, F, Weinberg RA. Growth suppression by p16INK4 requires functional retinoblastoma protein. *Proc Natl Acad Sci USA* 1995;92:6289–6293.
12. Serrano M, Gomez-Lahoz E, DePinho RA, Beach D, Bar-Sagi D. Inhibition of ras-induced proliferation and cellular transformation by p16[INK4]. *Science* 1995;267:249–252.

13. Parry D, Bates S, Mann DJ, Peters G. Lack of cyclinD-cdk complexes in Rb-negative cells correlates with high levels of p16$^{INK4/MTS1}$ tumor suppressor gene product. *EMBO J* 1995;14:503–511.

14. Guan K, Jenkins CW, Li Y, Nichols MA, Wu X, O'Keefe CL, Matera AG, Xiong Y. Growth suppression by p18, a p16$^{INK4-MTS1}$ and p14$^{INK4-MTS2}$-related cdk6 inhibitor, correlates with wild type pRb function. *Genes Dev* 1994;8:2939–2952.

15. Bardeesy N, Morgan J, Sinha M, Signoretti S, Srivastava S, Loda M, et al. Obligate roles for p16INK4A and p19(Arf)-p53 in the suppression of murine pancreatic neoplasia. *Mol Cell Biol* 2002;22:635–643.

16. Tannapfel A, Busse C, Weinans L, Benicke M, Katalinic A, Geissler F, et al. INK4a-ARF alterations and p53 mutations in hepatocellular carcinomas. *Oncogene* 2001;25:7104–7109.

17. Martinez-Delgado B, Richart A, Garcia MJ, Robledo M, Osorio A, Cebrian A, et al. Hypermethylation of p16INK4A and p15INK4B genes as marker of disease in the follow-up of non-Hodgkin's lymphomas. *Br J Hematol* 2000;109:97–103.

18. Faderl S, Kantarjian HM, Manshouri T, Chan CY, Pierce S, Hays KJ, et al. The prognostic significance of p16INK4/p14ARF and p15INK4B deletions in adult acute lymphoblastic leukaemia. *Clin Cancer Res* 1999;5:1855–1861.

19. Thullberg M, Bartkova J, Khan S, Hansen K, Ronnstrand L, Lukas J, et al. Distinct versus redundant properties among members of the INK4 family of cyclin-dependent kinase inhibitors. *FEBS Lett* 2000;470:161–166.

20. Gartel AL, Tyner AL. The growth regulatory role of p21 (waf1/cip1), in *Molecular and Subcellular Biology*. Vol. 20. Macieir-Coelho A, ed. Springer, Berlin, 1998, pp. 43–71.

21. Niculescu AB III, Chen X, Smeets M., Hengst L, Prives C, Reed SI. Effects of p21cip1/waf1 at both the G1/S and the G2/M cell cycle transition: pRb is a critical determinant in blocking DNA replication and in preventing endoreduplication. *Mol Cell Biol* 1998;18:629–643.

22. Zhang H, Hannon GJ, Beach D. p21-containing cyclin kinases exist in both active and inactive states. *Genes Dev* 1994;8:1750–1758.

23. Nevins JR. Towards an understanding of the functional complexity of the E2F and the retinoblastoma families. *Cell Growth Differ* 1998;9:585–593.

24. Asada M, Yamada T, Ichijo H, Delia D, Miyazono K, Fukumuro K, Mizutani S. Apoptosis inhibitory activity of cytoplasmic p21(cip1/waf1) in monocytic differentiation. *EMBO J* 1999;18:1223–1234.

25. Caelles C, Helmberg A, Karin M. p53-dependent apoptosis in the absence of transcriptional activation of p53-target genes. *Nature* 1994;370:220–223.

26. Polyak K, Kato JY, Solomon MJ, Sherr CJ, Massague J, Roberts JM, Koff A. p27kip1, a cyclin-cdk inhibitor, links transforming growth factor-beta and contact inhibition to cell cycle arrest. *Genes Dev* 1994;8,9–22.

27. Fero ML, Rivkin M, Tasch M, Porter, P, Carow, CE, Firpo, E, et al. A syndrome of multi-organ hyperplasia with features of gigantism, tumorigenesis, and female sterility in p27kip1-deficient mice. *Cell* 1996;85:733–744.

28. Kiyokawa H, Kineman RD, Manova-Todorova KO, Soares VC, Hoffman ES, Ono M, et al. Enhanced growth of mice lacking the cyclin-dependent kinase inhibitor function of p27kip1. *Cell* 1996;85:721–732.

29. Millard SS, Yan JS, Nguyen H, Pagano M, Kiyokawa H, Koff A. Enhanced ribosomal association of p27kip1 mRNA is a mechanism contributing to accumulation during growth arrest. *J Biol Chem* 1997;272:7093–7098.

30. Muller D, Bouchard C, Rudolph B, Steiner P, Stuckmann I, Saffrich R, et al. Cdk2-dependent phosphorylation of p27 facilitates its myc-induced release from cyclin E/cdk2 complexes. *Oncogene* 1997;15:2561–2576.

31. Leone G, DeGregori J, Sears R, Jakoi L, Nevins JR. Myc and Ras collaborate in inducing accumulation of active cyclin E/cdk2 and E2F. *Nature (London)* 1997;387:422–426.

32. Reynisdottir I, Massague J. The subcellular locations of p15INK4B and p27kip1 coordinate their inhibitory interactions with cdk4 and cdk2. *Genes Dev* 1997;11:492–503.

33. Orend G, Hunter T, Ruoslahti E. Cytoplasmic displacement of cyclinE-cdk2 inhibitors p21Cip1 and p27kip1 in anchorage-independent cells. *Oncogene* 1998;16:2575–2583.

34. Fero ML, Randel E, Gurley KE, Roberts JM, Kemp CJ. The murine gene p27kip1 is haplo-insufficient for tumour suppression. *Nature* 1998;396:177–180.

35. Spirin KS, Simpson JF, Takeuchi S, Kawamata N, Miller CW, Koeffler HP. p27kip1 mutation found in breast cancer. *Cancer Res* 1996;56:2400–2404.

36. Matsuoka M, Edwards M, Bai C, Parker S, Zhang P, Baldini A, et al. p57^{kip2}, a structurally distinct member of the p21cdk inhibitor family, is a candidate tumor suppressor gene. *Genes Dev* 1995;9:650–662.

37. Koi M, Johnson LA, Kalikan LM, Little PF, Nakamura Y, Feinberg AP. Tumor cell growth arrest caused by subchromosomal transferable DNA fragments from chromosome 11. *Science* 1993;260:361–364.

38. Thompson JS, Reese KJ, DeBaun MR, Perlman FJ, Feinberg AP. Reduced expression of the cyclin-dependent kinase inhibitor gene p57kip2 in Wilm's tumor. *Cancer Res* 1996; 56: 5723–5727.

39. Lai S, Goepfert H, Gillenwater AM, Luna MA, El-Naggar AK. Loss of imprinting and genetic alterations of the cyclin-dependent kinase inhibitor p57kip2 gene in head and neck squamous cell carcinoma. *Clin Cancer Res* 2000;6:3172–3176.

40. Feinberg AP. Imprinting of a genomic domain of 11p15 and loss of imprinting in cancer: an introduction. *Cancer Res* 1999;59 (7 Suppl):1743s–1746s.

41. Stiegler P, Kasten M, Giordano A. The RB family of cell cycle regulatory factors. *J Cell Biochem* 1998;30/31:30–36.

42. Slansky JE, Farnham PJ. Introduction to the E2F family: protein structure and gene regulation. *Curr Top Microbiol Immunol* 1996;208:1–30.

43. La Baer J, Garret MD, Stevenson LF, Slingerland JM, Sandhu C, Chou HS, et al. New functional activities for the p21 family of CDK inhibitors. *Genes Dev* 1997;11:847–862.

44. Wu X, Levine A. p53 and E2F-1 cooperate to mediate apoptosis. *Proc Natl Acad Sci USA* 1994;91:3602–3606.

45. Fong LY, Nguyen VT, Farber JL, Huebner K, Magee PN. Early deregulation of the p16INK4a-cyclinD1/cyclin-dependent kinase 4-retinoblastoma pathway in cell proliferation-driven esophageal tumorigenesis in zinc-deficient rats. *Cancer Res* 2000;60:4589–4595.

46. Alexander K, Hinds PW. Requirement for p27(KIP1) in retinoblastoma protein-mediated senescence. *Mol Cell Biol* 2001;21(11):3616–3631.

47. Baldi A, De Luca A, Claudio PP, Baldi F, Giordano GG, Tommasino M, et al. The RB2/p130 gene product is a nuclear protein whose phosphorylation is cell cycle regulated. *J Cell Biochem* 1995;59:402–408.

48. Nevins J. Toward an understanding of the functional complexity of the E2F and retinoblastoma families. *Cell Growth Differ* 1998;9:585–593.

49. Howard, C M, Claudio, P P,De Luca, A, Stiegler, P, Jori, FP, Safdar NM, et al. Inducible pRb2/p130 expression and growth-suppressive mechanisms: evidence of a pRb2/p130, p27^{Kip1}, and cyclin E negative feedback regulatory loop. *Cancer Res* 2000;60:2737–2744.

50. Zhang D, Vuocolo S, Masciullo V, Sava T, Giordano A, Soprano DR, Soprano KJ. Cell cycle genes as targets of retinoid induced ovarian tumor cell growth suppression. *Oncogene* 2001;20(55):7935–7944.

51. King R, Deshaies R, Peters J, Kirschner M. How proteolysis drive the cell cycle. *Science* 1996;274:1652–1659.

52. Pagano, M. Cell cycle regulation by the ubiquitin pathway. *FASEB J* 1997;11(13): 1067–1075.

53. Ciechanover A, Schwartz AL. The ubiquitin proteasome pathway: the complexity and myriad functions of proteins death. *Proc Natl Acad Sci USA* 1998;95:2727–2730.

54. Glotzer MA, Murray A, Kirschner M. Cyclin is degraded by the ubiquitin pathway. *Nature* 1991;349:132–138.
55. Maki C, Hulbregtse J, Howley P. In vivo ubiquitination and proteasome-mediated degradation of p53. *Cancer Res* 1996;56:2649–2654.
56. Ciechanover A, Orian A, Schwartz AL. The ubiquitin-mediated proteolitic pathway: mode of action and clinical implications. *J Cell Biochem* (suppl) 2000;34:40–51.
57. Ciechanover A, Hod Y, Hershko A. A heat-stable polypeptide component of an ATP-dependent proteolytic system from reticulocytes. *Biochem Biophys Res Commun* 1978; 81:1100–1105.
58. Wilkinson KD, Urban MK, Haas AL. Ubiquitin is the ATP-dependent proteolysis factor of rabbit reticulocytes. *J Biol Chem* 1980;255,7529–7532.
59. Goldstein G, Scheid M, Hammerling U, Schlesinger DH, Niall HD, Boyse EA. Isolation of a polypeptide that has lymphocyte-differentiating properties and is probably represented universally in living cells. *Proc Natl Acad Sci USA* 1975;72(1):11–15.
60. Hough R, Pratt G, Rechsteiner M. Ubiquitin-lysozime conjugates. Identification and characterization of an ATP-dependent protease from rabbit reticulocyte lysates. *J Biol Chem* 1986;261:2400–2408.
61. Varshavsky A. The N-end rule: functions, mysteries, uses. *Proc Natl Acad Sci USA* 1996;93:12142–12149.
62. Lanker S, Valdivieso MH, Wittenberg C. Rapid degradation of the G1 cyclin Cln2 induced by CDK-dependent phosphorylation. *Science* 1996;271:1597–1601.
63. Yaglom J, Linskens HK, Sadias S, Rubin DM, Futcher B, Finley D. p34-Cdc28-mediated control of Cln3 degradation. *Mol Cell Biol* 1995;15:731–741.
64. Verma R, Annan R, Huddleston M, Carr S, Reynard G, Deshaies R. Phosphorylation of Sic1 by G1 Cdk required for its degradation and entry into S phase. *Science* 1997;278:455–460.
65. Diehl J, Zindy F, Sherr C. Inhibition of cyclin D1 phosphorylation on threonine 286 prevent its rapid degradation via the ubiquitin proteasome pathway. *Genes Dev* 1997;11:957–972.
66. Clurman BE, Sheaff RJ, Thress K, Groudine M, Roberts JM. Turnover of cyclin E by the ubiquitin proteasome pathway is regulated by cdk2 binding and cyclin phosphorylation. *Genes Dev* 1996;10:1979–1990.
67. Carrano AC, Eytan E, Hersko A, Pagano M. SKP2 is required for ubiquitin mediated degradation of the CDK inhibitor p27kip1. *Nature Cell Biol* 1999;1:193–199.
68. Yaron A, Gonen H, Alkalay I, Hatzubai A, Jung S, Beyth S, et al. Inhibition of NF-KB cellular function via specific targeting of the IkBa-ubiquitin ligase. *EMBO J* 1997;16:6486–6494.
69. Rubinfeld B, Robbins P, El-gamil M, Albert I, Porfiri E, Polakis P. Stabilization of β-catenin by genetic defects in melanoma cell lines. *Science* 1997;275:1790–1792.
70. Nishizawa M, Furuno N, Okazaki K, Tanaka H, Ogawa Y, Sagata N. Degradation of Mos by tye N-terminal proline (Pro2)-dependent unbiquitin pathway on fertilization of Xenopus eggs: possible significance of natural selection for Pro2 in Mos. *EMBO J* 1993;12:4021–4027.
71. Dimmeler S, Breithschopf K, Haendeler J, Zeiher AM. Dephosphorylation targets bcl-2 for ubiquitin dependent degradation: a link between the apoptosome and the proteasome pathway. *J Exp Med* 1999;189:1815–1822.
72. Visintin R, Prinz S, Amon A. CDC20 and CDH1: a family of substrate-specific activators of APC-dependent proteolysis. *Science* 1997;278:460–463.
73. Zhu Y, Carrol M, Papa FR, Hochstrasser M, D'Andrea AD. DUB-1, a deubiquitinating enzyme with growth-suppressing activity. *Proc Natl Acad Sci USA* 1996;93:3275–3279.
74. Blagosklonny MV, Wu GS, Omura S, El-Deiry WS. Proteasome-dependent regulation of p21$^{wafl/cip1}$ expression. *Biophys Res Comm* 1996;227;564–569.
75. Maki CG, Huibregtse JM, Howley PM. *In vivo* ubiquitination and proteasome mediated degradation of p53. *Cancer Res* 1996;56:2649–2654.
76. Maki CG, Howley PM. Ubiquitination of p53 and p21 is differentially affected by ionizing and UV radiation. *Mol Cell Biol* 1997;17:355–363.

77. Cayrol C, Ducommun B. Interaction with cyclin-dependent kinases and PCNA modulates proteasome-dependent degradation of p21. *Oncogene* 1998;12,17(19):2437–2444.
78. Rousseau D, Cannella D, Boulaire J, Fitzgerald P, Fotedar A, Fotedar R. Growth inhibition by CDK-cyclin and PCNA binding domains of p21 occurs by distinct mechanisms and is regulated by ubiquitin proteasome pathway. *Oncogene* 1999;18:3290–3302.
79. Yu Z, Gervais JLM., Zhang H. Human CUL-1 associates with the SKP1/SKP2 complex and regulates p21[CIP1/WAF1] and cyclin D proteins. *Proc Natl Acad Sci USA* 1998;95: 11324–11329.
80. Fukuchi K, Tomoyasu S, Nakamaki T, Tsuruoka N, Gomi K. DNA damage induces p21 protein expression by inhibiting ubiquitination in ML-1 cells. *Biochim Biophys Acta* 1998;1404:405–411.
81. Sheaff RJ, Singer JD, Swanger J, Smitherman M, Roberts JM, Clurman BE. Proteosomal turnover of p21[cip1] does not require p21[cip1] ubiquitination. *Mol Cell* 2000;5:403–410.
82. Hirai H, Roussel MF, Kato J, Ashmun RA, Sherr CJ. Novel INK4 proteins, p19 and p18, are specific inhibitors of the cyclin D-dependent kinases CDK4 and CDK6. *Mol Cell Biol* 1995;15:2672–2681.
83. Thullberg M, Bartek J, Lukas J. Ubiquitin/proteasome-mediated degradation of p19[INK4d] determines its periodic expression during the cell cycle. *Oncogene* 2000;19:2870–2876.
84. Yan Y, Frisen J, Lee MH, Massague J, Barbacid M. Ablation of the cdk inhibitor p57[kip2] results in increased apoptosis and delayed differentiation during mouse development. *Genes Dev* 1997;11(8):973–983.
85. Nishimori S, Tanaka Y, Chiba T, Fujii M, Imamura T, Miyazono K, et al. Smad-mediated transcription is required for transforming growth factor-beta 1-induced p57(Kip2) proteolysis in osteoblastic cells. *J Biol Chem* 2001;6,276(14):10700–10705.
86. Urano T, Yashiroda H, Muraoka M, Tanaka K, Hosoi T, Inoue S, et al. p57(Kip2) is degraded through the proteasome in osteoblasts stimulated to proliferation by transforming growth factor beta1. *J Biol Chem* 1999 Apr 30;274(18):12197–12200.
87. Pagano M, Tam SW, Theodoras AM, Beer-Romero P, Del Sal G, Chau V, et al. Role of the ubiquitin proteasome pathway in regulating abundance of the cyclin-dependent kinase inhibitor p27[kip1]. *Science* 1995;269:682–685.
88. Vlach J, Hennecke S, Amati B. Phosphorylation-dependent degradation of the cyclin-dependent kinase inhibitor p27[kip1]. *EMBO J* 1997;16(17):5334–5344.
89. Sheaff RJ, Groudine M, Gordon M, Roberts JM, Clurman BE. Cyclin E/cdk2 is a regulator of p27[kip1]. *Genes Dev* 1997;11:1464–1478.
90. Tsvetkov LM, Yeh K, Lee S, Sun H, Zhang H. p27[kip1] ubiquitination and degradation is regulated by the SCF[Skp2] complex through phosphorylated Thr187 in p27. *Curr Biol* 1999;9:661–664.
91. Carrano AC, Eytan E, Hershko A, Pagano M. SKP2 is required for ubiquitin-mediated degradation of the CDK inhibitor p27[kip1]. *Nat Cell Biol* 1999;1(4):193–199.
92. Montagnoli A, Fiore F, Eytan E, Carrano AC, Draetta GF, Hersko A, Pagano M. Ubiquitination of p27 is regulated by cdk dependent and trimeric complex formation. *Genes Dev* 1999;13(9):1181–1189.
93. Sutterluty H, Chatelain E, Marti A, Wirbelauer C., Senften M, Muller U, Krek W. p45SKP2 promotes p27[kip1]degradation and induces S phase in quiescent cells. *Nat Cell Biol* 1999;1(4):207–214.
94. Podust NV, Brownell JE, Gladysheva TB, Luo R, Wang C, Coggins MB, et al. A Nedd 8 conjugation pathway is essential for proteolytic targeting of p27[kip1] by ubiquitination. *Proc Natl Acad Sci USA* 2000;97,9:4579–4584.
95. Tomoda K, Kubota Y, Kato J. Degradation of the cyclin-dependent kinase inhibitor p27[kip1] is instigated by Jab1. *Nature* 1999;398:160–165.
96. Hu W, Bellone CJ, Baldassarre JJ. RhoA stimulates p27[kip1] degradation through its regulation of cyclin E/cdk2 activity. *J Biol Chem* 1999;274:3396–3401.

97. Kawada M, Yamagoe S, Murakami Y, Suzuki K, Mizuno S, Uehara Y. Induction of p27^{kip1} degradation and anchorage independence by Ras through the MAP kinase signaling pathway. *Oncogene* 1997;15:629–637.

98. O'Hagan RC, Ohh M, David G, de Alboran IM, Alt FW, Kaelin WG, De Pinho RA. Myc enhanced expression of Cul1 promotes ubiquitin-dependent proteolysis and cell cycle progression. *Genes Dev* 2000;14,17:2185–2191.

99. Borriello A, Della Pietra V, Criscuolo M, Oliva A, Tonin GP, Iolascon A, et al. p27^{kip1} accumulation is associated with retinoic-induced neuroblastoma differentiation: evidence of a decreased proteasome-dependent degradation. *Oncogene* 2000;19:51–60.

100. Mammilapalli R, Gavrilova N, Mihaylova VT, Tsyetkov LM, Wu H, Zhang H, Sun H. PTEN regulates the ubiquitin-dependent degradation of the cdk inhibitor p27kip1 through the ubiquitin 3 ligase SCF (SKP2). *Curr Biol* 2001;11,4:263–267.

101. Sgambato A, Cittadini A, Faraglia B, Weinstein IB. Multiple functions of p27kip1 and its alterations in tumor cells: a review. *J Cell Physiol* 2000;183:18–27.

102. Zhang H, Kobayashi R, Galaktionov K, Beach D. p19Skp1 and p45Skp2 are essential elements of the cyclinA-cdk2 S phase kinase. *Cell* 1995;82:915–925.

103. Nakayama K, Nagahama K, Minamishima YA, Matsumoto M, Nakamichi I, Kitagawa K, et al. Targeted disruption of SKP2 results in accumulation of cyclin E and p27^{kip1} polyploidy and centrosome overduplication. *EMBO J* 2000;19(9):2069–2081.

104. Hara T, Kamura T, Nakayama K, Oshikawa K, Hatakeyama S, Nakayama K. Degradation of p27^{Kip1} at the G(0)-G(1) transition mediated by a Skp2-independent ubiquitination pathway. *J Biol Chem* 2001;276(52):48937–48943.

105. Piva R, Cancell I, Cavalla P, Bortolotto S, Dominguez J, et al. Proteasome dependent degradation of p27^{kip1} in gliomas. *J Neuropathol Exp Neurol* 1999;58:691–696.

106. Esposito V, Baldi A, De Luca A, Groger AM, Loda M., Giordano GG, et al. Prognostic role of the cyclin dependent kinase inhibitor p27 in non small cell lung cancer. *Cancer Res* 1997;57:3381–3385.

107. Loda M, Cukor B, Tam SW, Lavin P, Fiorentino M, Draetta GF, et al. Increased protesome-dependent degradation of the cyclin-dependent kinase inhibitor p27 in aggressive colorectal carcinomas. *Nature Med* 1997;3:231–234.

108. Lloyd VR, Erickson LA, Jin L, Kulig E, Qian X, Cheville JC, Scheithauer BW. p27kip1: a multifunctional cyclin-dependent kinase inhibitor with prognostic significance in human cancer. *Am J Pathol* 1999;154:313–323.

109. Masciullo V, Sgambato A, Pacilio C, Pucci B, Ferrandina G, Palazzo J, et al. Frequent loss of expression of the cyclin-dependent kinase inhibitor p27 in epithelial ovarian cancer. *Cancer Res* 1999;59:3790–3794.

110. Adams J, Palombella VJ, Sausville EA, Johnson J, Destree A, Lazarus DD, et al. Proteasome inhibitors: a novel class of potent and effective antitumor agents. *Cancer Res* 1999;59: 2615–2622.

111. Teicher BA, Ara G, Herbst R, Palombella VJ, Adams J. The proteasome inhibitor PS-341 in cancer therapy. *Clin Cancer Res* 1999;5:2638–2645.

112. Murray RZ, Norbury C. Proteasome inhibitors as anti-cancer agents. *Anticancer Drugs* 2000;11:407–417.

12 Synthetic Oligopeptides as Cancer Cell Cycle Modulators

Anna Severino, PhD, Armando Felsani, PhD, Antonio Giordano, MD, PhD, and Marco G. Paggi, MD, PhD

CONTENTS

1. INTRODUCTION

In higher eukaryotes, many important biological processes, such as cellular differentiation, apoptosis, embryonic development, and finally cancer onset and progression, are closely related to the modulation of the cell cycle.

In the past decade, the basic knowledge on the machinery controlling the cell cycle has been unquestionably improved. Many cell cycle-related key genes have been recognized, and their importance has been carefully evaluated *(1–8)*. Usually, we represent the cell cycle as a circle, where major protein effectors are symbolized in correlation with the phases of the cell cycle in which their function is primarily documented. Nevertheless, the whole picture is far from being completely understood. The key goal of increasing the overall comprehension of the homeostasis governing the cell cycle can be reached by gradually transfering the initial knowledge obtained thus far, mainly analytical, to a new synthetic and integrated awareness of the molecular pathways involved.

From: *Cancer Drug Discovery and Development:*
Cell Cycle Inhibitors in Cancer Therapy: Current Strategies
Edited by: A. Giordano and K. J. Soprano © Humana Press Inc., Totowa, NJ

One of the modern and specific approaches to influence the cell cycle is through the alteration of specific protein-protein interactions that govern the internal equilibrium of the whole process. Nowadays, the possible molecular fine-tuning of the cell cycle is a realistic and appealing challenge for scientists aiming to modify the patho-physiological processes that depend on the cell cycle.

A consistent number of amino acid sequences involved in protein-protein interactions that specifically modulate the cell cycle have been identified, and their functional role investigated. Some of these sequences, reproduced as synthetic oligopeptides, are potentially interesting for their ability to interfere with specific protein-protein interactions and, consequently, for their effect on cell cycle modulation.

2. CLASSIFICATION BY MOLECULAR MOTIFS

Most of these oligopeptide sequences belong to nuclear proteins and will be classified and illustrated in the following paragraphs.

2.1. INK4 Family-Related Peptides

The INK4 family of cell cycle inhibitors (named after "Inhibitors of CDK4") is composed of four members (p16^{INK4a}, p15^{INK4b}, p18^{INK4c}, and p19^{INK4d}), whose main activity is to inhibit selectively CDK4 and CDK6, the D-type cyclin-dependent kinases, via a direct binding (for a review *see [9]*). The result of this binding is the block of the cell cycle, with accumulation of cells in the late G_1 phase. This effect is attributed chiefly to the lack of phosphorylation of pRb—the product of *RB*, the prototype of the tumor suppressor genes—and of the related proteins p107 and pRb2/p130 *(3)*. In fact, during the early/mid G_1 phase, the RB family proteins become substrates of both CDK4 and CDK6, activated by the presence of the D-type cyclins. Subsequently, in late G_1, the RB proteins will become substrates of Cyclin E/CDK2 activity, thus allowing, in their "hyper-phosphorylated" form, the transition through the restriction point between the G_1 and S phases of the cell cycle. In the presence of the INK4 family of proteins, due to the consequent inhibition in CDK4 and CDK6 activities, the RB family proteins remain in their "under-phosphorylated" form, and the cell is unable to make the transition between the G_1 and S phases.

All the INK4 genes and their products have been implicated in human cancer *(10)*, but a major role is attributed to *p16^{INK4a}* *(p16) (11,12)*, mainly in tumors arising from neuro-ectodermal tissues, such as melanoma *(13)*, malignant glioma *(14)*, and neuroblastoma *(15)*. The p16 protein is a potent and specific inhibitor of CDK4 and CDK6 activity. p16 acts by direct interaction with these CDKs *(16)*, thus competing actively for their binding with the D-type cyclins, which represent the positive effectors. The overall effect is a dramatic, but strictly temporally defined, inhibition of CDK4 and CDK6 activities, and a consequent accumulation of the cells in G_1, mainly due to the presence of pRb and related proteins in their active, under-phosphorylated forms. As a corollary, p16 inactivation in cancer cell lines or in specific tumors is rarely accompanied by pRb inactivation and vice versa *(17)*, as this would represent a redundant alteration in the same pathway. Nevertheless, exceptions have been described *(12)*.

Molecular analysis of the p16 protein led to the identification of the 20-amino acid sequence [84]DAAREGFLDTLVVLHRAGAR[103], which still interacts with CDK4 and CDK6, inhibiting the in vitro phosphorylation of pRb mediated by Cyclin D_1/CDK4 and thus blocking entry into the S phase *(18)*. Further dissection of this 20-aa peptide led to the identification of the 10-aa sequence [90]FLDTLVVLHR[99], which retains the ability to inhibit Cyclin D1/CDK4 activity and to block the progression of the cell cycle to the S phase in a pRb-dependent manner *(19–21)*. The specificity of these peptides also appears from their ineffectiveness in inhibiting Cyclin E/CDK2 activity *(19)*. In addition, in human diploid fibroblasts, the cells arrested by such peptides display several phenotypic features characteristic of senescent cells, such as a reduced proliferative capacity, an altered size and shape, the presence of underphosphorylated pRb, increased expression of plasminogen activator inhibitor, and the appearance of senescence-associated β-galactosidase activity *(22,23)*.

Overexpression of the *p16* gene has been shown to be associated with apoptosis *(24–26)*. Moreover, when wild-type *p16* is overexpressed via viral infection, p16-defective cells demonstrate increased sensitivity to apoptosis when compared to p16-positive cells *(27)*.

Making a reasonable parallel between the effects of the p16-mimicking oligopeptides and those of *p16* gene overexpression, these oligopeptides are now proposed as a powerful and selective tool against cancer cells lacking p16 function. At this point, further experimentation, also in vivo, is unquestionably appealing.

2.2. Cip/Kip Family-Related Peptides

The second class of CKI includes three members, p21[Cip1/Waf1/Sdi1] (p21), p27[Kip1] (p27), and p57[Kip2] (p57). These proteins display a broader interfering activity on cyclin/CDK complexes compared to the INK4 class, since they are capable of binding various cyclins, including cyclins A, E, and D, and the corresponding CDK subunits. The effect of the binding on the activity of the cyclin/CDK complexes is different according to their composition and stoichiometry. The kinase activity of cyclin A/CDK2 and cyclin E/CDK2 complexes is completely inhibited by saturating amounts of the Cip/Kip proteins, whereas cyclin D-CDK4/6 complexes are more resistant to Cip/Kip inhibition, and can actually act as a sort of molecular storage of these proteins.

The Cip/Kip proteins possess, within their N-terminal region, amino acids—motifs that mediate the direct binding to both cyclin and CDK moieties *(28–30)*.

Most p21-containing complexes are quaternary; in fact, they contain, besides cyclins and CDKs, the proliferating cell nuclear antigen (PCNA), a subunit of DNA polymerase delta. In this way, p21 can coordinate the effects of the inhibition of CDK activity with the control of the process of DNA replication and repair. The inhibition of CDKs and the PCNA-binding of p21 are activities functionally and structurally distinct and are localized on different parts of the p21 molecule, at the N- and C-terminus, respectively. The CDK-inhibiting region is included in the first 71 N-terminal amino acids of p21, whereas the PCNA-binding motif is located between residues 141 and 160. More recently, a CDK-inhibiting activity has been found in the C-terminal part of the molecule (31–33).

The function of PCNA is essential for the replication of nuclear DNA, cooperating with the DNA polymerases delta and epsilon. Three PCNA molecules, each containing two topologically identical domains, form a ring that acts as a sliding clamp, which tethers the DNA polymerase to its template, enhancing the enzyme's processivity (34–37). In addition, PCNA is required for nucleotide excision repair (38,39). Interestingly, the interaction of p21 with PCNA blocks DNA replication but does not impair nucleotide excision repair (40,41). The region of PCNA that interacts with p21 is also the target of another PCNA-binding protein, Fen1 (42). Presumably, p21 competes with Fen1 for PCNA binding, and the prevention of the Fen1-PCNA interaction could result in the inhibition of DNA replication by p21 (42). A conserved PCNA-binding motif has been identified in a number of PCNA-binding proteins, among which the *Drosophila Melanogaster* Dacapo protein, homologous to mammalian p21, and the Pogo family of transposases (43).

2.2.1. Use of Peptides Containing Cyclin/CDK-Binding Motifs from p21

The interaction between cyclin/CDK complexes and p21 has been studied in detail using peptides derived from the p21 sequence. A first characterization of p21 functional domains by this technique has been reported by Chen et al. (30). They synthesized a series of overlapping peptides spanning the entire p21 sequence, and used them as antagonists of p21 either in experiments of coimmunoprecipitation of p21 with cyclin E/CDK2 or of inhibition by p21 of cyclin E/CDK2 kinase activity. Two peptides, [15]SKACRRLFGPVDSEQLSRDCDALMAG[40] and [58]PLEGDFA WERVRGLGLPKLY[77], showed the strongest activity in antagonizing p21 activity, leading to the identification of two possible cyclin/CDK interaction domains in the N-terminus of p21. Interestingly, these two peptides have no significant inhibitory activity against cyclinE/CDK2 by themselves. The first 6 amino acids of the 15-40 peptide are important for blocking p21 binding to cyclin E/CDK2. The regions including both peptides are highly conserved in human and mouse p21, human p27 and human p57, suggesting that the N-terminal regions of these proteins might interact and inhibit CDK activity by a similar mechanism.

Chen et al. *(31)* and Adams et al. *(32)* showed in human p21 two copies of a cyclin-binding motif necessary and sufficient for binding cyclin A- and cyclin E-CDK2 complexes. One copy is located at the N-terminus (^{16}KACRRLFGF^{24}) and the other at the C-terminus (^{152}HSKRRLIF^{159}). Synthetic peptides derived from these sequences inhibited the cyclin-CDK kinase activity in vitro and DNA replication in *Xenopus* egg extracts. This cyclin-binding motif has been found in a number of other cell cycle regulatory proteins that bind cyclin A and E-CDK2 complexes, among which E2F, p107, pRb2/130, p27, and p57. The core of this cyclin-binding motif is represented by the sequence Z-Arg-X-Leu, where Z is a basic or cysteine and X is a basic residue *(32)*.

With the aim of developing small peptides as leads to drug design, Lane and coworkers carried out a systematic scanning of the p21 sequence using 11 overlapping 20-mer peptides *(33)*. Each peptide was examined for its ability to bind CDK4 and cyclin D_1. They identified three domains of p21 that form stable complexes with cyclin D_1 and/or CDK4. Domain 1 peptide (^{16}KACRRLF GPVDSEQLSRDCD^{35}), able to bind cyclin D_1 only, coincides with the region described earlier as a recognition site for cyclins A and E. Domain 2 peptide (^{46}RERWNFDFVTETPLEGDFAW^{65}), able to bind CDK4 only, corresponds to a region of p21 implicated in the interaction with CDK2 *(28)*. The C-terminal domain 3 peptide (^{141}KRRQTSMTDFYHSKRRLIFS^{160}) interacts both with cyclin D_1 and CDK4. Using an in vitro Retinoblastoma protein (pRb)-phosphorylation assay, the authors demonstrate that both domain 1 and domain 3 possess a kinase inhibitory activity. The C-terminal domain peptide had the highest activity, with a concentration for half-maximal cyclin D_1-CDK4 inhibition ($I_{0.5}$) of 0.1 µ*M*. This peptide showed no inhibitory activity against cyclin B-Cdc2 histone H1 kinase, while its activity against cyclin E-CDK2 was 40 times lower ($I_{0.5}$ = 4 µ*M*). Using alanine-scan mutations, it has been possible to define a minimal 8-amino acid peptide (^{154}KRRLIFSK^{161}) still retaining the ability to inhibit pRb phosphorylation, although with a higher $I_{0.5}$ of 100 µ*M*. The full-length domain 3 peptide and the truncated one have been coupled to a carrier peptide sequence, derived from the homeodomain of the Antennapedia protein (*see* below). The carrier-coupled peptides were then added to cultures of human-keratinocyte-derived cells (HaCaT, with mutated p53), and of human breast cancer (MCF7) and fibroblast (MRC5) cells (with wild-type p53). Both peptides were able to significantly reduce the number of cells entering S phase and concomitantly increase the number of those in G_1. The G_1 arrest induced by the full-length peptide treatment was associated with pRb hypophosphorylation.

2.2.2. Use of Peptides Containing PCNA-Binding Motifs from p21

The interaction between p21 and PCNA has been investigated using a genetic two-hybrid screen and with arrays of synthetic peptides derived from the p21 protein sequence. The interaction between p21 and PCNA involves the C-terminal region of p21 and the central loop of PCNA, which connects the two domains of the PCNA monomer. The interaction was finely mapped using peptides derived from the entire sequence of the p21 protein, and the critical residues were found to be [144]QTSMTDFY[151] (amino acids 144-151 of p21). A 20-residue peptide containing this sequence ([141]KRRQTSMTDFYHSKRRLIFS[160], designated p21PBP, for p21 PCNA-Binding Peptide) was able to inhibit the in vitro replication of Simian Virus 40 (SV40) DNA and could precipitate PCNA from whole cell extracts *(44)*.

The same 20-residue peptide was used successfully to dissociate the Fen1-PCNA complex, with PCNA binding preferentially to the p21PBP peptide *(42)*. As reported above, this fact may account for the observed inhibition of DNA replication by the p21PBP peptide *(44)*.

The p21PBP peptide has been used as the starting point for further development of p21 peptidomimetics. A competitive PCNA binding assay has been set up by using p21PBP peptides linked to agarose beads and highly purified, fluorescein-labeled, recombinant PCNA molecules *(45)*. This assay, together with the isothermal titration calorimetry (ITC) method, has been used to quantify and investigate at the molecular level the formation of complexes between PCNA and various peptides derived from the C-terminus of p21. This technical approach has been used by Lane and coworkers to screen rationally designed peptides for their ability to bind PCNA and to inhibit the PCNA-p21PBP complex. A 16-residue peptide (consensus motif 1 peptide) has been identified, with the following sequence: SAVLQKKITDYFHPKK. Consensus motif 1 peptide and p21PBP (141-160) have similar affinities for binding PCNA and abilities to inhibit in vitro replication of DNA originating from SV40 *(45)*.

2.2.3. CDK2 Inhibition by Peptide Aptamers

A different approach has been used to identify small peptides capable of interacting with cell cycle regulatory proteins. The active-site loop of *E. coli* thioredoxin (TrxA) can be used as a scaffold to display conformationally constrained random-variable peptide sequences. These proteins, called peptide aptamers, are capable of specific and high-affinity molecular recognition. Peptide aptamers able to bind different target proteins can be selected genetically in a yeast two-hybrid system from combinatorial libraries *(46)*. Using this technique, Brent and coworkers *(47)* isolated a 20-mer peptide aptamer (pep8; the variable region is: YSFVHHGFFNFRVSWREMLA) capable of binding CDK2 and inhibiting its kinase activity. The pep8 aptamer binds CDK2 at or near its active site and its mode of inhibition is competitive. Unlike the natural CDK2 inhibitor p21, it shows marked substrate specificity; in fact, it can inhibit histone H1 but not retinoblastoma protein phosphorylation. The pep8 aptamer's variable region is sufficient for this activity, since the same results were obtained in vitro using the free peptide. Moreover, SAOS-2 cells, transiently transfected with a

CMV-pep8 expression plasmid, showed a significant and reproducible increase in the G_1 cell fraction, although less effectively than that induced by the transfection of CMV-p21 *(48)*.

2.3. RB Family Protein-Related Peptides

The Retinoblastoma *(RB)* gene is the "founder" of the *RB* family of tumor and growth-suppressor genes, which also comprises *p107 (49,50)* and *Rb2/p130 (51–53)*. Their gene products, the RB proteins (pRb, p107, and pRb2/p130), possess the common ability to negatively control the cell cycle *(50,54–56)*. These proteins, in fact, can inhibit the transition between the G_1 and S phases via the inactivation of mitosis-promoting transcription factors, such as those of the E2F family *(1,3,6,57)*. Consequently, the RB proteins play a strategic role in regulating differentiation, embryonic development, and apoptosis, and in restraining cancer onset and progression *(58–62)*.

Molecular dissection has made it possible to define most of the epitopes responsible for RB family protein tasks in cellular homeostasis (for reviews *see* refs. *3,63,64*). Most of these functions are inevitably related to specific protein-protein interactions. Now, some specific cases deserve particular mention. It has been shown that specific domains of the RB family proteins can inhibit CDK2 kinase activity *(65–69)*. This implies that portions of these molecules are able *per se* to negatively control the kinase activities responsible for their own inactivation as cell cycle regulators. Further molecular dissection and characterization of these amino acid sequences will possibly indicate synthetic oligopeptides able to inhibit CDK activities, a promising tool in cell cycle modulation.

The "pocket" domain is considered the core of all three RB proteins *(3)*. This multi-functional domain governs most of the protein-protein interactions that involve the RB proteins, such as those with the E2F-DP families of transcription factors, with the E1A, E7, and large T antigen viral oncoproteins and with the D-type cyclins. Indeed, the sequence considered responsible for the interaction with proteins harboring the LXCXE domain (D-type cyclins, E1A, etc.) is the 6-mer [649]LFYKKV[654], which, interestingly, is also able to bind insulin in vitro *(70)*. Peptides reproducing the LFYKKV sequence, or the extended 14-mer sequence spanning between amino acids [645]TSLSLFYKKVYRLA[658], show the capability to inhibit cancer cell cycle in vitro, with particular emphasis in pRb-defective lineages, in contrast with the less striking effect in non-neoplastic cells *(71)*. It would be interesting to investigate the effects of these oligopeptides in inhibiting cancer growth in vivo by systemic or intra-tumor administration, as well as to evaluate their side effects on normal tissues and on the whole organism.

2.4. DP Family-Related Peptides

E2F transcription factors are central players in controlling the cell cycle, differentiation, and transformation. They consist of heterodimers formed by the interaction between two members of the E2F and DP protein families *(72–75)*. These heterodimers bind the promoter of their target genes, thus modulating their transcriptional activity.

To interfere with E2F activity, peptide aptamers specifically interacting with E2F DNA-binding and dimerization domains were isolated from combinatorial libraries using genetic screening in yeast *(46)*. The aptamer library was constituted of constrained 20-residue peptides displayed in the active loop of the *E. coli* thioredoxin molecule *(47,48,76)*. Using this approach, a 20-mer peptide (RCVRCRFVVWIGLRVRCLV), corresponding to the variable region of one of the selected aptamers, was synthesized and its capacity to interfere with E2F functions in vivo and in vitro was evaluated. When transfected in CCL39 cells, this peptide specifically disrupts the DNA binding activity of E2F/DP complexes and inhibits the activity of a co-transfected E2F responsive reporter gene, in a concentration-dependent manner. Moreover, the peptide was also able to delay or block the entry of the cells into the S phase, as judged by the reduction of the incorporation of BrdU. It is worthwhile to notice that this peptide mimics a region of DP1 that binds E2F, since the WIGL motif (underlined in the aforementioned peptide sequence) is present in the sequences of the peptide as well as of the helix 3 of the DP heterodimerization domain. Human DP1 molecules in which the WIGL motif was mutated, showed a significantly reduced DNA binding capacity as compared to the wild-type DP1, suggesting a reduced ability to heterodimerize with E2F.

3. PROTEIN TRANSDUCTION: INTERNALIZING MOTIFS AND NUCLEAR TARGETING

Protein transduction, an emerging technology with potential applications in gene therapy, can be best described as the internalization of proteins into the cell, from the external environment. Short peptide sequences, such as those that will be described later, are able to translocate efficiently through the plasma membrane. This property makes it possible to consider them as useful vectors for the intracellular delivery of molecules that do not spontaneously cross the cellular membranes; these molecules can be drugs, antisense oligonucleotides or peptides, indifferently, and can carry with them their pharmacological properties.

3.1. Antennapedia

Antennapedia is a transcription factor in *Drosophila Melanogaster*. A polypeptide of 16 amino acids in length derived from the third helix of the Antennapedia DNA binding domain (RQIKIWFQNRRMKWKK) is capable of translocating through the biological membranes of the cells. This phenomenon is also evident at temperatures below 10°C, thus supporting its independence from endocytosis or other cellular energy-dependent processes *(77,78)*. This

Antennapedia-derived 16-amino acid peptide, used as a high-efficiency carrier to the cytoplasm and nucleus for oligopeptides and oligonucleotides, is non-cell-type-specific and offers several potentially interesting applications *(79)*. It has been chimerized with several biologically active peptides, in order to allow their maximum intracellular and intranuclear accumulation. As Antennapedia is *per se* virtually devoid of any biological activity *(21)*, the effects of these chimeric peptides are attributed to the intracellular accumulation of the biologically active moiety chimerized with Antennapedia. An example is the CDK4/6-inhibiting peptide sequence derived from the p16^{INK4a} protein, conjugated with the Antennapedia internalizing sequence, highly effective in inhibiting the cell cycle *(19–21)*.

3.2. HIV-1 Tat

Tat is an 86-amino acid protein involved in the replication of Human Immunodeficiency Virus type 1 (HIV-1). Similarly to Antennapedia, Tat can traverse biological membranes and perform the transduction of chimerized proteins or peptides. Recent data demonstrate that chemical coupling of a Tat-derived peptide to several proteins allows their internalization into several cell lines or tissues. The Tat sequence necessary and sufficient for an efficient internalization process can be as short as 10 amino acids ^{48}GRKKRRQRRR^{57} *(80,81)*. Also in the case of Tat-derived peptides, no inhibition of their intracellular uptake is observed at low temperatures.

4. CONCLUSIONS

This section describes some examples of peptides interfering with mechanisms that control the cell cycle. Nevertheless, we learned from these data that it is possible to engineer synthetic oligopeptides, which are actually able to generate a specific pharmacological effect via their direct interference in molecular processes within live cells or tissues. However, as for more conventional active drugs, the key question is whether or not the translation of these exciting experimental results "from bench to bedside" will occur without any loss of efficiency or specificity of their biological effects. In fact, while these peptides appear to be very powerful biological tools, they are capable, on the other hand, to generate potentially relevant side effects.

We are deeply interested in reaching efficient cures for cancer patients, and this can be "simply" epitomized as the way to kill cancer cells while sparing the normal ones in the whole organism. From a theoretical point of view, we can engineer active peptides such that they can deal with genotypic or phenotypic differences between cancer and normal cells. However, the final assessment of the selectivity in killing their target, i.e., cancer cells, is to be considered empirically. A potentially interesting example of such speculations comes from the p16-mimicking peptides. Among the reported effects of *p16* gene transduction, we have growth arrest and induction of apoptosis, both more evident in p16-negative than in p16-positive cells *(24,27)*. Because the p16-mimicking peptides reproduce a number of effects of the p16 protein, it can be argued that, in some instances, the same selectivity of the effect in different cells attributed to the p16 protein could apply to the p16-mimicking peptides. Such a discrepancy would represent a pivotal point in order to encourage the use of such peptides, as substitutes of gene therapy, to cure cancer in vivo. The effect of these peptides in vivo could be selectively directed towards p16-negative cancer cells, in this way sparing normal tissues and organs. In fact, normal cells have at least the possibility to downmodulate the endogenous p16 protein levels, thus giving a specific response against the toxicity induced by the p16-mimicking peptides. Anyway, it should be taken into consideration that such p16-mimicking peptides would lack efficacy towards cancer cells that do not display any genetic or epigenetic impairment of p16 function. Following this kind of hypotheses, we should perform specific molecular analyses in advance, in order to predict if the cancer patient would be responsive to such specific therapies with a considerable therapeutic index.

Despite these limitations, the novelty and the envisaged specificity of these peptide approaches to inhibit the cell cycle in cancer cells make these topics extremely appealing and worthy of further in vivo development.

ACKNOWLEDGMENTS

Research in our laboratories is supported by AIRC and Ministero della Sanità grants to M.G.P. and A.F.; by Progetto Strategico CNR-MIUR "Oncologia" to A.F.; and by NIH RO1 CA 60999-01A1 and PO1 CA 56309 grants to A.G. who is a recipient of a FIRC fellowship.

REFERENCES

1. Weinberg RA. The retinoblastoma protein and cell cycle control. *Cell* 1995;81:323–330.
2. MacLachlan TK, Sang N. Giordano A. Cyclins, cyclin-dependent kinases and Cdk inhibitors: implications in cell cycle control and cancer. *Crit Rev Eukariot Gene Expr* 1995;5:127–156.
3. Paggi MG, Baldi A, Bonetto F, Giordano A. Retinoblastoma protein family in cell cycle and cancer: a review. *J Cell Biochem* 1996;62:418–430.
4. Bernards R. E2F: a nodal point in cell cycle regulation. *Biochim Biophys Acta Rev Cancer* 1997;1333:M33–M40.
5. Bartek J, Bartkova J, Lukas J. The retinoblastoma protein pathway in cell cycle control and cancer. *Exp Cell Res* 1997;237:1–6.
6. Mulligan G, Jacks T. The retinoblastoma gene family: cousins with overlapping interests. *Trends Genet* 1998;14:223–229.
7. Johnson DG, Walker CL. Cyclins and cell cycle checkpoints. *Annu Rev Pharmacol Toxicol* 1999;39:295–312.
8. Ekholm SV, Reed SI. Regulation of G(1) cyclin-dependent kinases in the mammalian cell cycle. *Curr Opin Cell Biol* 2000;12:676–684.

9. Carnero A, Hannon GJ. The INK4 family of CDK inhibitors. *Curr Top Microbiol Immunol* 1998;227:43–55.

10. Roussel MF. The INK4 family of cell cycle inhibitors in cancer. *Oncogene* 1999; 18: 5311–5317.

11. Lukas J, Sorensen CS, Lukas C, Santoni-Rugiu E, Bartek J. p16[INK4a], but not constitutively active pRb, can impose a sustained G1 arrest: molecular mechanisms and implications for oncogenesis. *Oncogene* 1999;18:3930–3935.

12. Ruas M, Peters G. The p16[INK4a]/CDKN2A tumor suppressor and its relatives. *Biochim Biophys Acta Rev Cancer* 1998;1378:F115–F177.

13. Bartkova J, Lukas J, Guldberg P, Alsner J, Kirkin AF, Zeuthen J, Bartek J. The p16-cyclin D Cdk4-pRb pathway as a functional unit frequently altered in melanoma pathogenesis. *Cancer Res* 1996;56:5475–5483.

14. Srivenugopal KS, Ali-Osman F. Deletions and rearrangements inactivate the p16[INK4] gene in human glioma cells. *Oncogene* 1996;12:2029–2034.

15. Takita J, Hayashi Y, Nakajima T, Adachi J, Tanaka T., Yamaguchi N, et al. The *p16(CDKN2A)* gene is involved in the growth of neuroblastoma cells and its expression is associated with prognosis of neuroblastoma patients. *Oncogene* 1998;17:3137–3143.

16. Hall M, Bates S, Peters G. Evidence for different modes of action of cyclin-dependent kinase inhibitors: p15 and p16 bind to kinases, p21 and p27 bind to cyclins. *Oncogene* 1995;11:1581–1588.

17. Shapiro GI, Rollins BJ. p16[INK4A] as a human tumor suppressor. *Biochim Biophys Acta Rev Cancer* 1996;1242:165–169.

18. Fahraeus R, Paramio JM, Ball KL, Laín S, Lane DP. Inhibition of pRb phosphorylation and cell-cycle progression by a 20-residue peptide derived from p16[CDKN2/INK4A]. *Curr Biol* 1996;6:84–91.

19. Fahraeus R, Lain S, Ball KL, Lane DP. Characterization of the cyclin-dependent kinase inhibitory domain of the INK4 family as a model for a synthetic tumour suppressor molecule. *Oncogene* 1998;16:587–596.

20. Gius DR, Ezhevsky SA, Becker-Hapak M, Nagahara H, Wei MC, Dowdy SF. Transduced p16[INK4a] peptides inhibit hypophosphorylation of the retinoblastoma protein and cell cycle progression prior to activation of Cdk2 complexes in late G_1. *Cancer Res* 1999;59: 2577–2580.

21. Fujimoto K, Hosotani R, Miyamoto Y, Doi R, Koshiba T, Otaka A, et al. Inhibition of pRb phosphorylation and cell cycle progression by an antennapedia-p16(INK4A) fusion peptide in pancreatic cancer cells. *Cancer Lett* 2000;159:151–158.

22. McConnell BB, Starborg M, Brookes S, Peters G. Inhibitors of cyclin-dependent kinases induce features of replicative senescence in early passage human diploid fibroblasts. *Curr Biol* 1998;8:351–354.

23. Kato D, Miyazawa K, Ruas M, Starborg M, Wada I, Oka T, et al. Features of replicative senescence induced by direct addition of antennapedia-p16INK4A fusion protein to human diploid fibroblasts. *FEBS Lett* 1998;427:203–208.

24. Sandig V, Brand K, Herwig S, Lukas J, Bartek J, Strauss M. Adenovirally transferred p16[INK4/CDKN2] and p53 genes cooperate to induce apoptotic tumor cell death. *Nature Med* 1997;3:313–319.

25. Schreiber M, Muller WJ, Singh G, Graham FL. Comparison of the effectiveness of adenovirus vectors expressing cyclin kinase inhibitors p16[INK4A], p18[INK4C], p19[INK4D], p21[WAF1/CIP1], and p27[KIP1] in inducing cell cycle arrest, apoptosis and inhibition of tumorigenicity. *Oncogene* 1999;18:1663–1676.

26. Plath T, Detjen K, Welzel M, von Marschall Z, Murphy D, Schirner M, et al. A novel function for the tumor suppressor p16(INK4a). Induction of anoikis via upregulation of the alpha(5)beta(1) fibronectin receptor. *J Cell Biol* 2000;150:1467–1478.

27. Kim M, Katayose Y, Rojanala L, Shah S, Sgagias M, Jang L, et al. Induction of apoptosis in p16INK4A mutant cell lines by adenovirus-mediated overexpression of p16INK4A protein. *Cell Death Differ* 2000;7:706–711.

28. Goubin F, Ducommun B. Identification of binding domains on the p21^{Cip1} cyclin-dependent kinase inhibitor. *Oncogene* 1995;10:2281–2287.

29. Nakanishi M, Robetorye RS, Adami GR, Pereira-Smith OM, Smith JR. Identification of the active region of the DNA synthesis inhibitory gene p21Sdi1/CIP1/WAF1. *EMBO J* 1995;14:555–563.

30. Chen IT, Akamatsu M, Smith ML, Lung FDT, Duba D, Roller PP, et al. Characterization of p21$^{Cip1/Waf1}$ peptide domains required for cyclin E/Cdk2 and PCNA interaction. *Oncogene* 1996;12:595–607.

31. Chen JJ, Saha P, Kornbluth S, Dynlacht BD, Dutta A. Cyclin-binding motifs are essential for the function of p21^{CIP1}. *Mol Cell Biol* 1996;16:4673–4682.

32. Adams PD, Sellers WR, Sharma SK, Wu AD, Nalin CM, Kaelin WG, Jr. Identification of a cyclin-cdk2 recognition motif present in substrates and p21-like cyclin-dependent kinase inhibitors. *Mol Cell Biol* 1996;16:6623–6633.

33. Ball KL, Lain S, Fahraeus R, Smythe C, Lane DP. Cell-cycle arrest and inhibition of Cdk4 activity by small peptides based on the carboxy-terminal domain of p21WAF1. *Curr Biol* 1997;7:71–80.

34. Prelich G, Kostura M, Marshak DR, Mathews MB, Stillman B. The cell-cycle regulated proliferating cell nuclear antigen is required for SV40 DNA replication in vitro. *Nature* 1987;326:471–475.

35. Prelich G, Tan CK, Kostura M, Mathews MB, So AG, Downey KM, Stillman B. Functional identity of proliferating cell nuclear antigen and a DNA polymerase-delta auxiliary protein. *Nature* 1987;326:517–520.

36. Bravo R, Frank R, Blundell PA, MacDonald-Bravo H. Cyclin/PCNA is the auxiliary protein of DNA polymerase-delta. *Nature* 1987;326:515–517.

37. Krishna TS, Kong XP, Gary S, Burgers PM, Kuriyan J. Crystal structure of the eukaryotic DNA polymerase processivity factor PCNA. *Cell* 1994;79:1233–1243.

38. Shivji KK, Kenny MK, Wood RD. Proliferating cell nuclear antigen is required for DNA excision repair. *Cell* 1992;69:367–374.

39. Nichols AF, Sancar A. Purification of PCNA as a nucleotide excision repair protein. *Nucleic Acids Res* 1992;20:2441–2446.

40. Shivji MK, Grey SJ, Strausfeld UP, Wood RD, Blow JJ. Cip1 inhibits DNA replication but not PCNA-dependent nucleotide excision-repair. *Curr Biol* 1994;4:1062–1068.

41. Shivji MK, Ferrari E, Ball K, Hubscher U, Wood RD. Resistance of human nucleotide excision repair synthesis in vitro to p21Cdn1. *Oncogene* 1998;17:2827–2838.

42. Warbrick E, Lane DP, Glover DM, Cox LS. Homologous regions of Fen1 and p21Cip1 compete for binding to the same site on PCNA: a potential mechanism to co-ordinate DNA replication and repair. *Oncogene* 1997;14:2313–2321.

43. Warbrick E, Heatherington W, Lane DP, Glover DM. PCNA binding proteins in Drosophila melanogaster: the analysis of a conserved PCNA binding domain. *Nucleic Acids Res* 1998;26:3925–3932.

44. Warbrick E, Lane DP, Glover DM, Cox LS. A small peptide inhibitor of DNA replication defines the site of interaction between the cyclin-dependent kinase inhibitor p21WAF1 and proliferating cell nuclear antigen. *Curr Biol* 1995;5:275–282.

45. Zheleva DI, Zhelev NZ, Fischer PM, Duff SV, Warbrick E, Blake DG, Lane DP. A quantitative study of the in vitro binding of the C-terminal domain of p21 to PCNA: affinity, stoichiometry, and thermodynamics. *Biochemistry* 2000;39:7388–7397.

46. Vidal M, Braun P, Chen E, Boeke JD, Harlow E. Genetic characterization of a mammalian protein-protein interaction domain by using a yeast reverse two-hybrid system. *Proc Natl Acad Sci USA* 1996;93:10321–10326.

47. Colas P, Cohen B, Jessen T, Grishina I, McCoy J, Brent R. Genetic selection of peptide aptamers that recognize and inhibit cyclin-dependent kinase 2. *Nature* 1996;380:548–550.
48. Cohen BA, Colas P, Brent R. An artificial cell-cycle inhibitor isolated from a combinatorial Library. *Proc Natl Acad Sci USA* 1998;95:14272–14277.
49. Ewen ME, Xing YG, Lawrence JB, Livingston DM. Molecular cloning, chromosomal mapping, and expression of the cDNA for p107, a retinoblastoma gene product-related protein. *Cell* 1991;66:1155–1164.
50. Zhu L, van den Heuvel S, Helin K, Fattaey A, Ewen ME, Livingston DM, et al. Inhibition of cell proliferation by p107, a relative of the retinoblastoma protein. *Genes Dev* 1993;7:1111–1125.
51. Mayol X, Graña X, Baldi A, Sang N, Hu Q, Giordano A. Cloning of a new member of the retinoblastoma gene family (pRb2) which binds to the E1A transforming domain. *Oncogene* 1993;8:2561–2566.
52. Hannon GJ, Demetrick D, Beach D. Isolation of the Rb-related p130 through its interaction with CDK2 and cyclins. *Genes Dev* 1993;7:2378–2391.
53. Li Y, Graham C, Lacy S, Duncan AM, Whyte P. The adenovirus E1A-associated 130-kD protein is encoded by a member of the retinoblastoma gene family and physically interacts with cyclins A and E. *Genes Dev* 1993;7:2366–2377.
54. Goodrich DW, Wang NP, Qian YW, Lee EY, Lee WH. The retinoblastoma gene product regulates progression through the G1 phase of the cell cycle. *Cell* 1991;67:293–302.
55. Starostik P, Chow KNB, Dean DC. Transcriptional repression and growth suppression by the p107 pocket protein. *Mol Cell Biol* 1996;16:3606–3614.
56. Claudio PP, Howard CM, Baldi A, De Luca A, Fu Y, Condorelli G, et al. p130/pRb2 has growth suppressive properties similar to yet distinctive from those of retinoblastoma family members pRb and p107. *Cancer Res* 1994;54:5556–5560.
57. Ewen ME. The cell cycle and the retinoblastoma protein family. [Review]. *Cancer Metastasis Rev* 1994;13:45–66.
58. Riley DJ, Lee EYHP, Lee W-H. The retinoblastoma protein: more than a tumor suppressor. *Annu Rev Cell Biol* 1994;10:1–29.
59. Sidle A, Palaty C, Dirks P, Wiggan O, Kiess M, Gill RM, et al. Activity of the retinoblastoma family proteins, pRB, p107, and p130, during cellular proliferation and differentiation. *Crit Rev Biochem Mol Biol* 1996;31:237–271.
60. Herwig S, Strauss M. The retinoblastoma protein: a master regulator of cell cycle, differentiation and apoptosis. *Eur J Biochem* 1997;246:581–601.
61. Stiegler P, Kasten M, Giordano A. The RB family of cell cycle regulatory factors. *J Cell Biochem* 1998;30–36.
62. Paggi MG, Giordano A. Who is the boss in the retinoblastoma family? The point of view of *Rb2/p130*, the little brother. *Cancer Res* 2001;61:4651–4654.
63. Kaelin WG, Jr. Functions of the retinoblastoma protein. *Bioessays* 1999;21:950–958.
64. Stiegler P, Giordano A. The family of retinoblastoma proteins. *Crit Rev Eukaryot Gene Expr* 2001;11:59–76.
65. Adams PD, Li XT, Sellers WR, Baker KB, Leng XH, Harper JW, et al. Retinoblastoma protein contains a C-terminal motif that targets it for phosphorylation by cyclin-cdk complexes. *Mol Cell Biol* 1999;19:1068–1080.
66. Lacy S, Whyte P. Identification of a p130 domain mediating interactions with cyclin A cdk2 and cyclin E cdk2 complexes. *Oncogene* 1997;14:2395–2406.
67. Woo MSA, Sánchez I, Dynlacht BD. p130 and p107 use a conserved domain to inhibit cellular cyclin-dependent kinase activity. *Mol Cell Biol* 1997;17:3566–3579.
68. De Luca A, MacLachlan TK, Bagella L, Dean C, Howard CM, Claudio PP, et al. A unique domain of pRb2/p130 acts as an inhibitor of Cdk2 kinase activity. *J Biol Chem* 1997;272:20971–20974.
69. Castaño E, Kleyner Y, Dynlacht BD. Dual cyclin-binding domains are required for p107 to function as a kinase inhibitor. *Mol Cell Biol* 1998;18:5380–5391.

70. Radulescu RT, Bellitti MR, Ruvo M, Cassani G, Fassina G. Binding of the LXCXE insulin motif to a hexapeptide derived from retinoblastoma protein. *Biochem Biophys Res Commun* 1995;206:97–102.
71. Radulescu RT, Jaques G. Selective inhibition of human lung cancer cell growth by peptides derived from retinoblastoma protein. *Biochem Biophys Res Commun* 2000;267:71–76.
72. Bernards R. E2F: a nodal point in cell cycle regulation. *Biochim Biophys Acta Rev Cancer* 1997;1333:M33–M40.
73. Helin K. Regulation of cell proliferation by the E2F transcription factors. *Curr Opin Genet Dev* 1998;8:28–35.
74. Macleod K. pRb and E2f-1 in mouse development and tumorigenesis. *Curr Opin Genet Dev* 1999;9:31–39.
75. Nevins JR. The Rb/E2F pathway and cancer. *Hum Mol Genet* 2001;10:699–703.
76. Gyuris J, Golemis E, Chertkov H, Brent R. Cdi1, a human G1 and S phase protein phosphatase that associates with Cdk2. *Cell* 1993;75:791–803.
77. Derossi D, Joliot AH, Chassaing G, Prochiantz A. The third helix of the Antennapedia homeodomain translocates through biological membranes. *J Biol Chem* 1994; 269: 10444–10450.
78. Derossi D, Calvet S, Trembleau A, Brunissen A, Chassaing G, Prochiantz A. Cell internalization of the third helix of the Antennapedia homeodomain is receptor-independent. *J Biol Chem* 1996;271:18188–18193.
79. Derossi D, Chassaing G, Prochiantz A. Trojan peptides: the penetratin system for intracellular delivery. *Trends Cell Biol* 1998;8:84–87.
80. Vives E, Brodin P, Lebleu B. A truncated HIV-1 Tat protein basic domain rapidly translocates through the plasma membrane and accumulates in the cell nucleus. *J Biol Chem* 1997; 272:16010–16017.
81. Schwarze SR, Hruska KA, Dowdy SF. Protein transduction: unrestricted delivery into all cells? *Trends Cell Biol* 2000;10:290–295.

Index